DIMENSION

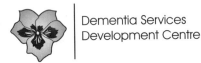 Dementia Services
Development Centre

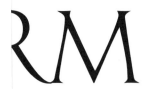 **UNIVERSITY OF STIRLING**

RM

This book is due for return on or before the last date stamped below.
To renew your loan online, please go to www.shelcat.org/pdem and log on

D1388713

ENT

A

TION

Please return this book to:

Library & Information Service
Dementia Services Development Centre
Iris Murdoch Building
University of Stirling
FK9 4LA

Tel: 01786 467740
Email: dementia@stir.ac.uk

DIMENSIONS of LONG-TERM CARE MANAGEMENT

AN INTRODUCTION

MARY HELEN McSWEENEY-FELD AND REID OETJEN, EDITORS

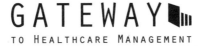

GATEWAY
TO HEALTHCARE MANAGEMENT

AUPHA

Health Administration Press, Chicago, Illinois
Association of University Programs in Health Administration, Arlington, Virginia

16   15   14   13   12   5   4   3   2   1

Library of Congress Cataloging-in-Publication Data

Dimensions of long-term care management : an introduction / Mary Helen McSweeney-Feld and Reid Oetjen, editors.
  p. cm.
 ISBN 978-1-56793-383-3 (alk. paper)
 1. Long-term care facilities--United States--Administration. 2. Long-term care of the sick--United States--Administration. 3. Long-term care of the sick--United States--Finance. 4. Long-term care of the sick--Moral and ethical aspects. 5. Long-term care of the sick--Law and legislation. 6. Older people--Long-term care. I. McSweeney-Feld, Mary Helen. II. Oetjen, Reid M.
 RA997.D56 2012
 362.16068--dc23
                    2011051595

The paper used in this publication meets the minimum requirements of American National Standard for Information Sciences—Permanence of Paper for Printed Library Materials, ANSI Z39.48-1984. ⊗ ™

Acquisitions editor: Janet Davis; Project manager: Sam Raue Hebert; Cover designer: Scott Miller; Layout: Scott Miller

Health Administration Press
A division of the Foundation
   of the American College of
   Healthcare Executives
One North Franklin Street
Suite 1700
Chicago, IL 60606
(312) 424-2800

Association of University Programs
   in Health Administration
2000 14th Street
Suite 780
Arlington, VA 22201
(703) 894-0940

Brief Contents

Preface

The delivery system for long-term care services, as well as the variety of these services, has grown considerably over the past decade. External forces such as changes in demographics and population diversity, the creation of new laws and regulations, and the development of new technologies for the provision of healthcare services have ushered in new job opportunities for individuals interested in caring for people with chronic illness and long-term care needs. At the same time, older individuals have redefined retirement as a time to contribute to their families and surrounding communities or discover a new career path. These forces are not unique to the United States—they have become a global phenomenon affecting the healthcare and economic systems of many countries. They require instructors to take a new look at long-term care services so that they may offer students an opportunity to study this dynamic, rapidly growing sector and train for new career paths.

This book was written at an introductory level so that it may be used by undergraduates and other students new to healthcare management. Readers will gain a broad overview of the market for long-term care services. One of the premises of the book is that approaches to providing for individuals' long-term care needs must bring more flexibility to the delivery system and reimbursement. Another prominent issue addressed is the role of technology and the management of resources in the delivery of long-term care services. These factors will continue to grow in importance as the pressures of providing services to an increasingly aged and chronically ill population collides with society's limited resources.

Dimensions of Long-Term Care Management is organized in three sections. Part I provides an overview and definitions of long-term care, long-term care services, and delivery systems for these services. Also included are perspectives on who provides these services and who uses them and discussion of systems for reimbursement.

Part II looks at the spectrum of long-term care services, including residential care, home and community-based care, technology and long-term care, hospice and end-of-life care, care for individuals with chronic illnesses (with special emphasis on Alzheimer's disease and dementia), and the impact that growing cultural diversity in the population needing these services is having on long-term care delivery.

Part III is an overview of the management issues affecting long-term care service delivery. These chapters consider management issues unique to the long-term care field, the design of long-term care services and environmental considerations, human resources issues, the marketing of long-term care services, legal and ethical issues, and regulation of long-term care and provide further details on financing and reimbursement of long-term care services.

This book also provides international perspectives on long-term care services and concludes with an epilogue that identifies factors affecting the future of long-term care service delivery.

This book is accompanied by an instructor's resources component that includes the answers to the end-of-chapter questions, the answers to the case studies, a test bank of examination questions, sample course syllabi, and instructional PowerPoint slides. Written and developed with significant contributions by Dr. Carol Molinari, the instructor's resources take into account instructors' need for flexible coverage of the topic; the growing use of classroom technology and online/hybrid course delivery systems; and varying course length, from 5-week intensives to traditional 14-week, semester-based classes. For access to the instructor's resources, e-mail hap1@ache.org.

We hope this book inspires people to enter the long-term care field and consider a career path in this dynamic and evolving global market. We also hope that readers develop the same enthusiasm and passion for long-term care services that we have. We look forward to your feedback on the book.

Mary Helen McSweeney-Feld, PhD
Associate Professor
Office of Collaborative Programs
Towson University
Towson, Maryland
ltcbook@yahoo.com

Reid M. Oetjen, PhD
Associate Professor and Program Director
Department of Health Management & Informatics
University of Central Florida
Orlando, Florida
reid.oetjen@ucf.edu

ACKNOWLEDGMENTS

This book could not have been written without the unique contributions of a number of scholars in the field who graciously agreed to share, in their respective chapters, their knowledge and expertise. We are deeply indebted to them and are grateful for their willingness to work with us to make this project a success.

We would especially like to thank Carol Molinari, associate professor of health systems management at the University of Baltimore. In addition to contributing an excellent chapter titled "Diversity and the Delivery of Long-Term Care Services," Carol provided invaluable help by reviewing and editing chapters, suggesting revisions and additions, researching various topics, and brainstorming ways to reorganize sections. She also developed the instructor's resources package, including writing significant portions. We gratefully acknowledge the time, insight, and experience that Carol brought to this book.

Mary Helen McSweeney-Feld
Reid Oetjen

PART I

Overview of Long-Term Care

Our definitions of long-term care and long-term care services have changed considerably throughout the twenty-first century. These changes were prompted by major shifts in society: the aging of the baby boomers, increased diversity in the population, changes in reimbursement for healthcare services, use of new technologies, and an evolution in attitudes toward aging and retirement. These issues will continue to evolve over time. Part I provides basic definitions, statistics, and trends in long-term care and describes the larger environment that influences the demand for and consumption of long-term care services. A model of long-term care service is discussed that emphasizes a fluid, single point of entry to long-term care services, which include the key elements of residential services, home and community-based care, and technology and how they relate to each other. The authors encourage readers to use this introduction to become culturally competent on the issues of aging and long-term care and to incorporate concepts and knowledge learned here into their classrooms, their career choices and workplaces, and their personal interactions with others.

CHAPTER 1

Introduction to the Dimensions of Long-Term Care

Mary Helen McSweeney-Feld, PhD; Reid Oetjen, PhD; and G. Dale Welch, PhD

LEARNING OBJECTIVES

After completing this chapter, you should be able to

➤ explain the demographics of aging in the United States and their impact on an individual's retirement decision;

➤ define long-term care, long-term care services, and the models for long-term care service delivery;

➤ explain the role of caregivers and caregiving in the delivery of long-term care services; and

➤ define the providers and payers of long-term care services.

THE AGING TSUNAMI: AN OVERVIEW OF OLDER AMERICANS

Aging tsunami
The aging Baby Boomers' huge impact on society.

A recent publication by the Federal Interagency Forum on Aging Related Statistics (2010) states that in the United States people aged 65 or older are living longer and are more prosperous than those in previous generations. In 2008, this group numbered 39 million people, representing more than 13 percent of the total population. Rapid growth in this segment is predicted to continue, primarily due to the aging of baby boomers. By 2030, older adults are estimated to reach 72 million—nearly 20 percent of the total population (Federal Interagency Forum on Aging Related Statistics 2010). This is evidence of the well-known age wave or **aging tsunami** predicted by Ken Dychtwald (1990) in his seminal book *The Age Wave*.

Older Americans over 65 are better educated than ever before. In 1965, only 24 percent of older people had a high school diploma; in 2008, that number rose to 77 percent, and 21 percent had gone on to earn a bachelor's degree or higher (Federal Interagency Forum on Aging Related Statistics 2010). With higher levels of education, older Americans enjoy higher incomes and net worth levels. Furthermore, an increasing share of their income comes from earnings as more work past age 65, either from a desire to remain active in the workforce or out of economic necessity. However, lingering inequalities based on differences in gender, social and economic status, education, and race and ethnic background exist among this population.

When compared with the rest of the US population, older Americans without high school diplomas and elderly African Americans generally earn less and have fewer means to support themselves financially. The life expectancy of elderly Americans lags that of the elderly in other developed nations. This lag exists despite the fact that older Americans' healthcare expenditures, especially prescription drugs, nearly doubled between 1992 and 2006. Arthritis, hypertension, and other chronic ailments plague a large portion of the elderly in the United States. However, statistics from the past several years indicate a decrease in disability and other impairments that restrict the functioning of seniors.

The increasing longevity of older Americans, combined with higher educational levels and a desire to preserve standards of living despite the need to manage chronic health conditions, has redefined the notion of retirement in the United States. Active elders desire to remain engaged in life—they prefer to be self-sufficient and not burden their families. This "third age" (the third stage of life: the years after retirement but before the onset of any major disabling health problems) must be recognized to fully comprehend the needs of older Americans.

CHANGING DEFINITIONS OF RETIREMENT

Retirement
Withdrawing from one's occupation, business, or office and pursuing new activities.

To understand the environment surrounding long-term care (LTC) and the individuals who need LTC services, the term *retirement* must first be defined. Retirement is formally defined as a state of separation from an occupation or a position; traditionally in retirement, a person left the workforce to pursue activities such as traveling, engaging in personal hobbies, and visiting family and friends. People going into the new third age assumed that they and other retirees would have (1) a steady stream of income from a government system such as Social Security, (2) pension income from their employers, and (3) private savings to finance these activities. This collection of funding sources is sometimes referred to as the **three-legged stool of economic security**. However, recent economic downturns affecting investment returns, combined with increasing costs of healthcare services, have forced many retirees to return to the workforce so that they do not outlive their financial resources. Adding employment income to the three-legged stool has led to a new reality for many older Americans: the **four pillars of retirement income** (Geneva Association 2011).

The extent to which retirees are able to pay for LTC services has traditionally depended on government healthcare plans such as Medicare, government pensions from Social Security, private employer-sponsored pensions, and personal savings. This relationship has also held for retirees in many other industrialized countries around the world. However, flat economic growth is now testing many governments' abilities to fund the public portions of this mix, and in many countries initiatives to raise the retirement age and the eligibility age for public health insurance and pension programs have started. Combined with the effect of the aging tsunami, the large numbers of retirees who will become eligible for services from these public systems in the near future will test the abilities of policymakers to continue to provide benefits. New models and options for delivery of care will be important pieces of the LTC service delivery system, as will a reliance on seniors to care for themselves and become informed consumers as they age in their communities.

Three-legged stool of economic security
A concept used by financial planners to describe the three most common sources of retirement income: Social Security retirement benefits, employee pensions, and personal savings.

Four pillars of retirement income
The idea that postretirement employment provides additional income when the traditional three sources—Social Security, pensions, and savings—are insufficient.

EMPLOYMENT IN RETIREMENT: THE NEW CHALLENGE

While the solution of returning to the workforce to supplement income seems logical, this transition can be difficult for individuals who had decided much earlier to begin their golden years. Limited jobs for older individuals exist (especially if retirement was chosen because of serious health conditions), and fewer resources are available for them to turn to for advice, coaching, and job leads. The notion of **encore careers**, where retirees from one industry pursue jobs in new fields, is a relatively recent development; websites such as www .encore.org cater to that market. Websites such as www.retirementjobs.com provide advice and information to older job seekers and a rating system for age-friendly employers. However, age discrimination is prevalent, especially in job markets with limited openings and large numbers of available younger workers. Nevertheless, employment in retirement may become a new norm for seniors across the globe, providing them with income to help pay for their LTC needs.

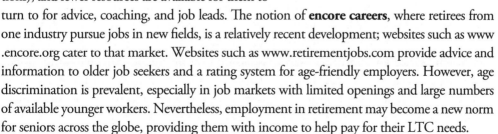

KEY POINT
New Retirement Options

Economic downturns and the increasing cost of healthcare have led many of today's retirees to return to the workforce.

Encore career
Employment in the second half of life, often in positions of greater meaning and social impact in not-for-profit or public-interest fields.

Defined benefit plan
A retirement plan, typically funded by an employer, that pays a retiree a set amount of money on a predictable schedule.

Defined contribution plan
A retirement plan to which an employer contributes money, such as a 401(k), while the person is employed there. Once that employee leaves the company, the company's obligation is over.

Social Security
A federal government program that pays benefits to senior citizens and certain other individuals. Social Security often serves as the primary source of retirement income for low income elderly persons.

Long-term care
A wide range of health services, supportive services, and other assistance, provided informally or formally to individuals who have a chronic illness or disability and are unable to function independently on a daily basis.

EMPLOYER-SPONSORED RETIREMENT PLANS

Employer-sponsored pensions were introduced as a benefit after World War II. At retirement, individuals working for many years could rely on a pension provided by their employer (a **defined benefit plan**) and, often, on employer-paid healthcare benefits. Thus, they could pursue retirement with the feeling of financial security. The role of these plans has greatly changed since their inception. Economic concerns have prompted many organizations to change the model of their pension plan to a **defined contribution plan**. A defined contribution plan differs from a defined benefit plan in that the company contributes money to an employee's retirement plan, such as a 401(k), while the person is employed there, but once that employee leaves the company, the company's obligation is over.

THE CHANGING ROLE OF PUBLIC PENSION PLANS

For many individuals older than 65, **Social Security** benefits are a primary source of retirement income. Since 1950, the portion of Social Security designated for retirees—the Old Age and Survivors Income (OASI) trust fund—has operated under a pay as you go structure referred to as current-cost financing. Significant increases in the elderly population, lower birthrates, and decreased labor force due to economic downturns could compromise Social Security's capability to provide the largest portion of retirement income for retirees; even if Social Security remains at its current level, many retirees will have to work to supplement their income. This aging tsunami is not exclusive to the United States; the situation is the same in many European and Asian nations. With increasingly older populations and tighter budgets, policymakers may seek more cost-effective approaches to providing LTC services (Huber et al. 2009). For example, Germany and Sweden have developed model return-to-work programs for individuals with disabilities in an attempt to curb potential increases in pension fund expenditures (Sim 1999).

WHAT IS LONG-TERM CARE?

Long-term care consists of a wide variety of health and support services and other assistance provided informally or formally to individuals who have a chronic illness or disability and are unable to function independently. **Long-term care services** may be offered to consumers (at any age and in various settings) who need help performing **activities of daily living (ADLs)**, such as bathing, dressing, eating, toileting, and transferring (e.g., walking), and **instrumental activities of daily living (IADLs)**, including cooking, cleaning, buying groceries and other essentials, administering medication, handling money or finances, and using the telephone. Individuals with Alzheimer's disease or dementia have additional, specialized needs. LTC services can be tailored to the physical, mental, emotional, social, spiritual, and financial demand and capacity of the client, and the service may evolve over time as the needs and resources of the client change. LTC is oriented toward managing and living with chronic illness or disabilities, not curing them. As such, it aims to ensure continuity of care rather than episodic interventions (Hooyman and Kiyak 2011).

THE HISTORY OF LONG-TERM CARE SERVICE DELIVERY

To understand the structure of the LTC delivery system today, look at its rich history and heritage in the United States. Research by Smith and Feng (2010) suggests a timeline of cycles and concerns in LTC that consists of five distinct periods of approximately 20 years each over the past century. Each period focused on a specific concern and supposed solution that added to an inadequate safety net of care that still exists today.

DID YOU KNOW?
Pensions Evolve

In some instances, the threat of bankruptcy or closure forced large companies to terminate their pension plans, leaving many long-serving employees with a fraction of their planned retirement income. In addition, the introduction of the pension accounting rule (Financial Accounting Standards Board Rule 106) in the 1990s led many employers to end healthcare coverage for future retirees and pass along cost increases to individuals already receiving benefits from the plans. These trends will continue, and current members of the workforce will be less able to rely on the resources of their employers to finance their retirement income needs.

THE FIRST AND SECOND PERIODS

During the first period, which lasted until 1930, all infirmed were put together in almshouses, sometimes referred to as poor farms for elderly "inmates." When the Social Security Act was passed in 1935, pensions were provided to older people, but with the stipulation that anyone housed in a public facility such as an almshouse could not receive one. While the intent of this legislation was to bring about the end of almshouses, it helped establish voluntary and proprietary nursing homes that accepted people with physical and mental infirmities (Mara 2008). Residing in these private boarding homes allowed those with LTC needs to be eligible for federal Old Age Assistance, which started the second period—Old-Age Income Security Solution.

THE THIRD PERIOD

By the 1950s, much more legislation emerged, establishing the next phase of public financing for nursing-home facility construction and public payment for LTC services. This period expanded access to affordable health insurance and lasted until 1970. Changes to the Social Security Act permitted payments to public LTC institutions and direct government payments

Long-term care services
Services provided to consumers at any age and in a wide range of settings that correspond to problems in performing activities of daily living and instrumental activities of daily living.

Activities of daily living (ADLs)
Routine daily activities; the basic ADLs are eating, bathing, dressing, toileting, and walking. A person's ability to perform ADLs is a determining factor in the level of long-term care he needs.

CURRENT ISSUE
The Widespread Use of Long-Term Care Services

According to a recent study, LTC services are used by 10.9 million noninstitutional-ized people (50 percent of whom are not elderly) and 1.8 million people who live in nursing homes (most of whom are elderly). This study revealed that 92 percent of noninstitutionalized elderly receive unpaid help with their care, while only 13 percent receive paid help (Kaye, Harrington, and LaPlante 2010). These statistics indicate that a significant portion of the US population is already consuming LTC services and that a formal paid system of caregiving support that would allow them to continue to live in the community would be limited.

Instrumental activities of daily living (IADLs) Activities such as shopping, house cleaning, cooking, and managing finances that are not necessary for fundamental functioning but allow people to function independently.

to LTC facilities, which made the industry appealing to small-business owners. In addition, during this period, state-licensure programs for nursing homes started to appear.

The Hill-Burton Act of 1946 was amended in 1954, which made federal grants (along with construction and design guidelines) available to both public and not-for-profit companies interested in building nursing homes. However, the amendments stipulated that these homes be affiliated with hospitals, thereby promoting the medical model of care within a nursing home environment. In the late 1950s, the American Association of Nursing Homes was formed, and this group successfully lobbied Congress to pass legislation allowing for-profits to obtain nursing-home funding from the Small Business Administration (SBA) and the Federal Housing Administration (FHA). The Kerr-Mills Act of 1960 followed, which provided federal–state matching funds for the medically needy, such as nursing home residents, and federal money for home care services.

The tradition of federal oversight and financing of LTC carried over into the Great Society legislation of the 1960s. Medicare and Medicaid were signed into law in 1965, and a provision in Medicare covered post-hospital "extended care" of 100 days. Then, in 1968, the Moss amendments to the Social Security Act established new rules and regulations for Medicaid-funded nursing homes to follow.

THE FOURTH PERIOD

From the early 1970s through 1990, the fourth period of government program options and enforcement ensued, further expanding government attempts to control provider abuses. The Social Security amendments were extended to offer Medicare coverage to individuals with disabilities; the Supplemental Security Income (SSI) program was instituted;

and, by the late 1970s, certificate-of-need programs and amendments to the Medicare and Medicaid anti-fraud and abuse provisions were passed. In 1983, concern about escalating healthcare costs led to the creation of Medicare diagnosis-related groups (DRGs), which limited payments to hospitals and helped move post-acute care to ambulatory care and nursing home facilities where there were few payment limitations. The familiar theme of federal oversight of LTC services emerged again in 1987 when the Omnibus Reconciliation Act created the State Survey and Enforcement System for nursing homes.

THE FIFTH PERIOD

The 1990s to the present can be characterized as a phase of market reforms, innovative demonstration programs, and expansion of private insurance for LTC expenses. In 1997, Congress passed the Balanced Budget Act, which established the Prospective Payment System for Medicare-funded post-hospital services; in 2004, quality indicators were established for nursing homes that accept Medicare payments. The 1999 Supreme Court *Olmstead* decision, which prohibited unnecessary institutionalization of persons with disabilities, provided the impetus for expansion of home and community-based services, and by 2007, nearly 40 percent of Medicaid expenditures were for services provided in noninstitutional settings. New homelike models of care evolved, such as assisted living, Eden Alternative housing, and Green House cottages. Despite the innovations of the past decades, financial challenges remain. The cost of LTC services for all individuals who need them, regardless of their geographic location or income, continues to strain government and family budgets.

THE AGING PROCESS AND LONG-TERM CARE SERVICE DELIVERY

Knowledge of the **aging process** is essential to understand the LTC delivery system. Changes in the functions and capabilities of the body are natural and are critical determinants of service provision and reimbursement.

Aging process
The changes in the functions and capabilities of people's bodies over time; influenced by genetic and environmental factors.

GENETIC AND ENVIRONMENTAL FACTORS

How an individual ages depends on genetic and environmental factors. Genetics, more than the environment, may account for the difference in the way people age; however, lifestyle choices such as diet, exercise, tobacco use, and outlook are also important to consider.

PHYSICAL SIGNS OF AGING

The body is the window to aging. Over the years, height can shrink due to poor posture, bending of the spine, and foot problems. The fat proportion of the body can double between

Early Indicators Project
A long-term study of Union Army members that put forth a theory of "technophysio evolution," which posits that humans have gained a degree of control over their environment that has permitted rapid improvements in morbidity and mortality.

ages 25 and 75 (American Geriatrics Society 2005). One consequence of the change in fat proportion is that drugs that dissolve in fat tissues remain in the body longer in older bodies than in younger bodies.

The way the body regulates its various systems (e.g., circulatory, nervous, respiratory, digestive) is also affected by age. For example, a weakened heart or clogged arteries impede the body's method of pumping blood throughout the systems. Older individuals regulate the amount and makeup of body fluids more slowly, which makes them more susceptible to infections.

The body is not affected by genetics alone; it can adapt to environmental stimulants and rejuvenate itself. The **Early Indicators Project**, a study of Union Army soldiers, most of whom lived to age 65 and even 70, put forth the theory of technophysio evolution. This theory suggests that over time, humans have gained a progressively higher degree of control over their environment, which has permitted rapid improvements in morbidity and mortality. Consequently, disability rates may decline with future aging cohorts, which could lead to an era in which the elderly have fewer limitations (Fogel 2004).

MODELS OF LONG-TERM CARE DELIVERY

Continuum of long-term care
A holistic system comprising services and mechanisms that assist individuals over time through a wide range of physical health, mental health, and social services needs, across all levels of care intensity.

The opportunities for provision of LTC services have evolved; a growing proportion of services are now provided in the home and other community-based settings, rather than in traditional residential or acute care environments such as nursing homes or hospitals. To facilitate reimbursement, many providers of LTC services have organized their activities around a **continuum of long-term care**. This continuum "is defined as a [holistic] system of services and integrating mechanisms that guide and track [clients] through an array of health, mental health, and social services spanning all levels of intensity of care. It includes mechanisms for organizing services and operating them as an integrated system" (Evashwick 2007). This continuum helps individuals understand and organize their thinking about the provision of LTC services. However, growing issues of treatment and payment for chronic illness, and the increasing complexity of the reimbursement system for LTC (especially services provided on an informal basis), may require different approaches as the boomer population and generations that follow move into retirement and their third age.

Single point of entry (POE) model
A model of long-term care in which patients can obtain all the services they need through a single agency or organization.

Since the 1990s, many states have moved to a **single point of entry (POE) model** for LTC service. The POE model is known by various names, such as single-entry point and aging single-access point. Regardless of the terminology used, the POE model means that patients can obtain all LTC services through just one provider organization. This movement has also grown in an attempt to comply with the US Supreme Court *Olmstead* decision requiring individuals receiving LTC to obtain services in the least restrictive setting possible (Mollot and Rudder 2008). Because only one provider coordinates and delivers the care, decreasing inefficiencies and red tape, the expectation is that the POE model saves the consumer time and money.

Exhibit 1.1
Dimensions of
Long-Term Care
Model

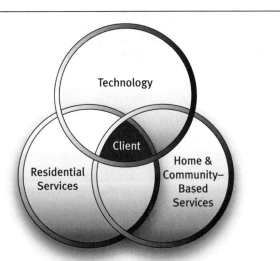

© Mary Helen McSweeney-Feld

Another approach to the delivery of LTC services is the **dimensions of care model**, shown in Exhibit 1.1, which acknowledges the services identified in the continuum of care model, allows the consumer to have a single point of entry into the LTC delivery system, and emphasizes the need for the consumer to use technology in administering self-care and to use services within the community in a cost-effective fashion. The technology component in the model is important, as the growth in the size of the aging population in the twenty-first century will require seniors to use technology to age in their communities in a cost-effective fashion as the availability of caregivers (especially unpaid) declines. This approach is also nonlinear in that it acknowledges that individuals may consume services in acute and post-acute care environments as well as in community-based settings.

While no model of LTC service provision is ideal in explaining the consumption of services, the dimensions model gives consumers greater flexibility to determine the combinations of services that best allow them to age with dignity and enjoy a greater quality of life. It is also the basis for the organization of this book.

Dimensions of care model

A nonlinear approach to long-term care that acknowledges the services identified in the continuum of care model, allows the consumer to have a single point of entry into the LTC delivery system, and encourages consumers to use technology in administering self-care and to use services within the community.

CURRENT ISSUE
Long-Term Care Settings: Rural Versus Urban Communities

Rural areas present special challenges to the delivery of LTC services. Approximately 22 percent of people aged 65 or older reside in rural areas (2000 US Census figures), and rural seniors make up a larger proportion of their community's population than urban seniors do.

(continued)

CURRENT ISSUE (continued)
Long-Term Care Settings: Rural versus Urban Communities

A large population of seniors live in the rural areas of the South and Midwest (Ricketts 1999). Rural elders are older than their urban counterparts, with many seniors belonging in the oldest-old (older than 85) category. Often, elder-focused healthcare and LTC services in rural areas are more expensive, inconveniently located, and not widely available (Ricketts 1999). Among rural seniors' challenges are insufficient transportation options, a limited number of care providers (especially physicians), and inadequate funding for community-based social and health services. In addition, poor seniors in rural areas often suffer from substandard living conditions marked by nutritional deficiencies, dilapidated housing, and overall poor health (Rogers 1999).

The mix of residential and community-based providers for LTC services is also different in rural areas. Rural elderly people are more likely to use a nursing home than an assisted living facility (ALF), due to income constraints and limited availability. They are more likely to rely on Medicaid than are urban elderly people, which means rural nursing homes generally have fewer services and higher utilization rates than urban nursing homes do. The same situation exists with rural ALFs; they tend to offer less privacy and fewer services than their urban counterparts. Many LTC services, such as skilled nursing care, are provided in institutional settings such as rural and critical access hospitals. Choices for nonresidential care services are also limited in rural areas. Home health care agencies are fewer in number, are more likely to use nursing aides, and offer a smaller variety of services. However, the growth of telehealth services (healthcare services provided through the use of telecommunication, Internet, or other assistive technology) has helped spread knowledge and use of community-based services in remote areas.

In 2008, the Rural Long Term Care Workgroup (a nongovernmental organization that consists of governmental and private long-term care providers) convened a national workshop to identify strategies for building rural eldercare services. Resource and referral programs, day care–based PACE (Programs of All-Inclusive Care for the Elderly), telehealth, and care management were identified as options. Community infrastructure building—which relies on the participation of churches, faith-based groups, and community organizations such as colleges and universities—and more flexible funding strategies from state Medicaid programs were identified as critical factors in the provision of quality services in rural settings (Rural Long-Term Care Workgroup 2008).

KEY ASPECTS OF LONG-TERM CARE

WHAT ARE LONG-TERM CARE SERVICES?

LTC services are provided in six distinct settings:

- ◆ Acute care
- ◆ Ambulatory care
- ◆ Home
- ◆ Residential
- ◆ Outreach and linkage
- ◆ Technological

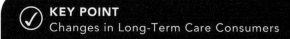

KEY POINT
Changes in Long-Term Care Consumers

While most people envision the consumers of LTC services as aged or elderly, many are nonelderly with physical or intellectual disabilities.

This list represents a consolidation and extension of earlier service models and incorporates new developments in residential care alternatives and the use of technology to link service providers to consumers of LTC who live in remote areas.

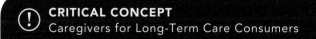

CRITICAL CONCEPT
Caregivers for Long-Term Care Consumers

While not direct consumers of LTC services, caregivers influence the decision to use LTC programs and services. Caregiving—which is performed by either a paid employee or unpaid family members or friends—is a complex concept that covers a wide range of care.

The population being served may be children, all adults (aged 18 years or older), older adults (aged 50 to 64), the elderly (aged 65 to 85), or the oldest-old (aged over 85). The reason for providing care may be physical impairments from birth, disability after an accident, complications resulting from a chronic illness, or Alzheimer's disease or other dementia—a range of conditions, causes, and ages of onset.

The care may be informal (provided by a spouse, child, sibling, or other family member), formal (provided by a trained professional), or a combination of the two. The caregiver may live far away from the recipient, in the same community or neighborhood, or in the recipient's residence. The concept of caregiving is also complicated by the fact that some individuals providing care do not identify themselves as caregivers. Sometimes, caring for an older parent or spouse is not a role that adult children or spouses expect, but when the need arises, they attempt to provide some level of care.

WHO ARE FAMILY CAREGIVERS?

Caregivers
Individuals who provide healthcare and/or supportive long-term care services. Caregivers are an important part of the system of support that allows consumers to continue to live in the community.

Caregivers provide a variety of supportive services for loved ones or other consumers. The caregiver for an older adult male is most likely to be his spouse. Older women, however, are more often cared for by another family member—usually an adult child—because many women outlive their spouses. Spousal care declines with a person's age, but care provided by an adult child and other relatives increases with age (Novak 1989, 354). Estimates of the number of family caregivers vary. In the United States, an estimated 34 million family caregivers, the majority of them women, provide 75 to 80 percent of LTC in the community; the estimated value of their unpaid labor is $375 billion a year. Note that this unpaid contribution is usually not considered when researchers estimate the costs of LTC or healthcare (Gibson and Houser 2007). In America's fragmented LTC delivery system, formal caregivers come and go, and family caregivers are often the only people who witness a family member's entire illness (Levine et al. 2010).

Policymakers who are attempting to save money and provide better quality care through healthcare reform should consider four main areas of concern with respect to caregiving and caregivers: (1) the collection of comprehensive information about family caregivers; (2) continued funding for training and support of caregivers; (3) recognition of the needs of caregivers in programs that transition individuals from institutional to noninstitutional settings; and (4) financing reforms (Levine et al. 2010).

WHAT KINDS OF ORGANIZATIONS PROVIDE LONG-TERM CARE SERVICES?

Hospitals, nursing homes, and other residential care organizations provide a large proportion of LTC services. However, a growing proportion of LTC services are delivered through home-based and community-based programs. These providers may be privately owned; for-profit or not-for-profit; governmental, such as the Area Agencies on Aging or Veterans Affairs; or faith-based. As the use of assistive technology in the provision of long-term care services grows, the list of organizations providing such technology may include technology start-ups as well as large, established computer, telecommunications, and pharmaceutical firms looking to expand their markets and services.

WHO PAYS FOR LONG-TERM CARE SERVICES?

Payment for formal LTC services in the United States comes primarily from government sources such as Medicare and Medicaid. In 2007, of the total $190.4 billion in estimated spending for nursing home and home health care, Medicare paid for 25 percent, Medicaid and other public funds paid for 42 percent, out-of-pocket funds (i.e., payments for services directly by individuals) paid for 22 percent, and private insurance and other sources paid for 11 percent (excluding hospital-based spending on skilled nursing care) (Hartman et al. 2010). Private sources of payment include commercial insurance providers such as traditional and managed care insurance plans, private LTC insurance, and private pay initiatives.

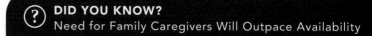

DID YOU KNOW?
Need for Family Caregivers Will Outpace Availability

Soon, there will be more older persons in need of family caregivers than there will be family members who can fill the responsibility. The need for family caregivers will increase in the future, because the proportion of the population that is older than 65 is expected to increase at a rate of 2.3 percent, while the number of available caregivers in the family will increase at a rate of just 0.8 percent (Mack 2005).

A LOOK AHEAD

The outlook for healthcare reform and its impact on LTC services is mixed. Only a small number of LTC program initiatives have been included in the current legislation. The LTC delivery system remains fragmented and patched together, and an increasing number of clients will likely enter the system as America ages. The situation is similar in many European and Asian countries that are facing the strains of declining tax revenues, the need to fund expensive public health and retirement programs, and the rapid growth in the proportion of people in their 60s who are eligible to collect benefits from these programs. However, LTC providers are looking at new options for provision of care, such as greater use of technology and shared resources in community settings. These options have created growth in new industries and new job opportunities for individuals interested in providing care to the growing senior market.

FOR DISCUSSION

1. What is the aging tsunami, and why is it an important factor in understanding the delivery of LTC services?

2. What are the four pillars of retirement income, and how are they related to retirement?

3. What are encore careers?

4. What are the periods of care in the history of LTC service delivery, and why are they important?

5. Describe two important physiological factors in the aging process.

6. What are activities of daily living, and why are they used as determinants of need for LTC services?

7. Why is the role of unpaid caregivers an important factor in the provision of LTC services?

8. What are some limitations faced by agencies and community organizations that provide LTC services in rural areas?

9. Who are the consumers of LTC services, and are they all aged 65 or older?

10. What is the role of employer-sponsored health and pension plans in the retirement of individuals, and why are these plans important?

PART II

Care Settings for Long-Term Care Services

Long-term care services are delivered in two settings: (1) residential care, where individuals live in specialized housing to receive services; and (2) community-based and home-based care, where clients receive services or engage in self-care but live in their own homes. A third (and growing) option for LTC service delivery is the use of technology, such as information systems and assistive technologies. Technology often allows consumers to care for themselves as they age in the community. The variety of these technology-based services and the volume of services provided have grown tremendously in recent years.

The premise of this book is that the structure of LTC service delivery has evolved from a predictive, linear continuum of care process to a more flexible model. This model, called the dimensions of long-term care model, emphasizes that consumers move fluidly between all three care settings—residential, home and community, and technological.

Part II of this book provides information on each of these care settings and shows how the dimensions model operates for specialized issues of chronic disease management and end-of-life care. Chapter 2 focuses on the range of residential care settings, from independent living to assistive living to the skilled nursing facility, and reviews the continuing care retirement community, which incorporates aspects of all other residential settings in one location. The chapter also makes a comparison between residential LTC services in this country and those in other countries. New directions in care settings, as well as their impact on tomorrow's service delivery, also are discussed.

Chapter 3 is an overview of LTC services provided within community-based and home-based settings—a growing portion of the LTC industry. Chapter 4 looks at the use of technology—that is, information systems to manage residential, home-based, and community-based services and assistive technology to support consumers with LTC needs. Chapter 5 examines the special needs of individuals with chronic disease and illness within a case study of Alzheimer's disease and dementia. Chapter 6 provides a review of care settings by discussing hospice and palliative care—interventions offered at the end of life. Chapter 7 completes the overview by discussing cultural competency issues related to long-term care.

CHAPTER 2

Residential Settings for Long-Term Care Services

Mary Helen McSweeney-Feld, PhD; Reid Oetjen, PhD; and Lawanda D. Warthen, PhD

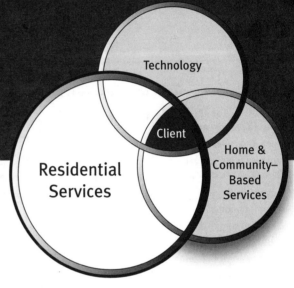

LEARNING OBJECTIVES

After completing this chapter, you should be able to

➤ define the terms *independent living, assisted living, skilled nursing facility,* and *continuing care retirement community*;

➤ describe the history and development of residential long-term care settings in the United States;

➤ explain the types of long-term care services delivered in residential settings;

➤ describe the factors driving the demand for long-term care services provided in residential care settings and the demand for high quality services in those settings;

➤ compare residential care settings in the United States with those in other countries; and

➤ discuss new developments for the provision of residential long-term care services.

INTRODUCTION

The term *residential care* is used to describe a variety of LTC services typically provided to individuals within a specific housing setting. The primary industry segments are (1) independent living and congregate care community, (2) assisted living facility, and (3) skilled nursing facility. A fourth industry segment is the continuing care retirement community, which integrates aspects of the three other segments, typically on one campus or in one geographic area. While some of these residential options have distinct service components, the lines between skilled nursing facilities and less intense residential alternatives are blurring.

INDEPENDENT LIVING

Independent living
A category of housing options for individuals who are able to live without assistance, including adult communities and congregate housing arrangements. These residences often impose age restrictions and offer social activities, supportive services, and increased security.

The term ***independent living*** covers a broad range of settings in which individuals, as a matter of preference and lifestyle, move into adult communities or congregate housing arrangements that impose age restrictions, offer social activities, and usually provide increased security. The target age for these residences is 50 or older. Typically, no healthcare services are offered as part of the residential contract, although individuals may be able to pay for outside assistance as necessary. The size of these arrangements can vary from a high-rise apartment building or townhouse condominium development to entire city settings, such as Sun City, Arizona, an independent living community of more than 100,000 individuals that features large recreational facilities and a wide range of activities. Other independent living arrangements include less structured community options—in some of these cases, individuals seeking services pay a fee for access; in others, local governments subsidize the provision of supportive services.

THE HISTORY OF INDEPENDENT LIVING

Section 202
A specialized housing subsidy program under the US Department of Housing and Urban Development that provides financing for construction of housing for low-income senior citizens and those with disabilities.

Independent living in the United States has its historical roots in two movements: the public housing movement of the 1930s and the development of age-segregated communities in Arizona in the 1950s. The foundation for independent housing arrangements within public housing was first developed during the New Deal era with the passage of the National Housing Act of 1934. City slums were demolished, public housing authorities were established, and waves of public housing were built in all of America's large cities.

This movement resumed with President Truman's American Housing Act of 1949, which set off a second wave of public housing construction. As adults older than 65 with lower incomes became eligible for public housing in the 1950s, projects started to provide for the needs of the active senior. In 1959, the **Section 202** program created a specialized housing program for older adults and those with disabilities. Many of these housing projects were built for ambulatory, independent seniors and included features such as emergency call buttons and grab bars. Under Section 202, rent subsidies are offered to low-income residents and interest-free funding is available to private or nonprofit organizations that build apartment dwellings for seniors in close proximity to other LTC residences. The program has been shown to be a cost-effective alternative to moving seniors into institutional settings before they need that level of services (Haley and Grey 2008).

In 1970, President Nixon signed a federal housing initiative called **Section 8**. This program has two components: (1) project-based vouchers given to a landlord who has reserved a portion of an existing, newly constructed, or rehabilitated housing to low-income (Section 8) renters; and (2) housing-choice vouchers given to individuals (elderly, disabled, and low-income) to use in renting a place that they select. The housing-choice voucher empowers those under the program to live outside housing projects.

At the same time as the public housing market for seniors was growing out of New Deal programs, the passage of the Social Security Act in 1935 was helping breed a new category of people—retirees. Retirement was an evolving concept, and it led to a novel idea: communities where active seniors could enjoy a full life without the obligations of children and work. These **age-segregated communities**, where seniors live with their peers, grew in popularity.

While religious and fraternal organizations had created retirement communities as early as the 1920s, the first age-segregated community—Youngtown—was created in 1954 in Arizona by Benjamin Schleifer. The philosophy behind age segregation was that supporting schools is costly, and one of Schleifer's main objectives was to ensure that Youngtown's residents could afford to live with dignity, even if their sole income came from Social Security benefits (Blechman 2008). Because only seniors lived in these communities, they did not need to raise tax dollars for schools.

This concept attracted the attention of real estate developer Del Webb, who conducted market research that suggested that retirees would welcome the opportunity to distance themselves from their offspring and that high on their priority list was good weather and something to do (Blechman 2008). He opened Sun City, Arizona, on New Year's Day in 1960, sold 2,000 homes by the year's end, and was heralded by *Time* magazine as the man who put "active" into retirement. By 1977, Sun City became Arizona's seventh-largest community, with 40,000 inhabitants. Webb's company eventually committed all its resources to building retirement communities. Sun City also became the model for other age-segregated communities in California, Florida, Texas, the Carolinas, and other states.

NEW DEVELOPMENTS IN INDEPENDENT LIVING

The notion of independent living communities has evolved into numerous community-based models, such as **naturally occurring retirement communities (NORCs)**, planned virtual retirement communities, cohousing communities, and livable communities.

Section 8
An affordable housing assistance program under the US Department of Housing and Urban Development that provides funds to landlords who designate a portion of their property for Section 8 tenants and rental vouchers to individuals who then select their own housing.

Age-segregated communities
Also known as age-restricted communities, this is housing, frequently gated, that restricts ownership of units to individuals over a set age, such as age 50 or 55, in order to provide a living area without the perceived problems of having children around.

Naturally occurring retirement communities (NORCs)
Communities with a large proportion of older persons residing within a specific geographical area. These communities frequently offer supportive service programs administered under the US Administration on Aging.

Planned virtual retirement community (PVRC)
A community in which the elderly live in their own homes, but receive information and services to help them remain independent.

Cohousing community
A type of collaborative community designed and operated by the residents. The community may be multigenerational or exclusively for people aged 55 and older.

Livable community
A community that includes features such as reasonably priced housing, access to public transportation, easy navigation, and supportive services that help residents remain independent and engaged, civically and socially.

NORCs are locales (e.g., neighborhoods, districts) in which more than 50 percent of the population is made up of elderly people. Even a building filled with senior citizens can be considered a NORC. These communities are called "naturally occurring" because they were not initially designated to be areas for older individuals; rather, they turned this way as a result of residents aging in the homes they occupied for many years or seniors moving into the area.

NORCs were officially recognized beginning in 1985, when the United Jewish Communities in New York City developed a supportive services model for such communities. This led to a new federal program, Community Innovations for Aging in Place, which was created by the 2006 reauthorization of the Older Americans Act. Under this program, more than 45 communities in 26 states received demonstration grant funding for NORCs. The NORC supportive services programs are designed to prevent service fragmentation and create healthy, integrated communities in which seniors can age in place. These programs fund social workers and healthcare workers and may involve ancillary services, ranging from adult daycare and transportation to a variety of supportive services (Bedney and Goldberg 2009).

Planned virtual retirement communities (PVRCs), sometimes referred to as villages, are self-help groups that link the elderly to community services to enable them to age in place successfully. Examples of successful PVRCs are the Community Without Walls in Princeton, New Jersey; Beacon Hill Village in Boston; and Capitol Hill Village in Washington, DC. PVRCs charge their members a nominal fee in exchange for resource information or small services, such as dog walking, meal preparation, or picture hanging (Gleckman 2009).

Cohousing communities are collaborative places in which residents actively participate in the design and operation of their own neighborhoods. The cohousing idea originated in Denmark and was promoted in the 1980s by the architects Kathryn McCamant and Charles Durett. Community members often eat meals together and collectively decide how to allocate resources within the community. The communities may be intergenerational or may be specific to seniors. Many communities are organized as clusters of housing units, intended to encourage walking and socialization, and have a common house as the center of the community where optional meals are shared and other activities take place. They may be organized around themes of sustainability or shared resources (Cohousing 2010).

According to AARP (Pandya 2005), "a livable community is one that has affordable and appropriate housing, supportive community features and services, and adequate mobility options, which together facilitate personal independence and the engagement of residents in civic and social life." **Livable communities** have developed grassroots organizations that study and provide support for seniors aging in their communities; the concept has been applied in a variety of LTC arrangements, such as communities for adults with disabilities and transportation systems and the elderly.

CRITICAL CONCEPT
Community Attachment and Community Engagement

Beyond 50.05: A Report to the Nation on Livable Communities contains results from a 2004 survey conducted by AARP and the Roper Public Affairs group. The report presents scales for two key concepts and indexes related to livable communities: community attachment and community engagement. The Community Attachment Index, which measures ties to neighbors and community, is drawn from questions about knowing neighbors by name, perceptions of community, and the desire to remain in the same community. The Community Engagement Index provides a summary measure across a range of activities that actively engage a person in the community around him, including volunteering, visiting neighbors, working on local issues, and political participation. The study found that community attachment is highly linked to successful aging, and options that facilitate community engagement, especially transportation and housing that are affordable and meet the healthcare needs of seniors, influence the livability of a community for elders (AARP 2005a).

Congregate care facilities
Facilities typically designed for those aged 75 to 82 that offer social activities and homemaker services such as meals, housekeeping services, and transportation. These homes also provide assistance with the instrumental activities of daily living.

Congregate care facilities offer social activities, security, and homemaker services such as meals, housekeeping services, and transportation. The target population of these facilities is typically persons aged 75 to 82. Their focus is to provide companionship, organized activities, and, in the event of a health-related event, some temporary personal care. Congregate care facilities typically assist residents with the instrumental activities of daily living, such as preparing meals, doing housework, shopping, and going to healthcare appointments. These facilities are typically regulated by the state agency responsible for supervision of healthcare services. They are known across the United States by a variety of names, such as adult foster care, board and care homes, congregate care homes, personal care homes, and enriched housing.

DID YOU KNOW?
Professional Associations for Long-Term Care Administrators

As the US population continues to grow and the demand for LTC services expands, owners and administrators of organizations that provide such services and support will be looking for individuals who are knowledgeable about the field of LTC administration. Professional associations such as the American College of Health Care Administrators (www.achca.org) and the National Association of Long Term Care Administrator Boards (www.nabweb.org) recognize that today's students are tomorrow's leaders. Check out their websites for more information.

INDEPENDENT LIVING: SETTINGS, CLIENTS, OWNERSHIP, AND FINANCING

The characteristics of independent living are highly varied, as seen in Exhibit 2.1. They range from high-end communities for the affluent—some of which have age restrictions and require the residents to purchase their living units—to group housing arrangements or government-subsidized housing options. Some clients served in independent living have substantial financial assets and income and seek socialization or the security of living in a supportive community. Other independent living residents have limited incomes. Many clients of subsidized housing options are older, widowed women in their late 70s and 80s with limited income.

With the aging of the US population, the need for this type of housing option may rapidly increase. Like the communities and clients themselves, the owners or operators of independent living communities have a wide financial range. Some are for-profit senior living companies that cater to the needs of the affluent, while others are not-for-profit entities or municipalities that seek to serve older adults who have limited financial means. Consequently, the fees for living in these communities vary greatly. Higher-end community units can cost from $1,000 to $4,500 a month; sometimes, residents pay an entrance fee (ranging from $30,000 to nearly $400,000) and monthly maintenance fees, which typically range from $400 to $3,000 or more. Congregate housing costs from $500 to $4,000 a month and may include housekeeping and activities (Pratt 2010). Wealthier seniors typically pay for these living arrangements themselves (especially for services in higher-end independent living complexes), while residents of subsidized senior apartment complexes rely on government assistance. Individuals who reside in the community and are members of living community networks may pay a membership fee for access to services, or their membership may be subsidized by their community, which is the case with NORCs.

EXHIBIT 2.1 Independent Living: Settings, Clients, Ownership, and Financing	*Settings*	High-end, diverse living complexes with multiple services/socialization opportunities Apartment complexes with basic services Service networks supported by members or government programs
	Clients	Affluent elderly people with financial resources Lower-income seniors with limited resources
	Ownership	For-profit senior housing or hospitality companies Not-for-profit, faith-based, or local communities
	Financing	Rental or unit purchase with monthly maintenance; out-of-pocket payments Subsidized monthly rates based on means-testing and federal government program guidelines Membership fees, sometimes subsidized by government programs

ASSISTED LIVING

There is no uniform definition of assisted living in the United States, as each state uses different terminology and determines the standards and arrangements for its local **assisted living facilities (ALFs)**. In general, however, assisted living supports individuals who have restricted functionality (due to advanced age, disability, or some other factor) while encouraging them to live with some degree of independence. ALFs provide residents a broad array of services, such as the following:

◆ Help with activities of daily living, such as eating, bathing, toileting, or getting around

◆ Around-the-clock supervision or monitoring without breaching residents' privacy

◆ Organized social activities in a safe and controlled environment

◆ Prepared meals, laundry service, healthcare services, and referrals to medical and health information and resources

> *Assisted living facilities (ALFs)*
> Facilities in which staff help residents with the activities of daily living, coordinate services from outside providers, and monitor activities to help to ensure residents' health, well-being, and safety.

THE HISTORY OF ASSISTED LIVING

Assisted living was introduced in the United States in the 1970s. It was viewed as an alternative to nursing homes for consumers who needed some personal care services, but not 24-hour medical care. Keren Brown Wilson, who began an assisted living program in Oregon, and Paul Klaussen, who started Sunrise Senior Living, were pioneers of homelike communities that offered a noninstitutional alternative to nursing homes.

In 2001, the Assisted Living Workgroup, a consortium of nearly 50 national organizations representing all aspects of assisted living, came together to develop consensus recommendations to improve the quality of assisted living. The group's activities concluded in 2003 with a list of 110 recommendations presented before the US Senate Special Committee on Aging. Despite this, states continue to regulate assisted living facilities with a variety of definitions and standards.

Two distinct stages mark the development of assisted living. The first stage was characterized by pioneering efforts to create a new kind of service where the physical plant, service delivery model, and approach to staffing support the ideas of privacy, dignity, and consumer choice. The policy discussion during this stage attempted to distinguish assisted living from other choices, such as skilled nursing homes or board and care homes. The second stage took these first principles and made them a primary driver of culture change in long-term care, resulting in more private rooms, residential living environments, greater choice of services (especially for those with disabilities), and staffing models that enhance the role of direct care workers (Redfoot 2008).

THE PHILOSOPHY OF ASSISTED LIVING

Many executives and providers of assisted living housing emphasize that assisted living is not an institution or a stopping point on a continuum but a philosophy of care. It is resident-centered and supports a resident's decision-making capabilities and right to direct his own care and activities (ALFA 2008).

Here are some common themes in assisted living:

◆ Individuals are referred to as residents or clients.

◆ Residents (along with their family) make the choice to move into and out of the facility.

◆ The facility itself is viewed as a community.

◆ Rooms or suites are viewed as standalone apartments or condominium units that cannot be accessed without permission from or knowledge of the resident, except for emergency purposes.

◆ Services are amenities offered to the resident, not parts of a treatment plan.

ASSISTED LIVING: SETTINGS, CLIENTS, OWNERSHIP, FINANCING

About 1 million Americans live in approximately 20,000 ALFs across the country. This number includes an estimated 115,000 people who receive assistance from state Medicaid programs (ALFA and NCAL 2008). Exhibit 2.2 shows the main features of assisted living.

As mentioned, assisted living is intended for those with limited functionality—whether they are older people or young adults with a disability. The diversity does not end there. ALF residents come from all income levels (from the wealthy to recipients of federal subsidies) and suffer from all types of medical and healthcare ailments (from knee problems to complications from a stroke). One of the most common ALF residents is an elderly woman who is widowed (ALFA 2008).

Costs for assisted living vary widely across states and regions. For example, the monthly fee in New York is between $1,000 and $5,800, while in California the monthly range is from $600 to $6,400 (AssistedLivingFacilities.org 2011). In some ALFs, the monthly fee pays for all services rendered to the resident, but other ALFs operate under an a la carte model, whereby separate charges for specialized services are added to the base fee. Residents typically pay for assisted living services out of pocket, but more and more people use LTC insurance or managed care insurance. The majority of state Medicaid programs offer reimbursement for a limited number of assisted living services (NCAL 2010).

EXHIBIT 2.2
Assisted Living:
Settings, Clients,
Ownership,
Financing

Settings	High-end complexes, may be freestanding or part of a continuing care community
	Apartment complexes with assistive services provided on-site
Clients	Affluent elderly people with financial resources
	Lower-income seniors with limited resources
Ownership	For-profit senior housing or hospitality companies
	For-profit mom-and-pop owners or entrepreneurs
	Not-for-profit, faith-based, or government-run communities
Financing	Rental or unit purchase with monthly maintenance; out-of-pocket payments
	Subsidized monthly rates based on means-testing and federal government program guidelines

SKILLED NURSING FACILITIES

Approximately 1.6 million Americans reside in about 17,000 **skilled nursing facilities**, and this number is expected to rise as the US population ages (AHCA 2010). Also called nursing homes, skilled nursing facilities are providers of custodial supervision and care, including short-stay rehabilitation and long-stay skilled nursing that may end in palliative and hospice care. The focus of these services is different from the hospital's focus on acute care episodes and surgical procedures.

Nursing home care revolves around chronic health conditions with no cure. While nursing care is the primary service, many skilled nursing facilities have diversified (such as by adding short-stay rehabilitation care) or have added special care units for younger residents or individuals who have Alzheimer's, AIDS, or brain injury; who use ventilators; or who need hospice care.

> **? DID YOU KNOW?**
> Perceptions of Nursing Homes
>
> According to a 2001 poll by PBS *NewsHour*, The Kaiser Family Foundation, and the Harvard School of Public Health, nearly 45 percent of the respondents believed they would be worse off after going into nursing homes than before they entered. Some gerontologists believe the traditional nursing home model will evolve into more innovative care delivery options.

Skilled nursing facilities
Facilities that provide medical, nursing, or rehabilitative services on an inpatient basis.

THE HISTORY OF NURSING HOMES

At the turn of the twentieth century, communities sent their elderly, impoverished citizens to almshouses to get care. Almshouses were charitable houses established to take care of the elderly; the conditions were often deplorable. The Social Security Act, passed in 1935, provided matching funds to states for assistance to older workers; this led to the development of private homes in which seniors could reside and collect these payments. In the 1950s, amendments to the Social Security Act required states to establish a system of licensing for nursing homes, and federal funding was also made available for building nursing homes. These regulations required that nursing homes follow a medical model of care, which sped the evolution of the industry from the welfare system to its current health-related system.

Nursing homes have long struggled with quality issues, and the federal government has historically used financial incentives to encourage compliance with quality regulations. The creation of Medicare and Medicaid in the 1960s led to the federal government paying for nursing home expenses. However, by the end of the 1960s, many facilities failed to comply with government regulations. As a result, in April 1969, the Department of Health and Human Services issued Intermediary Letter 371, which substantially reduced Medicare and Medicaid payments for nursing home services.

Nursing homes continued to have problems complying with federal regulations. In 1971, the Miller Amendment to the Social Security Act enabled the creation of intermediate-care facilities that provided less nursing care but still qualified for government reimbursement. In 1972, Public Law 92-603 allowed the Medicaid program to pay nursing homes on a reasonable cost basis. The expectation was that this would encourage skilled nursing facilities to improve their quality because providers would be reimbursed equitably for the care they delivered. However, by the 1980s, an Institute of Medicine (1986) report entitled *Improving the Quality of Care in Nursing Homes* concluded that the quality of life should be as important as the quality of care. At the time, long-term care facilities were plagued by reports of abuse and scandal. The report led to the 1987 passage of the Omnibus Reconciliation Act (OBRA 87), which instituted a top-to-bottom revision of skilled nursing facility regulations. OBRA 87 also allowed the creation of new services, such as subacute care.

Passage of the Health Insurance Portability and Accountability Act of 1996 (HIPAA) expanded the federal fraud and abuse law in the Medicare and Medicaid systems. Yet issues of quality of nursing home care continued, and in 2002, the Centers for Medicare & Medicaid Services (CMS) introduced the Nursing Home Quality Initiative (NHQI). This program established the Minimum Data Set for use in calculating reimbursement of nursing home services, set quality measures, and created Nursing Home Compare on Medicare.gov, where the public can view the results achieved by the NHQI. In 2008, CMS introduced the Five-Star Quality Rating system on Nursing Home Compare to allow consumers to distinguish high-performing facilities (five stars) from low-end performers (one star). Skilled nursing facilities are graded on the basis of various measures, such as staffing, health inspection rating, and performance on quality standards. However, the comparison feature is somewhat limited—it can only be used to compare facilities within the state, not across states (due to differences in health inspection regulations from state to state), and many of the measures used, such as staffing and quality, are self-reported by each facility.

The most recent CMS quality-monitoring initiative is the Nursing Home Value-Based Purchasing demonstration, which assesses how well or poorly skilled nursing facilities are performing against established quality standards. Facilities that show the best or improved performance are awarded incentive payments (CMS 2009). Nursing homes can also undergo accreditation and certification processes. To receive payments from Medicare and Medicaid, CMS requires nursing homes to be certified. The Joint Commission, a major accreditation organization for hospitals and other healthcare organizations, has an accreditation for skilled nursing facilities. The Commission on Accreditation of Rehabilitation Facilities (CARF) also has a certification program, but CMS does not recognize CARF accreditation as a replacement for its own certification process. Other organizations, such as Planetree, an internationally recognized leader in patient-centered care, offer designations for nursing homes for resident-focused care initiatives.

SKILLED NURSING HOMES: SETTINGS, CLIENTS, OWNERSHIP, FINANCING

Approximately 1.6 million Americans live in 17,000 nursing homes (AHCA 2010). The average number of beds in a nursing home is 107, with an average occupancy rate of 88 percent. Exhibit 2.3 provides an overview of nursing home characteristics.

Settings	Facilities, may be freestanding or part of a continuing care community	**EXHIBIT 2.3** Skilled Nursing Facilities: Settings, Clients, Ownership, Financing
	Diversified services, including short- and long-stay care	
Clients	Affluent elderly people with financial resources	
	Younger individuals who need short-stay rehabilitation care	
	Individuals who need specialty nursing care	
	Lower-income seniors who need intensive nursing care	
Ownership	For-profit senior housing or hospitality companies	
	For-profit mom-and-pop owners or entrepreneurs	
	Not-for-profit, faith-based, or government organizations	
Financing	Out-of-pocket payments, managed care insurance, and long-term care insurance payments	
	State Medicaid or other government program payments for residents who meet means-testing guidelines	

> ⓘ **CRITICAL CONCEPT**
> Nursing Homes by the Numbers
>
> Almost 90 percent of nursing home residents are older than age 65, and almost half of these are older than age 85 (*2004 National Nursing Home Survey: Facilities*, table 1). The average age of admission to a nursing home is 79, and women outnumber men three to one. The typical resident needs help with 3.75 activities of daily living (U.S. Bureau of Census 2000). Forty-two percent of residents have some form of dementia, and 33 percent have symptoms of depression (Gruber-Baldini et al. 2005). The average length of stay is two and a half years, but many nursing homes take shorter-stay residents (three months or less) for rehabilitation and other services reimbursed by Medicare or private insurance. Unlike hospitals, which are predominantly not-for-profit, for-profit skilled nursing facilities represented 67 percent of the marketplace in 2000. Only 26 percent of nursing homes were nonprofit, while 7 percent were government-run. Reimbursement for skilled nursing facility services is also different from hospitals, with 68 percent of services covered by Medicaid, 8 percent by Medicare, and 23 percent from private or out-of-pocket payments (NCHS 2004).

CONTINUING CARE RETIREMENT COMMUNITIES

Continuing care retirement communities (CCRCs)
Residential complexes for seniors that offer comprehensive nursing care and housing options to residents as they age and their needs change. Assisted living, skilled nursing, and independent living facilities, along with their respective nursing and service components, are all located in one community.

Continuing care retirement communities (CCRCs) are residential complexes for seniors that offer comprehensive nursing care and housing options to residents as they age and their needs change. Assisted living, skilled nursing, and independent living facilities, along with their respective nursing and service components, are all located in one community. This convenience allows seniors to age in place. Also called life care facilities, CCRCs often attract younger, active seniors, who move into the independent living facilities at first and then move to assisted living facilities within the campus if that need arises later in life. Active seniors may live in various independent living dwellings, such as a condominium or a single-family home.

THE HISTORY OF CONTINUING CARE RETIREMENT COMMUNITIES

CCRCs began to evolve in the early 1900s. Originally CCRCs were sponsored by churches and provided lifetime care for aging people without families in exchange for the person giving her assets to the church. Many nonprofit organizations continue to sponsor CCRCs. These nonprofits establish CCRCs that are intended for members of certain groups, such as those who share a religious belief, ethnic or racial background, and social or professional society. However, there are also CCRCs that do not cater to any groups (AAHSA 2008).

CCRCs: Settings, Clients, Ownership, Financing

The number of CCRCs has grown rapidly since 1960. According to LeadingAge (formerly the American Association of Homes and Services for the Aging), there were almost 1,900 CCRCs in the United States in 2012 (Maag 2012). The number increases by 15 to 20 percent each year. Exhibit 2.4 examines the characteristics of CCRCs (Ziegler Capital Markets 2009).

Virtually all seniors are candidates for a CCRC, including those who

◆   are physically able and well;

◆   like socializing with peers and others in the community;

◆   prefer a secure, quiet facility with easily accessible services;

◆   need help with activities of daily living; and

◆   can afford the high cost of being in the community.

Among the housing options for seniors, CCRCs are the most expensive, even though some individuals may qualify for a subsidy. For starters, there is an entrance fee, which costs between $20,000 and $500,000, depending on whether the senior buys or rents, what amenities are included, how big the living quarters are, and what type of contract is selected. Add to this cost the monthly fees, which range from $500 to $3,000 (SeniorHomes.com 2012).

Settings	Integrated community, frequently one campus, providing a wide array of services
	Diversified services, including independent living, assisted living, and skilled nursing care
Clients	Affluent elderly people with financial resources
Ownership	For-profit senior housing or hospitality companies
	For-profit mom-and-pop owners or entrepreneurs
	Not-for-profit, faith-based, or government organizations
Financing	Out-of-pocket payments, managed care insurance, and long-term care insurance payments
	State Medicaid or other government program payments for residents meeting means-testing guidelines

Exhibit 2.4
Continuing Care Retirement Communities: Settings, Clients, Ownership, Financing

According to LeadingAge, the typical kinds of CCRC contracts or fee schedules include the following (Mashburn 2011):

◆ Type A or extensive. This includes entrance and monthly fees to cover the housing, services, amenities, and freedom to transfer to another facility as needed.

◆ Type B or modified. This includes entrance and monthly fees to cover the housing. Assisted living/skilled nursing services are provided free or at a discount for a limited time.

◆ Type C or fee-for-service. This includes entrance and monthly fees to cover the housing. No free or discounted services are included, and residents pay for any service they need.

◆ Rental. This involves no entrance or monthly fees, and residents pay for any service they need.

✳ SPECIALIZED SETTINGS
Long-Term Care Services for Veterans

The US Department of Veterans Affairs (VA) provides an extensive variety of LTC services to veterans. These LTC services are provided under two key divisions: Veterans Health Care and Veterans Benefits.

Under the Health Care division, hospitals and healthcare services across the country are organized into 22 veterans integrated services networks (VISNs) (Allgov.com 2009). Nursing home care is provided by the VA Community Living Centers (formerly known as VA Nursing Home Care Units) to veterans who have functional challenges or inabilities. Veterans with dementia, those in need of short-term rehabilitation, and those in need of end-of-life care are also taken care of in these centers.

States may have their own veterans' homes, and the VA participates in two grant-in-aid programs to residents of these facilities. The VA provides construction grants to states that seek to build new state veterans homes or renovate existing facilities (Senior Veterans Service Alliance 2012c). The VA has an extensive system of community and home-based long-term care services, ranging from foster homes providing 24-hour supervision and personal assistance, adult day healthcare programs, home-based primary care, respite care, and hospice and palliative care programs. The VA has a well-established geriatric evaluation and management program known as GEM, which has been in existence since 1976. Recently, the VA introduced an extensive array of home and community-based services (Senior Veterans Service Alliance 2012b).

SPECIALIZED SETTINGS
Payment for VA Long-Term Care Services

VA Benefits Administration has a three-tiered program for payment of LTC benefits for veterans, their spouses, and their dependents known as Improved Pension. If the applicant meets specific service and income criteria, he may be eligible for a limited pension benefit under the Basic Benefits program. If he needs assistance with his daily routine due to physical limitations, he may qualify for the second tier of benefits under the Housebound program. The Aid and Attendance Special Pension is the third tier of this program, intended to pay for an aide who assists the veteran with activities of daily living and for services rendered to a veteran who has gone blind or has become mentally or physically impaired (MySeniorCare 2010).

Eligible veterans can also apply for disability benefits if the disability or illness was sustained or got worse during the veteran's military duty. The amount paid ranges, depending on the level of disability, and benefits are tax-free. Vocational rehabilitation benefits are available for qualified individuals. These benefits provide services that help veterans who suffered injury and disability during duty to find a job, keep a job, and live independently. Among the offerings under this program are job and career counseling, job-search assistance, education and training, financial aid, and medical and dental treatment. Special grants for special adaptive equipment and home modifications are also available (Senior Veterans Service Alliance 2012c).

New Developments in Residential Long-Term Care Services

Post-Acute Care Services

Post-acute care units or transitional care units (PACs and TCUs) help the transition of individuals needing additional support after a discharge from hospital-based, acute care settings. PACs and TCUs, which are generally part of a hospital or nursing home, offer nursing, home health, personal care, and many other services. These units improve the outcomes of individuals with rehabilitation care needs after complex surgical procedures such as hip and knee replacements or for individuals needing extensive hospital-like care for chronic illness or disease episodes. PACs and TCUs have financial and quality management benefits. Costs can be saved when patients who do not need full acute care can transition to a unit with a lower level of care intensity. Medicare, private insurers, and managed care organizations have been willing to pay for care in these "step-down" units to help reduce costs.

Post-acute care unit
A unit in a skilled nursing facility or hospital that provides healthcare services to individuals who need additional support after a discharge from acute care services in a hospital setting. Also referred to as transitional care units.

Culture change
An evolving philosophy of providing long-term care services that surpasses the traditional long-term care medical model by nurturing the human spirit while meeting medical needs. Also known as person-centered care or resident-directed care.

Eden Alternative
A philosophy of providing long-term care services in an environment that promotes quality of life for all involved, as opposed to the traditional institutional model.

CULTURE CHANGE, THE EDEN ALTERNATIVE, AND THE GREEN HOUSE PROJECT

In 2000, a number of LTC advocates established the Pioneer Network (see www .pioneernetwork.net) as an umbrella organization for the culture change movement. The Massachusetts Advocates for Nursing Home Reform (2008) defines the movement this way: "**Culture change** (also known as person-centered care or resident-directed care) transforms the long-term care medical model to one that nurtures the human spirit, as well as meeting medical needs. Culture change is not a finite destination—it is a work in progress, always evolving to meet the needs of the residents."

In addition, the Massachusetts Advocates for Health Reform put together the following goals of culture change:

◆ Restore control over daily living to residents of long-term care facilities, respecting the right of residents to make their own decisions.

◆ Involve all levels of staff in the care process, honoring those who work most closely with residents.

◆ Include families and friends in a comprehensive team-building approach to care.

◆ Provide a familiar and hospitable environment, a supportive workplace, and responsive, individualized care practices that focus on the needs and preferences of people, rather than those of the facility.

Two models of the culture change environment are the Eden Alternative and the Green House Project. In the early 1990s, Dr. Bill Thomas received a dementia care grant from the State of New York, and with it he developed an alternative to institutional nursing home care that emphasizes the introduction of nature (e.g., plants, animals), human support systems (e.g., family visitors, children), and homelike environments (e.g., neighborhoods of rooms, carpeted halls, non-institutional furnishings, communal dining centers). This is the principle behind the **Eden Alternative**.

Among the primary objectives of the Eden Alternative is to eliminate boredom, loneliness, and helplessness from the lives of nursing home residents, which Dr. Thomas calls the "three plagues" of nursing homes (Singh 2000). In this vein, the Eden Alternative calls for changes in management practice to an approach that encourages residents to participate in decisions regarding the provision of care and to provide feedback to the facility's administration about their practices. The staff, in turn, are encouraged to treat residents with respect, and many management decisions are decentralized. Under the Eden Alternative model, there is a facility-wide commitment to human growth through relationships.

The Eden Alternative influenced the development of the Green House Project. In this model, residents live in small groups (six to ten people) in freestanding cottages. The units are called **Green Houses**, and they are supported by the traditional administrative environment of the nursing home. The smaller unit size eliminates the need for nursing stations, medicine carts, and other institutional machinery. Services are typically provided by cross-trained, self-managed worker teams who support the small-scale care environment. It is based on a theory of "intentional community," where a natural bond exists between caregivers and residents.

INTERNATIONAL PERSPECTIVES ON RESIDENTIAL LONG-TERM CARE

In the European Union (EU), many LTC services are provided in residential care homes that provide nursing services or other forms of supportive care. These homes often provide custodial and nursing services for residents with extensive, long-term needs.

A key difference between the US and EU systems is payment for these services. EU governments typically provide heavy subsidies for their citizens' long-term care needs. However, ownership of care facilities follows a similar pattern as that in the United States, as many homes are owned privately in EU countries, and countries with previously dominant public healthcare systems are now seeking privatization.

A LOOK AHEAD

Residential options for providing LTC services in the United States have undergone tremendous expansion in recent years. As the healthcare system undergoes changes in its philosophy and reimbursement structure, the challenges of providing residential care in a homelike setting will continue to grow.

Green Houses
A deinstitutionalization movement for long-term care in which individuals who require care live in small homes and have access to clinical and personal care services on the level of those provided in high-quality nursing homes.

FOR DISCUSSION

1. Discuss the evolution of residential long-term care.

2. What was the role of legislation in the creation of residential care facilities?

3. What are the recent trends in independent living, and why are they important?

4. Discuss the concept of aging in place. What facet of long-term care embraces this concept fully?

5. What is the philosophy of care in assisted living? Is this different from other congregate care options?

6. What are the different payment mechanisms for long-term care services within the Veterans Affairs healthcare system?

7. Why are post-acute care units an important part of the transition process to residential long-term care?

8. Discuss the recent attempts to effect cultural change in long-term care. Be sure to address the Eden Alternative and the Green House Project.

CASE STUDY: CONGREGATE CARE

Don and Mary were happily married for 50 years and had two successful children and five grandchildren. Don and Mary met while serving in the US Army during the Korean Conflict. After their military service ended, they married and embarked on their careers. Don and Mary were healthcare professionals; Don was a professor at the local medical school, and Mary was a hospice nurse. Don and Mary were always active in their church and volunteered their time in the community. Both retired at age 65 to pursue their dreams of international travel and spending their children's inheritance.

During the early years of their retired life, the couple continued to work part time, travel extensively, and spend time with their grandkids. Their retirement plans seemed to be going swimmingly until Don noticed that his wife was having memory problems at the age of 78. Mary always kept up on the latest topics and was always the first to complete the crossword puzzles and other logic games in the newspaper. However, Mary seemed to become increasingly forgetful; she would run errands to purchase specific items and return home empty-handed. The couple decided to seek help from a gerontologist.

An extensive battery of cognitive and neuropsychological tests determined that Mary's language skills and mental abilities had markedly diminished. Mary was diagnosed with Alzheimer's disease, an incurable terminal brain disease. After the initial shock of the diagnosis, the couple developed a plan to cope with this disease—Don was going to be Mary's caregiver. The progression of the disease was tough for Don and the family to watch. At first Mary became confused, then she became progressively irritable and aggressive. Five years after the diagnosis, Mary became almost totally withdrawn. Her appetite was nonexistent, and she became incontinent. Additionally, Mary suffered from "sundowners syndrome"—a phenomenon whereby the individual experiences confusion and exasperation during the late afternoon or early evening hours.

Don struggled to care for her and keep an upbeat attitude; however, he too was experiencing the deterioration of aging. After years of being a competitive runner, his knees and other joints prevented him from fully assisting Mary. Don hired a home health aide to visit daily to assist Mary and also do some light household chores. As Mary's condition grew more serious, he had to make a decision. He was no longer able to care for her, and his own ailments were starting to severely impact his ability to take care of himself. Additionally, their retirement savings had dwindled to the point that they needed financial assistance from family members to get by. The case of Mary and Don is not uncommon, as many seniors experience the inevitable choice of long-term care.

CASE STUDY QUESTIONS

1. What long-term care options should Don consider for Mary and himself?

2. What are the requirements necessary to access the care you have chosen in Question 1?

3. What funding mechanisms are available to Don and Mary, and how does this affect the choice of care options?

4. What could Don and Mary have done to plan their care during their later years? What is your plan to prepare for the possibility of your need for long-term care?

Home and Community-Based Care Services

Mary Helen McSweeney-Feld, PhD,
and Karen Kopera-Frye, PhD

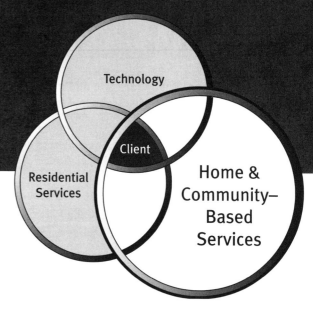

LEARNING OBJECTIVES

After completing this chapter, you should be able to

➤ define the terms *senior center*, *adult day services*, *home care*, and *medical home*;

➤ understand the history of the Older Americans Act, the development of the Aging Network, and the passage of Title XX, an amendment of the Social Security Act;

➤ discuss the types of long-term care delivered in home and community-based services (HCBS) settings;

➤ discuss new programs and regulatory initiatives for the provision of HCBS long-term care;

➤ discuss the impact of telehealth on HCBS;

➤ understand the special issues facing older disabled adults and their needs for HCBS; and

➤ compare HCBS and their settings in the United States with those in other countries.

INTRODUCTION

Developing home and community-based services (HCBS) alternatives for individuals needing long-term care continues to be a primary priority for many public healthcare programs. More and more consumers are opting to age in place in their community. The 1999 Supreme Court ruling in the *Olmstead* case (see Chapter 1) confirmed the discriminatory nature of government programs, which have favored institutional LTC over community-based solutions. These factors have prompted public healthcare programs to consider HCBS for their participants who need long-term care.

This chapter provides an overview of HCBS in the United States, starting with legislation that created the current networks of community-based services—the Older Americans Act and the Title XX program, which arose from an amendment to the Social Security Act. A description of HCBS services follows, including new initiatives that use technology in the provision of LTC services and programs developed under the Deficit Reduction Act. One section highlights the needs of older adults with disabilities. In addition, the chapter presents a comparison of HCBS in the United States with community-based services in other countries. Lastly, the outlook for providing HCBS in light of the current global economic downturn is addressed.

SOCIAL POLICY AND THE DEVELOPMENT OF COMMUNITY-BASED CARE SERVICES

Before the 1930s, the United States had few social programs designed specifically for older adults. Families, charitable organizations, and local governments were expected to provide these social services. Many factors—such as the low percentage of older adults, a strong belief in individual responsibility, and the free market economy—partially explain the slow response of the US government during this period (Hooyman and Kiyak 2011). The passage of the Social Security Act in 1935 ensured social insurance in retirement for qualified older Americans, and helped to protect the status of older adults in society. However, significant attention was not paid to the needs of older adults again by the federal government until the 1960s and 1970s.

Many Great Society programs instituted during this period, such as Medicare, Medicaid, Supplemental Security Insurance, Section 202 Housing, the Older Americans Act, and Title XX, laid the foundation for the provision of community-based care services in the United States. All of these developments helped older persons "age in place" (i.e., remain in their homes and in their community) while receiving needed LTC services.

AGING NETWORK

The aging network is a group of state, local, territorial, and tribal organizations, agencies, and individuals that provides services, support, resources, and advocacy for older Americans aged 60 and above. Its member organizations aim to encourage and strengthen independent living and avoid unnecessary institutionalization. Today's aging network includes the 655 Area Agencies on Aging (AAAs) operating on a local level, the state units on aging, more than 200 tribal and Native Hawaiian organizations, as well as thousands of nonprofit and for-profit organizations serving older Americans (Niles-Yokum and Wagner 2011).

FOUNDATION OF COMMUNITY SERVICES: THE OLDER AMERICANS ACT

Older Americans Act (OAA)
Legislation passed by the US Congress in 1965 that established the Administration on Aging and state agencies on aging to address the social services needs of older adults.

The **Older Americans Act (OAA)** was the product of many decades of mandates, proposals, and conferences designed to help the elderly and aging population in the United States. Enacted in 1965, the OAA ensures that funding and other resources are available to community-based programs that meet the complex needs of the aged and aging. Successive amendments to the OAA created additional programs that respond to specific issues. These programs include social, nutritional, housing, medical, mental health, training, and employment services and support to not only the elderly but also their caretakers. More important, the OAA protects the rights of vulnerable elders. For more information on the OAA, see www.aoa.gov/AoARoot/AoA_Programs/OAA/index.aspx.

Administration on Aging
A division of the US Department of Health and Human Services responsible for advancing the concerns and interests of older people and their caregivers.

The **Administration on Aging** (AoA) is the government agency that manages all funding, resources, and activities related to the provisions of the OAA. In this capacity, the AoA works with the organizations that make up the **Aging Network**. For more information on AoA, see www.aoa.gov.

The Older Americans Act consists of seven sections, or titles. The objectives of the act are stated in Title I, and they establish a unique role for the federal and state government in ensuring the well-being of older adults (O'Shaughnessy 2008).

Aging Network
Housed under the Administration on Aging, the Aging Network is a comprehensive and coordinated system of home and community-based long-term care services.

◆ Title I defines the objectives of the act.

◆ Title II establishes the AoA, the administrative agency for the Older Americans Act.

◆ Title III provides grants to fund and design state and community programs on aging. Four areas are funded under this Title: supportive services such as information and referral assistance, care management, and transportation; nutritional services such as congregate meal programs and home-delivered meals (e.g., Meals on Wheels); family caregiver services and assistance programs; and disease prevention and health promotion services geared to foster health in older adults through nutrition counseling, fitness, education, and health screening (Niles-Yokum and Wagner 2011).

♦ Title IV provides funding and support for aging research, as well as funding for new approaches (i.e., demonstration programs) in the delivery of aging services and training. Examples of these programs include the Aging and Disability Resource Centers (ADRCs), which help frail individuals remain in the community, and Chronic Disease Self-Management Programs (CDSMPs), which help individuals manage their own health services and chronic illnesses.

♦ Title V funds senior employment programs, providing part-time jobs for low-income, unemployed individuals who are older than 55 and have limited job prospects. These Senior Community Service Employment Programs (SCSEPs) are frequently essential sources of income for vulnerable seniors, as well as training programs for seniors to pursue new types of employment opportunities.

♦ Title VI provides supportive funds to Native Americans and Native Hawaiian organizations for social and nutrition services.

♦ Title VII addresses the rights of vulnerable elders by authorizing funds for elder rights protection programs, state ombudsman programs, and state legal assistance development.

Government funding of the OAA has been renewed by Congress multiple times, but not without difficulty. Through amendments to the OAA, the number of groups to which services must be provided has grown considerably, and the downturn in the global economy has expanded vulnerable populations that are in need of these services. Consequently, while programs with OAA funding retain their objective of universal participation, some have asked consumers in the programs to share some nominal cost of their services if they are able to do so.

SOCIAL SERVICES LEGISLATION: TITLE XX

In 1975, an amendment to the Social Security Act created **Title XX**, a program that provides block grants for social services. These grants are fixed amounts of funding given to states for various purposes, including community-based care for the elderly and disabled.

TYPES OF COMMUNITY-BASED SERVICES

SENIOR CENTERS

Senior centers, one of the most popular services funded by the OAA, are the gateway to the Aging Network, which connects older adults to community services that can help them stay healthy and independent. More than 60 percent of senior centers are designated focus

Title XX
A block grant program under the Social Security Act that provides community-based care for the elderly and disabled, as well as funding for child care and child abuse prevention programs.

Senior centers
Places where older adults come together for services and activities that reflect their experience and skills, respond to their diverse needs and interests, enhance their dignity, support their independence, and encourage their involvement in and with the center and the community.

points for OAA services, and nearly 11,000 senior centers are operating across the country. While the OAA provides most senior center funding, most centers receive additional funds from other governmental and private sources, with many centers receiving funds from three to eight different sources (NCOA 2011).

History of Senior Centers

Senior clubs have been around since the 1870s, but it was not until 1943 that a formal program began in New York City. This initiative, led by the New York City Welfare Department, spread quickly throughout the United States (Gelfand 2006). In 1973, OAA amendments (Title II and Title V) introduced the multipurpose senior center as it is known today (Gelfand 2006).

Senior Centers: Settings, Clients, Ownership, Financing

Three types of senior centers exist: (1) multipurpose centers, which offer comprehensive programs and services (Aday 2003); (2) intergenerational centers, which are sites where children and elders interact during scheduled activities and participate in the same programs (Generations United 2006); and (3) specialized centers, which provide a specific service, such as meals or healthcare (Gitelson et al. 2008). Exhibit 3.1 summarizes the key characteristics of the different types of senior centers.

Every day, approximately one million older adults receive services at senior centers. Seventy percent of these clients are female, and about half of them live alone. Research shows that older adults who participate in senior center programs can learn to manage and delay the onset of chronic disease and experience measurable improvements in their physical, social, spiritual, emotional, mental, and economic well-being (NCOA 2011). Because

Exhibit 3.1 Senior Centers: Settings, Clients, Ownership, Financing		
Settings	Multipurpose (nearly 75% of centers)	
	Intergenerational	
	Specialized center	
Clients	Typically older women between 70 and 79 years of age	
	Low to middle income	
	Desiring social interaction	
Ownership	Not-for-profit	
	May have national accreditation	
Financing	Home and community-based care block grants from the OAA	
	Private funding from businesses, foundations, donors	

senior centers are a gateway to the Aging Network (mentioned earlier), many centers are adjusting their programming to better appeal to aging baby boomers.

ADULT DAY SERVICES

Adult day services are community-based facilities for individuals who need supervised care during the day. Clients of adult day services include people who have physical and/or mental disabilities, who are elderly and cannot perform activities of daily living, or who have rehabilitation needs. In addition to serving the needs of the clients, adult daycare gives caregivers a break from their duties (NADSA 2011). Most adult day facilities are open only during the weekdays, but some operate on the weekends and during evening hours.

Adult day services Community-based facilities for individuals who need supervised care during the daytime, but who otherwise remain in their homes.

History of Adult Day Services

Adult day services evolved from the day-hospital concept developed in England after World War II. Many soldiers came back from the war with a variety of illnesses and injuries, overwhelming the existing hospital system (Hindman 2009). Hospitals simply could not handle the demand, some of which was for long-term stays. The day hospital was invented to enable soldiers who needed care to receive services during the day but leave by night to recuperate at home. This system freed up space for soldiers who had more major problems and needed to be admitted.

The concept did not reach the United States until the 1970s. At the time, reports about poor conditions in nursing homes were widespread. In response, adult daycares were positioned as viable options for families who did not want their loved ones to suffer nursing home mistreatment (CAADS 2010). The concept of adult daycares was further bolstered when federal reimbursement became available for their services (Hindman 2009).

Currently more than 4,600 centers provide care to nearly 150,000 recipients per day (NADSA 2011).

Adult Day Services: Settings, Clients, Ownership, Financing

Adult day services follow one of three models: medical, social, and specialty. The medical model offers clinical interventions and support, therapy, rehabilitation, and other health and wellness services. The social model revolves around organized activities (e.g., parties, games, field trips) that promote socialization among participants. The specialty model provides care that is tailored to a specific need, such as Alzheimer's and other types of dementia. All models emphasize safety and companionship while encouraging independence. Ultimately, adult day services allow families to defer expensive nursing home placement. Exhibit 3.2 summarizes the key characteristics of adult day services.

EXHIBIT 3.2
Adult Day Services:
Settings, Clients,
Ownership,
Financing

Settings	Medical model, providing healthcare and other supportive services
	Social model, providing meals and supervised group activities
	Specialty model, providing care for those with Alzheimer's, brain injuries, other chronic conditions
Clients	Nursing home–eligible clients who prefer to live in the community
	Consumers with chronic illnesses
	Predominantly females in their 70s
	High proportion of cognitively impaired individuals
Ownership	Not-for-profit, affiliated with hospitals, nursing homes, etc.
	For-profit, freestanding proprietary
Financing	State Medicaid programs
	Private foundation sources, private donors
	Out-of-pocket contributions from clients
	Private insurance

Following are findings from the Partners in Caregiving (2002) study on adult day centers:

◆ Adult day centers provide care for 150,000 care recipients each day.

◆ Nearly 78 percent of adult day centers operate on a nonprofit or public basis.

◆ Seventy percent of adult day centers are affiliated with larger organizations such as home care organizations, skilled nursing facilities, medical centers, or multipurpose senior organizations.

◆ The average age of the adult day center care recipient is 72, and two-thirds are women.

◆ Thirty-five percent of the adult day center care recipients live with an adult child, 20 percent with a spouse, 18 percent in an institutional setting, 13 percent with parents or other relatives, and 11 percent alone.

◆ Fifty-two percent of the adult day center care recipients have some cognitive impairment.

◆ The average daily rate for adult day services is $60, compared to an average rate of $19 an hour for home health aide care (Genworth Financial 2010).

◆ Medicare does not pay for any type of adult day care. However, in 35 states, Medicaid can be used to pay for adult day care services (Genworth Financial 2010).

Settings	High-tech, medical model, providing healthcare services (e.g., infusion therapy)
	Custodial or homemaker care
	Specialty model, providing care for HIV/AIDS, other chronic conditions
Clients	Nursing home–eligible clients who prefer to live in the community
	Consumers with chronic illnesses
Ownership	Not-for-profit, affiliated with hospitals, nursing homes, etc.
	For-profit, freestanding proprietary
Financing	Medicare and state Medicaid programs
	Commercial insurance, managed care plans

Exhibit 3.3
Home Care Services: Settings, Clients, Ownership, Financing

HOME CARE

Home care includes a variety of healthcare and supportive services provided by paid or unpaid caregivers to individuals with disabilities or illnesses. Home care can include specialized services such as **home infusion therapy**; custodial care services such as meal preparation, shopping, and cleaning; and assistance in paying bills. Approximately 12 million individuals receive care from over 33,000 home care providers. In 2009, annual expenditures for home care services were projected to be $72.2 billion (NAHC 2010). Exhibit 3.3 shows the key characteristics of home care services.

Home care
Healthcare or supportive services for individuals with a chronic disability or illness who live in the community.

Home infusion therapy
Drug therapy provided intravenously that is given to an individual at home.

Home Care: Settings, Clients, Ownership, Financing

Home care clients include people who have chronic illness (e.g., arthritis, diabetes), complex medical conditions (e.g., genetic disorders), physical and mental impairment, or incurable or terminal disease. In 2009, of the $72.2 billion spent on home health care, 41 percent was for Medicare-reimbursed home care services (NAHC 2010).

Types of professional providers (as opposed to unpaid caretakers) of home care services vary. They include home health care and nursing agencies, home care aide organizations, hospices, and a variety of independent businesses. Some providers are Medicare certified (i.e., they meet

(?) DID YOU KNOW?
Specialty Adult Day Services

Adult day services evening programs have been established to address the issue of sundowning (wandering, sleeplessness, and agitation in the late afternoon and evening hours) in adults with Alzheimer's disease and dementia. At the Hebrew Home for the Aged in Riverdale, New York, the Elder Serve at Night program provides all-night activities such as painting pictures, potting plants, dancing, engaging in discussions, and listening to music. The clients rest as they need, and return to their homes fed, showered, and typically relaxed from their night-long activities (*New York Times* 2009).

Medicare requirements for home care agencies) and are paid for their services by Medicare. State Medicaid programs also reimburse for home care expenses, and these payments fall under the mandatory traditional home health benefit, the personal care option, or the home and community-based waiver. Home care Medicaid reimbursement is still a small portion of total Medicaid expenditures, but it has the potential to increase substantially as the population ages and more and more families choose home care options.

Mhealth
The use of mobile technologies for healthcare purposes.

Telehealth
The delivery of health-related services and information via telecommunications technology.

TELEHEALTH AND HOME CARE SERVICES

Use of technology in the provision of home care and patient monitoring services is growing in popularity due to persistent shortages of trained home care providers, the increasing complexity and costs of transportation for providers to and from client homes, and limited reimbursement for home care services. Video phones and web-based technologies have been used to provide medical consultations, home telephone support, and follow-up care for many years. In recent years, a new field has emerged called **Mhealth**, which refers to the use of mobile technologies for healthcare purposes. Simple forms of Mhealth include mobile applications on a cell phone for patient education or management of chronic illness. More complex technologies include wireless sensors to monitor vital signs (*New York Times* 2011).

Electronic monitoring could significantly reduce medical costs. A 2008 Department of Veterans Affairs (VA) study of remote monitoring of patients through a home telehealth program showed a 25 percent drop in bed days and a 19 percent drop in hospital admissions for patients enrolled in the monitoring program (Darkins 2008). An extensive survey of the bibliography of home **telehealth** studies by the VA in 2010 confirmed the potential of cost savings and efficiencies in most research in this area (VA 2010). Another recent study of integrated telehealth and care management programs for Medicare recipients with chronic disease showed cost savings of $313 to $542 per person per quarter (Baker, Johnson, Macaulay, and Birnbaum 2011).

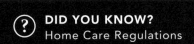

DID YOU KNOW?
Home Care Regulations

Every state sets its own home care licensing and certification rules. This makes it hard to determine how many providers nationwide are Medicare certified and how many practice without it. Providers (both individuals and organizations) who do not have Medicare certification cannot bill Medicare for reimbursement and are not required to abide by standards established by Medicare for home care services.

INNOVATIONS IN HCBS: CONSUMER-DIRECTED PROGRAMS

The Deficit Reduction Act (DRA) of 2005 introduced three innovative programs that give individuals the incentive to use HCBS for their long-term care needs. These state Medicaid-funded programs are (1) Cash and Counseling (section 6087), (2) HCBS State Plan (section 6086), and (3) Money Follows the Person "Rebalancing."

All DRA programs encourage individuals to age in place in the community. They promote that choice by offering reimbursement for self-directed personal assistance (**Cash and Counseling**), providing supportive services through Medicaid waiver programs (HCBS State Plan), or showing a Medicaid beneficiary discharged from a residential care facility the health and financial advantages of staying in the community for LTC services (**Money Follows the Person**). While the intent of these programs is consistent with research findings that elders prefer to age in place, the outcomes show mixed levels of success. Findings on cost savings have been inconclusive because the additional costs to family members are not always measurable (Brody 2009).

Following are other HCBS programs available to those who need LTC services:

- The **medical home** approach utilizes a primary care physician, in conjunction with a multidisciplinary team of healthcare providers, to coordinate the access to healthcare services when and where they are needed. Services are tailored to the specific needs and wants of the individual, and progress is tracked by all members of the multidisciplinary team through electronic records (Leland 2009; Rittenhouse et al. 2009). Medical home programs exist in more than a dozen states, and Medicaid provides the bulk of reimbursement for these services. Medicare has started a medical home demonstration that expands services to the elderly. The approach could also be expanded to rural areas, where virtual medical homes could be created through the use of telehealth technology and electronic medical record systems. In addition, Smart Medical Home prototypes have been investigated by numerous government agencies, including the Department of Veterans Affairs (see Chapter 4 for more on this discussion).

- **Program of All-Inclusive Care for the Elderly (PACE)** is targeted at elders who are eligible for Medicare and Medicaid funding to stay in nursing homes but prefer to age in the community. PACE is a nonresidential model that provides a variety of healthcare and social services and support for people (aged 55 or older) who have chronic conditions but can live in the community safely without 24-hour supervision. Reimbursement is a mixture of funds (sometimes a fixed or capitated amount) from Medicare and state Medicaid. Participants sign a contract that requires them to receive supplemental services (inpatient and outpatient) only through a PACE sponsor, which is

Cash and Counseling programs
Programs in which consumers direct and manage their personal assistance services, including long-term care, according to their specific needs and receive reimbursement for these services.

Money Follows the Person programs
A grant program that encourages a beneficiary discharged from an institutional care facility to remain in the community and receive services at home.

Medical home
A care approach whereby a primary care physician, in conjunction with specialists and other healthcare providers, coordinates the access to healthcare services when and where they are needed.

frequently a preidentified hospital or healthcare system. Research on PACE programs has shown their appeal to a variety of populations (including religious and ethnic groups) and in a variety of settings (both urban and rural communities). Studies tracking PACE enrollees over the years demonstrate that PACE provides better health outcomes than other traditional care and services arrangements for seniors with chronic care needs. The research also demonstrates that the staff serving these individuals are more satisfied working in a PACE environment, and that PACE programs are an effective use of taxpayer dollars (National PACE Association 2011). However, the process for starting a PACE program, as well as the training, is strenuous, and not all elders want to commit to receiving healthcare services from just one medical center or system.

◆ **Social Health Maintenance Organizations (SHMOs) or Lifecare** programs are similar to PACE in scope, but they provide healthcare and LTC services through Medicare in a managed care setting (unlike PACE's community-based setting). Membership offers other benefits currently not covered by Medicare or most other senior health plans. An evaluation report by CMS in 2002 of SHMOs found that the rate of hospitalization for SHMO participants was only reduced for a high-risk group (CMS 2002).

OLDER ADULTS WITH DISABILITIES: A SPECIAL ISSUE IN HCBS

Some older adults suffer from cognitive disabilities (e.g., mental retardation) and/or physical difficulties (e.g., inability to perform activities of daily living [ADLs]) that pose an additional challenge to healthcare providers. The variety and extent of these disabilities are staggering, and they may be classified under one of two types: (1) physical or mental impairment with ADLs and (2) cognitive disabilities, including lifelong genetic conditions such as Down's syndrome.

Older adults with dementia due to Alzheimer's disease, for example, must be constantly supervised to ensure that they do not hurt themselves or others in the process of performing daily routines. For example, they could boil a pot of water and leave the stove turned on, or they could cut their fingers but not know how to treat the wound. Furthermore, complications from chronic illness also set physical limitations on older individuals, preventing them from standing, walking, balancing, grasping objects, or seeing well. These movement problems require the healthcare provider to assist with ADLs, and the need for such help could be minor or major and occasionally or all the time, depending on the older adult's physical impairment and the availability of a family member who can assist. Note that not all older adults who need help with ADLs are physically challenged. Some are in good physical shape, but their cognitive problems are so severe that they cannot perform ADLs on their own. The bottom line is that the disability of an elderly person can be viewed on a continuum—usually, the greater the disability or impairment, the greater the need for and difficulty of services, and this need increases over time.

The best predictor of a person's need for long-term assistance is the ability to perform ADLs. Core ADLs, as explored in Chapter 1, are feeding, bathing, dressing, toileting, and transferring. The need could also be measured by the person's ability to perform instrumental activities of daily living, or IADLs—these activities require more cognitive skills, such as balancing a checkbook and shopping. Finally, the need is also defined by the duration of the condition: is the problem temporary (e.g., an elderly person fractured her hip), or permanent (e.g., an elderly person has dementia)? Whether the disability happened suddenly or has been present for some time, caregivers must be sensitive to the fact that the individual may be experiencing a significant loss of personal freedom because of her impairment (Agich 2009).

STATISTICS ON DISABLED OLDER ADULTS

Estimates of the numbers of disabled older adults in the United States vary depending on the data that are used. In 1990, approximately 1.6 million older adults had mild impairments—these are people who can mostly manage on their own with slight assistance from informal caregivers (often family members). In the 2000 Census, among males aged 65 or older, 40.4 percent reported some type of disability; among females of the same age group, the rate was 43 percent. Because of the increasing size of the future retirement population (due to the retirement of the boomers), the number of disabled older adults may soar in coming decades. By 2040, the number of older adults with disabilities is predicted to reach 21 million, and this population will grow faster than the younger population, with a likely rise in the economic burden of long-term care (Johnson, Toohey, and Wiener 2007).

SERVICE SETTINGS FOR DISABLED OLDER ADULTS

LTC support and services for elders with disabilities can be obtained in myriad settings, such as LTC hospitals, nursing homes, adult day service facilities, adult foster homes, respite care facilities, and other HCBS providers. These settings offer a rich continuum of care, such as a full menu of medical, therapeutic, and rehabilitative therapies; meals, transportation, and recreation; and adult education, advocacy, case management, and companion services, to name just a few. A recent study of disability assistance to working older adults showed that $357 billion of that assistance came from the federal government in 2008. The study also predicted that spending restraints by the federal government in the area of healthcare will directly affect the working age population with disabilities unless ways to make the delivery of healthcare services to this population become more efficient (Livermore, Stapleton, and O'Toole 2011).

Beginning in the early 1980s, Medicaid started funding long-term home and community-based services (Smith et al. 2000). In most states, the organizations providing such services must obtain a Medicaid waiver (i.e., a waiver of Medicaid regulations) to pay for a variety of specialty services.

INTERNATIONAL PERSPECTIVES ON HCBS

In the United States, the nursing home (and before this, almshouses and faith-based residences) used to be the traditional places to which the elderly who needed LTC services

---

⚠ CRITICAL CONCEPT
Practice Guidelines

Practice guidelines established by the American Association on Intellectual and Developmental Disabilities (known in the past as the American Association on Mental Retardation) are based on key assumptions that should be considered by healthcare professionals when working with older adults with disabilities (Janicki et al. 1996). While these guidelines are focused on mental and developmental disabilities, they could also apply to seniors with other disabilities. The recommendations include the following:

1. Care must be tailored to the individual's distinct needs.

2. Age-related decline is inevitable, such as reduced sensory functioning, but gross mental deterioration should not be expected.

3. Individuals with developmental disabilities are at greatest risk for Alzheimer's disease (AD).

4. Behavioral changes seen with AD may be present in an elder, but they could result from other causes, such as a urinary tract infection, and thus may be reversible.

5. Standard differential diagnosis procedures used in the general population with respect to intellectual disabilities and AD should be employed and should be adjusted for different skill levels.

6. Evaluation and changes in functioning should be compared to the individual's past performance, not norm groups, to properly monitor within-person changes.

In summary, an LTC organization's policy regarding disabled older adults should accommodate their varied levels of disabilities and needs so that they can be fully served.

were taken to receive live-in care. Societal changes and the passage of the Older Americans Act and other legislation have minimized this practice. US seniors with LTC needs and their families are now encouraged to take advantage of community-based alternatives to nursing homes and other residential settings.

In many other countries, it is more common for elders to be cared for at home. The belief system that underlies this practice in some countries is filial piety—care of aged and aging parents is the responsibility of the children (Hooyman and Kiyak 2011). Global family and life trends are changing that tradition, however.

Increased life expectancy, combined with lower fertility rates and the breakup of the family unit, has necessitated that many families investigate residential care options for its elders. Some industrialized countries have raised the retirement age, which gives older adults an incentive to keep working and diminish their use of long-term care services. However, cross-comparisons between the use of HCBS for long-term care in the United States and that in other countries remains difficult due to limited comparative studies in this area.

A Look Ahead

National healthcare reform initiatives and recent state court decisions have firmly supported individuals' choices to age in place and receive LTC services from HCBS. In addition, congressional healthcare reform bills include enhanced financial support for HCBS (Williams 2009). In Florida in 2008, roughly 8,500 Medicaid recipients filed a lawsuit against the state. They claimed they were improperly forced into nursing homes, which is in violation of a US Supreme Court case—the *Olmstead* decision—and the Americans with Disabilities Act. The recipients recently reached a $27 million settlement with the state, and these funds were to be used to improve education for nursing home residents about how they can transition from institutions to community-based care (Associated Press 2009).

The global economic downturn that began in 2008 has reduced the amount of money available to states to fund HCBS programs. In addition, the wide variations in state HCBS programs and the states' restrictive financial or functional eligibility standards for services may prevent community-based LTC providers from meeting the growing demand from consumers now and in the future. Policymakers need to continue to study and collect data on access, cost, and quality of HCBS as they continue to make these services a viable alternative for older consumers who want to age in place.

For Discussion

1. Discuss the history of social policy and the development of community-based services.

2. Explain the role of the Older Americans Act in the provision of services for elders in the United States.

3. List and detail the services provided by different types of HCBS.

4. Discuss the three models of delivery for adult day service programs.

5. Telehealth is a new development in providing LTC services. Discuss how telehealth may be used in the future to provide LTC services.

6. Discuss two options for elders to age in place in their homes and in the community in the United States. What are the advantages and disadvantages of each option?

7. What is the purpose of introducing a Medicaid waiver program for HCBS?

8. Discuss two challenges for adults with cognitive disabilities who live in the community.

9. In light of the current global economic turndown, what is the outlook for HCBS in the United States in the next five years?

CASE STUDY: AGING IN PLACE

Betty and Clayton Ross always dreamed of retiring to Upstate New York to escape the hustle and bustle of the big city. Their dreams of a serene retirement were dashed when Clayton was diagnosed with Parkinson's disease at age 55.

At first, Clayton was able to continue to work and deal with the tremors; however, it soon became unbearable, and he could no longer continue as the pastor in the church he founded. Clayton retired at age 59, and Betty was able to provide all of the care he needed at home for the next 15 years.

When Clayton reached age 74, the debilitating effects of his disease became too much for Betty to handle by herself. At that time, Betty and Clayton moved to rural Pennsylvania to be near one of their daughters and her family so that Betty could get assistance. For almost ten years, their daughter Sandy and her husband, Wally, provided assistance, including transporting them to all physician appointments and social outings. Sandy also visited each day to help her father with his activities of daily living. Wally oversaw their financial portfolio and often helped to meet any shortfalls due to the couple's dwindling funds. This arrangement worked well for almost ten years; however, it put a strain on the family relationship.

The next shoe dropped when Betty, at age 83, was diagnosed with chronic obstructive pulmonary disease, a progressive lung disease that made it difficult for her to breathe. Betty and Clayton were at a crossroads and discussed their dilemma with their daughter and her family. They maintained their desire to live at home rather than to be institutionalized and forgotten; however, they knew they could not live without assistance. As a result of the added stress of caring for Sandy's parents, Sandy and Wally's marriage and family life had suffered and they were feeling trapped. After all, Sandy and Wally had three children to take care of and often had to forgo family outings and miss their son's after-school activities. The family had tried to help the best they could, but when Wally was offered a job in another state, he could not turn down this opportunity for promotion and a fresh start on the family's life. As a result, Betty and Clayton were left to fend for themselves. They had always been able to live independently with the help of their family, but now what would they do?

The couple knew one thing: They wanted to be together and remain in their home. Their desire to age in place and stay together was emphatic; however, their savings had been almost entirely depleted, and they could no longer rely on their family's financial support because they had their own financial obligations.

Source: Oetjen and Oetjen (2006).

CASE STUDY QUESTIONS

1. Define aging in place.

2. What options are available to help Betty and Clayton age in place?

3. In light of their financial condition and their desire to live at home together, what is the best option for Betty and Clayton?

4. What could Betty and Clayton have done to plan better for the circumstances that they are currently facing?

Technology and Delivery of Long-Term Care Services

Barbara H. Edington, DPS, PMP;
Peter Gomori, PhD;
and Mary Helen McSweeney-Feld, PhD

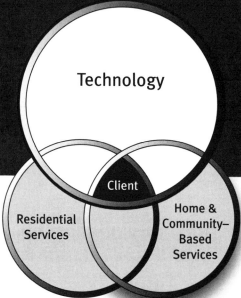

LEARNING OBJECTIVES

After completing this chapter, you should be able to

➤ understand the importance and role of technology in the provision of healthcare services and its unique contribution to the long-term care field;

➤ distinguish the two types of technology used in long-term care—information systems and applied technology;

➤ distinguish the parts of the systems development life cycle and the importance of enterprise-level management of a healthcare organization's technology systems;

➤ understand the role of technology in the development and implementation of an electronic medical record and other resident care systems; and

➤ understand the types of assistive technology that allow individuals to self-care as they age in place in their communities.

INTRODUCTION

Technology is a growing component in the delivery of healthcare services. It improves interoperational efficiencies within and between organizations, reduces the probability of medical errors, and improves the quality of care. Modern technology began affecting healthcare at the beginning of the twentieth century, when doctors in rural areas provided services over the telephone. Since then, the use of technology has vastly expanded to the use of computers, the web, and sophisticated systems for management and delivery of healthcare services.

These developments have also moved into long-term care facilities and home and community-based services (HCBS). Technology facilitates an individual's movement between the various dimensions of care and helps ensure quality. As global healthcare systems move toward a philosophy of consumer-driven care, where individuals are given more information and are encouraged to maintain their own health records and health outcomes, technology will become even more important. It will help consumers navigate the complex network of residential, HCBS, and other supportive services as they age in place in their communities.

LTC service providers have only recently started to use systems for electronic collection and management of health records and other patient information. Studies of electronic health record adoption in skilled nursing facilities and home health agencies yield wide variations in results.

However, a 2004 study by the American Association of Homes and Services for the Aging (AAHSA) of electronic information systems in US nursing homes found that 99.6 percent of homes had at least one information system for Minimum Data Set (MDS) reporting (96.4 percent) and billing (95.4 percent), and nearly 43 percent of US nursing homes had electronic information systems for medical records, including nurse's notes, physician notes, and MDS forms (Resnick et al. 2008). Some of this variation may be due to imprecise definition of terms.

The Office of the National Coordinator for Health Information Technology (ONC), a federal entity charged with coordination of nationwide efforts to implement and use the most advanced health information technology, was established through the passage of the HITECH Act of 2009. Long-term care organizations continue to work through ONC to develop a nationwide health information network and health information technology standards that can apply to a variety of healthcare settings and providers.

This chapter provides an overview of technology in LTC settings, starting with the foundations of information technology systems and enterprise-wide systems management. It also provides an overview of assistive technologies, emphasizing the new role of self-care technologies that help individuals maintain or improve their functional independence in the community. It concludes with an overview of the critical role that technology will play in the future delivery of LTC services.

FOUNDATIONS FOR INFORMATION TECHNOLOGY SYSTEMS IN LONG-TERM CARE

The aging of the population and increased regulation of the LTC industry have motivated service providers to become increasingly reliant on technology to deliver high-quality care at reasonable cost. An important part of this development has been the use of information systems that maintain client records and information, report information to reimbursement and regulatory agencies, and generate a variety of internal reports that help leadership manage the organization. Techniques for selecting projects and understanding how these systems are constructed are important components of the technology management process.

PROJECT MANAGEMENT

Organizations typically have more technology needs than money to fund them. Prioritizing projects is difficult. Before building or buying any new system, hardware, or software components, a committee composed of representatives from the various departments must analyze the technology needs of the organization and determine which projects will be allocated the necessary funds. The primary consideration for new projects is how well they align with the organization's strategic plan. The committee must also keep in mind the constraints of the existing system and the economic environment. Projects are then ranked on the investment and the expected return from that investment as well as the risk of not undertaking the project. The priority list may change if the regulatory environment or the economy changes.

Systems development life cycle
A cyclical, iterative approach to designing an information system that consists of four phases: analysis, design, implementation, and maintenance.

Iterative process
A process in an information system that can be repeated as needed to ensure that the outcome meets the business requirements of the user.

Life Cycle Approach

One approach to designing information systems for LTC organizations is to use the **systems development life cycle** (SDLC) (see Exhibit 4.1). This approach assumes that most information systems projects go through four phases: analysis, design, implementation, and maintenance. SDLC has many versions, and industries adapt the approach to meet their specific needs. While the process looks linear, in reality it is cyclical and is often applied as an **iterative process**. A process is iterative when the phases can be repeated as needed to ensure that the outcome meets the business requirements of the user. This cyclical nature allows for more interaction between the developers and the business users. Following is a detailed description of the SDLC project phases:

1. *Analysis phase.* After a systems project has been selected, the system designer analyzes the problem and how the system will address it. This information is reviewed in terms of what the end user of the system requires. Documentation of the end user's requirements is the major deliverable for this phase. The end user may review the requirements to ensure that they were correctly documented.

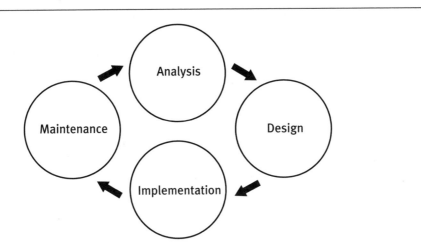

EXHIBIT 4.1
System
Development
Life Cycle

SOURCE: Project Management Institute, *A Guide to the Project Management Body of Knowledge (PMBOK® Guide)*, 4th ed., Project Management Institute, Inc., 2004. Copyright and all rights reserved. Material from this publication has been reproduced with the permission of PMI.

2. *Design phase.* During this phase, all of the components of the system, such as the architecture, the interfaces, and the integration with the database and other systems in the network, are designed and documented. A prototype is produced to verify with the end users that the project is adhering to their needs. A **prototype** is a physical or visual version of the components of the system; it does not have to be fully functional.

3. *Implementation phase.* In this phase, the prototype is developed with full functionality, incorporating the feedback from the end users. The software is developed, tested, and documented. The installation portion of the implementation often includes training on the new system for the end users. This is a critical juncture of the development life cycle because the end users are taking ownership of the system; if they do not understand how to use it, their misuse may be interpreted as a design flaw and the project may be considered to be less than fully successful.

4. *Maintenance phase.* Now the system is successfully implemented and in use, and the technology team must continue to keep it running efficiently and reliably. New employees may need to be trained periodically, and the system may require updates.

Managing the systems development project is the responsibility of the project manager. This individual works with a project team consisting of representatives of the departments and divisions that will use the new system. The **project manager** facilitates the development and monitors the progress to make sure deadlines are met and the budget is not exceeded. *A Guide to the Project Management Body of Knowledge* is often used as the

> **Prototype**
> A sample information system or model built to test a concept or a process before final implementation.

> **Project manager**
> An individual who manages a systems development project. The project manager facilitates the process of the development and monitors the progress to determine the possibility for schedule delays, cost overruns, or other risks that would affect the delivery of the system.

standard for project management. It is a collection of best practices, tools, and guidelines for project teams to use as they work through the systems development life cycle (Project Management Institute 2004). For more information on the Project Management Institute, which publishes these guidelines, visit its website at www.pmi.org.

Waterfall Method

A more traditional approach to designing systems is the **waterfall method**, in which each phase is completed before the next phase is started. In this approach, the end user typically does not see the finished product or system until the end of the project cycle and has little interaction with the development team. This leads to a high rate of dissatisfaction with systems because the end users only have one opportunity (the analysis phase) to explain their needs to the development team. If those needs are poorly documented or not fully described, the chance for an unsatisfactory outcome is high. Projects are not tested by the end user until the completion of the final phase, by which time a great deal of time and money has been allocated to the project (LaTour and Eichenwald-Maki 2006; Tan and Payton 2010).

ENTERPRISE-LEVEL TECHNOLOGY

Within an organization or enterprise, each department requires certain types of technology to support its operations. The clinical staff may need a mobile data-entry system, whereas the pharmacy does not rely on mobility for its data entry. However, both entry points must deliver data to a database that can be accessed by the inventory control department, which needs to link electronically to the suppliers for just-in-time delivery.

An **enterprise-wide technology management system** allows any department to access information and generate reports. It also allows the organization to link clinical and administrative components of the management process. The ability to transmit and read data regardless of the technology platform (or operating system) or the software language is referred to as **interoperability**. Interoperability is a challenge for many organizations because various departments often use incompatible systems or computer languages. When developing new systems, it is critical to take into account the interfaces, or links, between systems at the enterprise level, not just at the departmental level (LaTour and Eichenwald-Maki 2006).

THE ELECTRONIC MEDICAL RECORD

An **electronic medical record** (EMR) is a digital healthcare file that provides a historical view of an individual's healthcare information at a specific institution. The EMR is a good

---

Waterfall method
A traditional approach to information systems development in which each phase is completed before the next phase begins.

Enterprise-wide technology management system
A system that allows any division of an organization to access information and generate reports and to link clinical and administrative components of their management process.

Interoperability
The ability to transmit and read data regardless of the technology platform (or operating system) or the software language.

example of why interoperability is so important. Individuals needing LTC services or managing chronic health conditions frequently move through various parts of the service delivery systems, and an EMR that is able to follow them as they consume services can help optimize clinical outcomes. EMRs also are increasingly used to support clinical and administrative decision making (Wager, Lee, and Glaser 2009).

Theoretically, using a central source for all of the data relating to an individual is a common-sense approach to managing LTC information, but many factors can make EMR implementation a lengthy and difficult project. Most of the systems within an organization were built independently of each other, without much thought given to how they would integrate. For EMRs to manage all of an individual's data, they must be able to access the data stored on many types of platforms that were developed with many different applications. The integration of these various systems after they have been built is costly and time consuming. In addition, addressing the issues surrounding privacy and security of the data requires additional software, monitoring devices, and often specialized personnel.

The American Recovery and Reinvestment Act of 2009 (ARRA) earmarked nearly $2 billion for expansion of health information systems and the EMR. Although most of the ARRA funds were targeted for hospitals and physicians, a group called the Long Term & Post Acute Care Health Information Technology Collaborative has lobbied the Department of Health and Human Services to provide funds to LTC providers as well, considering that one-third of patients who leave the hospital are discharged to a long-term or post-acute care setting for further care (Wagner 2010).

DATABASES AND DATABASE MANAGEMENT OR DATA MINING

Data is the key element of the EMR. By combining data points, information is uncovered that can significantly affect the client's healthcare situation. The organization has multiple data-collection points, such as registration, nursing notes, and medical orders. Data from these disparate points of entry must be integrated into a system with a common platform and standards so that the data can be stored, maintained, secured, and accessed by different users in different formats according to the users' specific needs. The database must also be able to work with software that will provide clinical decision support, communication, and security for privacy and integrity (Haag and Cummings 2008).

Databases, generally speaking, are collections of data organized in a fashion that allows easy access to the data by various means, such as queries and reports. Databases take one of two common forms: relational or object oriented. **Relational databases** consist of tables of data and are designed in a logical structure for the storage and easy retrieval of the data. An **object-oriented database** stores the data and processing instructions, such as how to calculate certain quantities.

Electronic medical record

A digital healthcare file composed of various individual data elements that is typically a historical view of one individual's healthcare information.

Object-oriented database

A database that stores the data as well as the processing instructions, such as how to calculate certain quantities.

Relational database

A database that consists of related tables of data that are designed in a logical structure for storage and easy data retrieval.

Database management system
A software system that facilitates the creation, maintenance, and use of an electronic database.

Data mining
The analysis of data that has been stored in a data repository, such as a data warehouse.

Data warehouse
A repository of an organization's electronically stored data from which inquiries and analysis can be made.

Database management systems are used to enter, reorganize, and retrieve the data (Wager, Lee, and Glaser 2009). **Data mining** refers to the analysis of a database that has been stored in a data repository, such as a **data warehouse**. An organization stores its data in a data warehouse, where the data can be accessed and analyzed to support decision making. The growing LTC market will require companies to review huge volumes of data to interpret patterns, identify trends, and determine how to adjust expenses to maintain the organization's competitiveness. Data mining is beneficial for the following reasons:

◆ It provides access to historical data, such as patient outcomes and expenses, which in turn aid service providers in determining the most effective forms of treatment.

◆ It helps administrators understand their staffing needs.

◆ It guides administrators in managing organizational finances and ever-changing reimbursement levels, especially for clients covered by government plans.

BARRIERS TO INFORMATION TECHNOLOGY SYSTEMS ADOPTION

The LTC industry has been slow to adopt information technology systems, primarily due to the significant costs of upgrades and a failure to recognize the importance of information technology in the provision of quality care and reduction in medical errors. However, recent research has shown the significant benefits of EMR technology to providers that adopt it, particularly in the areas of accuracy in documenting patient acuity and compliance with government reporting and billing requirements (Connole 2010a). The implementation of EMR technology may also help with recruitment and retention of staff. A demonstration program implemented to determine the impact of EMRs on employment and labor relations in nursing facilities found that the adoption of EMRs attracted workers to nursing homes, reduced conflicts with fellow employees, improved communication with supervisors, and greatly reduced medical errors (Connole 2010b).

TECHNOLOGY APPLICATIONS IN LONG-TERM CARE

Applications of technology to provision of healthcare and LTC services have been occurring since the early twentieth century. The earliest form of telemedicine was physicians calling their patients who lived in remote areas to monitor their care. The field has expanded into the field of health promotion, health monitoring and surveillance systems, and robotics, and telemedicine is now used to aid consumers with their self-care.

TELEMEDICINE AND TELEHEALTH

As stated, **telemedicine**—the practice of monitoring the medical condition of a patient from far away or consulting with colleagues situated in different locations through the use of a technological device, such as the telephone, the computer, or medical equipment—has been around for a long time. **Telehealth** is a broader form of remote clinical intervention that works the same way as telemedicine but includes health promotion, consumer education, and administrative services related to patient care. Common applications of telehealth include monitoring systems, prescription ordering, emergency notification, and video and medical sensors attached to the patient. Home care providers have also used telehealth services to monitor clients remotely, thereby extending the reach of limited visiting nurse services in rural areas. These providers have seen an improvement in the quality of services provided to patients, reductions in costs, and reductions in unplanned hospitalizations and emergency department visits (Fazzi Associates 2008).

Research on telehealth has shown that adoption rates depend on the cost and adequacy of healthcare services in a region, the policies of state governments and insurers, and medical licensing requirements that may inhibit the provision of telehealth consultations by physicians or other licensed healthcare professionals (Maheu, Whitten, and Allen 2001).

ASSISTIVE TECHNOLOGIES

Assistive technology includes hardware and software that can help people with physical impairments or those managing chronic health conditions. Assistive items range from sophisticated computer system enhancements to home modifications and robots that can provide custodial care services to simple, inexpensive devices that can be used by anyone to enhance the quality of his life. The Assistive Technology Act of 1998 helped to increase access to and funding for assistive technology through state efforts and national initiatives. Large technology companies are demonstrating growing interest in funding and developing assistive technology applications for the senior and chronically ill population. Intel and General Electric corporations recently announced the formation of a new healthcare joint venture that will focus on telehealth, chronic disease management, and development of assistive technologies in these areas (Gelhaus 2010).

A LOOK AHEAD

Continued emphasis on individuals' responsibility for self-care as they age in place helps ensure that technology will continue to be an important player in the provision of LTC services. While significant financial barriers limit expansion of technology applications and health information systems, continuing research and demonstration programs show the

Telemedicine
The practice of using technology, such as a telephone or computer, to monitor the medical condition of a patient from a long distance or consult with colleagues in different locations.

Telehealth
The delivery of health-related services and information via telecommunications technology.

Assistive technology
Hardware and software applications that help people with physical impairments or those managing chronic health conditions.

importance of these systems in coordinating the care of individuals with chronic health conditions, in improving the quality of their care, and in reducing medical errors for individuals receiving LTC services. As health information systems expand and health information sharing continues among healthcare providers, the ideal scenario is that these efforts will extend to LTC services to ensure effective coordination of care for all individuals as they age in place.

CURRENT ISSUE
Nana Technology: Helping Seniors to Be Independent

Nana technology is a term developed by Andrew Carle, an assistant professor at George Mason University, to recognize the microchip-based technology available in the market that helps seniors remain independent in their community and improve the quality of their life. Carle wanted to close the "divide between Geeks and Grans" so that the older people who needed the technology could better understand and properly use the devices that could help them with self-care. Carle believed that federal and state governments could also listen more to the elder population's concerns about the care and services available to them.

He identified eight categories of Nana technology—health and wellness, safety, cognition, communication, sensory, mobility, lifestyle, and robotics/whole home systems. Examples of these technologies include a GlowCap that provides light and sound reminders to seniors to take their medications; a wireless cell phone with larger buttons and screen size; and integrated home-based, self-care systems that can monitor an individual's activity and document blood pressure, weight, and other vital signs. Carle believes that Nana technology has the potential to serve the entire senior population, whether living independently or in a community, and that we will continue to see the development of these products over the next two decades (*Senior Journal* 2006).

FOR DISCUSSION

1. Why is a database an important component of the information system in a healthcare setting?

2. Distinguish the concepts of telehealth and telemedicine.

3. Why is a systems development life cycle approach important in the implementation of information systems in LTC facilities and other healthcare organizations?

4. What is interoperability, and why is it an important component of systems development, especially in the LTC field?

5. What are assistive technologies? Why will they be used with greater frequency in the future by individuals with chronic illnesses and LTC needs?

6. Identify at least two advantages of having an electronic medical record in a nursing home.

7. Why are project managers important in the implementation and administration of information systems in the healthcare field?

8. What is data mining, and why is it an important component in the management of quality of LTC services?

9. Distinguish a relational database from an object-oriented database.

10. What is an enterprise-wide technology system, and why is it important if an LTC facility is interested in implementing an EMR for its clients?

CASE STUDY: THE SMART MEDICAL HOME

In a smart medical home, technological and medical innovations are integrated into a home or an apartment with the goal of creating a prototype that allows the residents to manage their health and illnesses at home.

A smart medical home is equipped with scanners, sensors, computers, cameras, and appliances that double as medical devices. Close monitoring, such as that provided in a smart medical home, enables the person living in the home and her physician and other caregivers to track vital statistics, onset of symptoms, medication intake, potential for injuries or falls, and exercise and sleeping patterns, among other health-related indicators. In this way, immediate intervention can be given or preventive measures taken. When completed and perfected, the smart medical home could be a prototype for independent senior living in the future.

SOURCE: Goh (2011).

CASE STUDY QUESTIONS

1. In the future, how receptive will seniors be to moving into and living in a smart medical home?

2. What legal or ethical issues could emerge, if any, related to individuals living and aging in place in a smart medical home?

3. What recommendation would you make to secure financing for expansion of the technologies being tested in smart medical homes?

CHAPTER 5

Chronic Care and Alzheimer's Disease

James Siberski and Margie Eckroth-Bucher, PhD, RN

LEARNING OBJECTIVES

After studying this chapter, you should be able to

➤ understand the chronic care model and the six components of effective chronic care services delivery;

➤ define Alzheimer's disease (AD), its three stages, and the implications of managing long-term care services for the AD population in nursing residential, home-based, and community-based (nursing home, personal care, and daycare) settings; and

➤ understand how care for individuals with AD can be facilitated through the use of the chronic care model, which emphasizes self-care.

INTRODUCTION

The world population is aging, and those who have chronic health conditions are living longer. This trend makes management of chronic illness one of the greatest challenges for the United States and other countries today and in the coming decades. In the United States alone, approximately 133 million people have a chronic illness, and that number may rise to 171 million by 2030 (Johns Hopkins University 2004). One important disease related to aging is Alzheimer's disease. The National Institute on Aging (2012) estimates that 5.1 million Americans are living with Alzheimer's disease. Insurance carriers, government agencies, and other medical care and LTC providers have taken great interest in coordinated care management for the chronically ill population. Toward this end, in 2011 Congress passed the National Alzheimer's Project Act, which aims to create a national Alzheimer's management plan.

CHRONIC CARE MODEL

Created by Edward Wagner with the MacColl Institute for Healthcare Innovation and Group Health Cooperative of Puget Sound, the chronic care model is a comprehensive, coordinated, and proactive approach to caring for people with chronic conditions. The model argues that excellent chronic care must include the following six components, which must work together to deliver safe and effective care (also see Exhibit 5.1):

EXHIBIT 5.1
The Chronic
Care Model

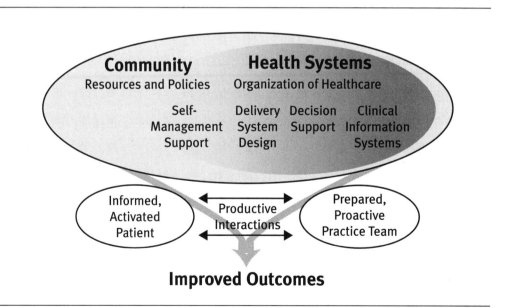

SOURCE: Figure 1 from Wagner, E. H. (1998). "Chronic Disease Management: What Will it Take to Improve Care for Chronic Illness?" *Effective Clinical Practice* 1 :2-4. Reprinted with permission from ACP-ASIM Journals and Books: found at http://www.doh.wa.gov/cfh/asthma/publications/plan/health-care.pdf.

1. The health system
2. Delivery system design
3. Decision support
4. Clinical information systems
5. Self-management support
6. The community

The effectiveness of this model was tested (and the model was improved) in the late 1990s. The demonstration project culminated in the creation of Improving Chronic Illness Care, a program funded by the Robert Wood Johnson Foundation. Innovations in team-based care management that links healthcare providers to the community, the evolution of patient-centered medical homes, and a focus on self-management of care using technology are all results of the application of the chronic care model, both in the United States and in many European countries.

ALZHEIMER'S DISEASE AND CHRONIC CARE SERVICES MANAGEMENT

Many chronic care service demonstrations have focused on **chronic illnesses** that affect individuals of all ages, such as diabetes, hypertension, and asthma, but other important chronic conditions, such as those that emerge as a result of aging and longevity, can be effectively managed with a similar approach. One of these conditions is **Alzheimer's disease** (AD), a degenerative brain disorder that leads to dementia, memory loss, and drastic changes in thinking and behavior. More than 5 million Americans and their loved ones are currently living with AD, and this number is estimated to nearly triple to 16 million by 2050 (Alzheimer's Association 2012). While AD can manifest in young individuals (i.e., those in their 30s), those typically diagnosed with AD are members of the elderly population. The incidence of AD among aging baby boomers is predicted to escalate (Alzheimer's Association 2012).

Among the aged 65 or older group, AD is the fifth leading cause of death (Alzheimer's Association 2011). Individuals with Alzheimer's may live with the condition for an extended period—in many cases, more than 20 years if early diagnosis and treatment are provided. As such, AD requires the long-term use of medical and long-term care services. Also essential to AD care are family members and other unpaid caregivers, who currently number about 15 million (Alzheimer's Association 2011).

Providers of LTC services have seen rapid growth in the number of clients and residents with Alzheimer's. Due to the complexity of the disease (i.e., deterioration of mental and physical status in later stages), home and community-based care services (see Chapter 3 discussion) have emerged that can monitor individuals with AD. These programs use a combination of home care approaches and technological systems. For individuals whose AD has progressed to the stage at which they require 24-hour care,

Chronic illness
A long-lasting or recurrent illness that needs to be managed on a long-term basis.

Alzheimer's disease
A progressive and fatal brain disorder that destroys brain cells and causes memory loss as well as problems with thinking and behaviors that can affect an individual's work and social activities.

Dementia

An acquired persistent impairment of intellectual function that compromises at least three of the following spheres of mental activity: language, memory, visual/spatial skills, emotion or personality, and cognition.

Diagnostic and Statistical Manual of Mental Disorders

A manual published by the American Psychiatric Association (APA) that provides the standard classification of mental disorders used by mental health professionals.

memory care units within residential facilities and freestanding residences for Alzheimer's care are available. The projected exponential increase in AD diagnosis in the future has necessitated targeted Alzheimer's education and training for a wide variety of healthcare providers, including facility administrators. Training is also offered and recommended to family and other loved ones who provide support and unpaid care to individuals with AD.

This chapter examines AD as a special case of chronic care management and argues that more fluid service delivery models, such as the dimensions of care model (see Chapter 1) and the chronic care model, which will be discussed in this chapter, can be effective approaches for people who suffer from AD and for those who take care of them.

THE ALZHEIMER'S DISEASE PROCESS

Dementia is defined by Dr. Robert Cummings as "an acquired persistent impairment of intellectual function with compromise in at least three of the following spheres of mental activity: language, memory, visual/spatial skills, emotion or personality, and cognition" (Cummings and Benson 1992). If an individual meets these criteria, he is said to be demented. Dementia has numerous causes, but Alzheimer's accounts for up to 75 percent of all dementia (Levine 2006; Cummings 2003). The other commonly diagnosed forms of dementia are (1) vascular dementia or small strokes, (2) Lewy bodies dementia, and (3) frontotemporal dementia (see Exhibit 5.2) (NINDS 2009).

Administrators of LTC facilities need to be aware that individuals who suffer from dementia have an acquired, persistent impairment of intellectual function and thus need specialized care. The level of such care varies according to the cause of the dementia and the stage of the illness and affects a facility's staffing requirements, training, need for resident supervision, and other factors. A reference that is helpful for those who work with clients with AD and other dementias is the fourth edition of the ***Diagnostic and Statistical Manual of Mental Disorders*** text revision (*DSM-IV-TR*). Published by the American Psychiatric Association and serving as a trusted reference book in the medical and mental health sectors, the *DSM-IV-TR* provides a classification of mental disorders, specific criteria for diagnosis, and a listing of the most important conditions to consider in a differential diagnosis for each category. This manual is a good resource for administrators and staff. When an administrator encounters a client who has not been diagnosed with a dementia but is experiencing memory complaints, displaying inappropriate social behaviors, or suffering hallucinations (for the first time), the administrator should refer the client to a qualified medical professional for a comprehensive assessment. A physician must assess the causes of dementia-like symptoms, as some of them can be reversed if they originated from a treatable condition such as depression, adverse drug interaction, thyroid problem, excessive use of substances, vitamin deficiency, or tumor.

Exhibit 5.2
Three Common
Causes of
Dementia

1. *Vascular dementia (VaD).* A syndrome of insufficient blood flow to the brain areas that causes cognitive problems and can be recognized by its step-wise progression. Some causes are hypertension, diabetes, heart disease, and tobacco smoking. It can begin after age 50 and accounts for approximately 10 percent to 20 percent of all dementias.

2. *Lewy bodies dementia (LBD).* * "The central feature of LBD is progressive cognitive decline, combined with three additional defining features: (1) pronounced 'fluctuations' in alertness and attention, such as frequent drowsiness, lethargy, lengthy periods of time spent staring into space, or disorganized speech; (2) recurrent visual hallucinations; and (3) Parkinsonian motor symptoms, such as rigidity and the loss of spontaneous movement. People may also suffer from depression."

3. *Frontotemporal dementia (FTD).* * "The symptoms of FTD fall into two clinical patterns that involve either changes in behavior or problems with language. The first type features behavior that can be either impulsive (disinhibited) or bored and listless (apathetic) and includes inappropriate social behavior; lack of social tact; lack of empathy; distractibility; loss of insight into the behaviors of oneself and others; an increased interest in sex; changes in food preferences; agitation or, conversely, blunted emotions; neglect of personal hygiene; repetitive or compulsive behavior; and decreased energy and motivation. The second type primarily features symptoms of language disturbance, including difficulty making or understanding speech, often in conjunction with the behavioral type's symptoms. Spatial skills and memory remain intact."

* Definitions reprinted with permission from NINDS, http://www.ninds.nih.gov.

RISK FACTORS

The risk of Alzheimer's disease is 1 percent at age 70 to 74, and the risk almost triples every five years after that: It is about 8.5 percent for those over age 85. A family history of AD with first-degree relatives (i.e., mother, father) increases the risk from 10 percent to 30 percent. Other risks include head trauma, depression, low education attainment, hyperlipidemia, diabetes, Down's syndrome, and gender. Women have a greater risk because they live longer than men, and as noted, age is a risk factor (Ford 2008).

SYMPTOMS

The signs and symptoms of dementia include personality change, difficulty coping with change, confusion, repetition (e.g., asking the same question), difficulty reading quickly, forgetfulness, poor decision making, difficulty with self-care (i.e., performing activities of daily living, as described in earlier chapters), and difficulty with the executive functions that allow independent living (i.e., performing instrumental activities of daily living, as described in earlier chapters).

THREE STAGES OF ALZHEIMER'S DISEASE

Understanding the three stages of AD is essential. These stages are not distinct or freestanding; instead, they are part of a continuum—symptoms initially appear mild and later become severe, thereby increasing the requirements for care. AD typically begins after age 50, and once the symptoms emerge they will only progress. The three stages are (1) preclinical, which lasts two to three years; (2) mild, which can last from one to ten years; and (3) severe, which can last one to ten years (National Institute on Aging 2010).

Preclinical Stage

In the preclinical stage, the symptoms are mild and commonly characterized by mild cognitive impairment. Individuals with preclinical AD are more likely to be at home or at a daycare. Forgetfulness is normally evident, and the forgetfulness can be problematic, depending on the client's position in the preclinical stage. Mild problems with speech, word-finding issues, and difficulty learning new information also occur. For example, a client with preclinical AD may demand lunch right after she eats, and she may repeat this pattern throughout the day, straining the patience of caregivers.

Mild Stage

In the mild stage, individuals may be at a daycare or, if they are further along in the mild stage, at a personal care facility. Because the mild stage represents a worsening of symptoms, caregivers may have to be trained to deal with the clients' restlessness, irritability, pacing, poor comprehension, delusions, and agitation. The progression to the mild stage also affects the activities of daily living, as discussed in Chapter 1. Therefore, depending on the individual's position in the mild stage, caregivers may encounter difficulty when the person attempts to dress and complete other basic functions. The mild stage also is marked by memory problems and increased confusion. As the confusion gets worse, wandering behavior occurs (discussed later in the chapter).

(?) DID YOU KNOW?
Four As of Cognitive Dysfunction

1. Amnesia is one of the first signs of dementia. It is the inability to learn new information and cannot be corrected by prompting or cueing.

2. Aphasia deals with both expressive and receptive communication. A person with aphasia gets lost in his words and fails to understand what someone is asking him to do.

3. Apraxia is the inability to follow commands.

4. Agnosia is the inability to identify persons, places, or things. A person with agnosia who fails to identify a fork will be unable to follow through on the directive "pick up your fork and eat."

Caregivers need to be educated on how to successfully deal with these four As so as not to challenge a person's disabilities and frustrate both parties.

Source: Alzheimer's Foundation of America (2011).

Severe Stage

In the severe stage, persons with AD reside in nursing homes because they require total care for all functions, including feeding. Individuals with severe AD are often incapable of communicating or recognizing themselves or family members. Individuals in this stage are bedridden most or all of the time and will sleep much of the time (Alzheimer's Foundation of America 2011). Staff should be skilled in caring for the incontinent resident, who will require frequent repositioning to prevent skin breakdown.

Excess disability
Disability caused not by a disease but by disuse of a skill, which may lead to atrophy of that skill and ultimately increase the workload of staff.

ACTIVITY THERAPY

At present, AD is not curable, but it is treatable. Therefore, the LTC administrator must not only understand the value of activity therapy, programming, and therapists but also adhere to the Centers for Medicare & Medicaid Services regulations for the activities and activity directors in the facility. Administrators are advised to consider activity therapy as the responsibility of both the activity therapy department and the nursing department, including the certified nursing assistants, as this needs to be a team effort to be successful. Activity therapists, in turn, need to provide meaningful, purposeful, and normalizing activities for residents. Activity therapy prevents excess disability from developing among residents with AD and other dementias. Individuals who benefit from activity programming include those who are severely disoriented;

⚠ CRITICAL CONCEPT
Preventing Premature Disability

LTC providers need to attempt to restructure a task when a client can no longer complete it; this ensures that providers do not take over the task and gives the client another chance to do it herself. For instance, a caregiver should place the fork in the person's hand to determine if she can still feed herself, instead of feeding her. By choosing to unnecessarily feed the client, the caregiver is creating **excess disability**— a disability caused by disuse, not by disease, that leads to atrophy of skills and ultimately increases workload.

Another example applies to a client who can no longer follow the sequence for brushing her teeth, even with prompts. Rather than brushing her teeth for her, the caregiver could lay out the toothbrush, toothpaste, rinse cup, and towel; hand the client the toothbrush; and gently guide her hand to imitate the act of brushing teeth. Caregivers should make all efforts to encourage individuals with AD to do what they can for themselves so that they do not lose their abilities prematurely.

who have a sensory deficit and cognitive impairment; who have intellectual disabilities; who practice self-stimulation; who avoid eye contact; and who are in constant motion, whether in a wheelchair or on foot.

The **Minimum Data Set** (MDS) is the standard assessment required for newly admitted individuals to any nursing home in the United States. This assessment includes an activities section that addresses the resident's lifelong interests and preferences so that they can be incorporated into her treatment plan. All levels of long-term care have some form of care planning. The resident's care plan, which is based on a comprehensive assessment that notes any issues that affect the resident's involvement in activities, is the vehicle by which the activity department addresses the resident's strengths, needs, interests, preferences, abilities, and short- and long-term goals.

The activity therapist is the individual who determines programming and interventions specific to the resident's capabilities. Activity programming needs to go beyond birthday parties and bingo; it must involve residents in activities that stimulate cognitive activity (Grandal 2008). Activities should enhance the cognitive abilities of all residents, whether they have normal cognition or have significant cognitive difficulties. Preventing, slowing the loss of, and restoring the cognitive abilities of those who suffer from excess disability not only benefit the residents but also translate into less work for the staff and decreased utilization of services. The use of computer simulations has shown promise in improving cognitive ability in individuals with normal cognitive functions, mild impairment, and moderate impairment. In fact, research indicates that such therapy generally has positive effects on cognitive and memory functioning scores (Jedrziewski, Lee, and Trojanowski 2007). As a result, future therapy, physical exercise, diet, and socializing opportunities in the treatment of AD will likely leverage the use of computer simulations (Eckroth-Butcher and Siberski 2009).

BEHAVIORAL DISORDERS AND PROGRESSIVELY LOWERED STRESS THRESHOLD

Many personal care, daycare, and nursing home staff are well trained, but they still lack expertise in managing the behavioral disturbances typically seen in the three stages of AD. The LTC administrator needs to be aware of the financial costs and the staff considerations, such as morale, related to managing these behavioral disturbances. In addition, the administrator must be aware of progressively lowered stress threshold. As individuals with AD progress through the stages, they find themselves less able to rely on their past coping skills, strategies, and knowledge base to deal with their present situation; thus, they experience an increase in stress. As this stress escalates into anxious behavior, it quickly progresses into dysfunctional behavior—a high level of anxiety, night awakenings, catastrophic response to a stimulus that may be trivial, sundowning syndrome, confusion, combative behavior, and other negative acts—that require significant staff time to control.

Minimum Data Set
A standardized screening, assessment, and data collection tool for determining the level of care need for long-term care expenses in nursing homes and hospitals.

! CRITICAL CONCEPT
Administrative Implications of Dementia

LTC facility administrators need to be aware of the symptomatic changes that can occur in older individuals that indicate some type of dementia. They also need to consider their plan to care for these clients. Issues they may consider include

- the responsiveness of the facility to the illness,

- the treatment,

- the responsibilities of the facility to provide services,

- the short- and long-term outcomes, and

- the planning around these outcomes.

These strategic considerations enable the administrator to budget, provide appropriate staffing levels, offer appropriate training, and meet the expectations of the client as well as the family or surrogate.

These negative behaviors have an effect on the milieu of the facility (if the individual is a resident) and on the stress levels of other people, including other residents, staff, and family. The sources of stress for individuals with AD include fatigue, multiple competing stimuli, medication side effects, pain, changes in routine, and demands that exceed ability (Smith et al. 2006). Following are several approaches to managing behavioral disorders.

ABC Approach

The A in the ABC approach represents either the activator or antecedent—that is, the situation that precipitated the behavior. The A may be identified by asking, Was the environment too noisy? Were the visitors upsetting? The B is the behavior that resulted. The behavior must be defined. Recognize that staff members can only deal with one behavior at a time. The C is the consequences of that behavior. The goal is to identify the activator (A) that stimulated the behavior (B) that triggered a response from someone (generally a staff member) in the environment. This response is the consequence that will either reward the behavior or help to extinguish it.

The ABC approach works in any of the stages of Alzheimer's and can be applied to other dementias with different presentations, such as frontotemporal dementia and Lewy bodies dementia (Brown and Hillam 2004).

Validation Therapy Approach

Validation therapy probably works better in the middle and later stages of dementia, specifically one caused by Alzheimer's disease. This approach relies on "going with the person" to her reality or place to better understand what she is experiencing. According to validation therapy, all behavior has meaning that needs to be understood. Consider the individual with AD in a daycare, personal care, or a nursing home who comes to a staff member to say, "I can't wait; my father is coming to visit me today." The staff could respond with a reality orientation and inform the 80-year-old that her father is dead, which may stimulate grief, searching and pining behavior, agitation, and questions of why she was not told of this death. Or using the validation approach, the staff could ask her about her father—his name, occupation, physical characteristics, and personal likes and dislikes—but should never comment on whether he is alive or dead. The staff could simply discuss the father, the client's feelings, and the significance of the fact that she misses her father.

Unmet Needs Approach

The unmet needs approach argues that the caregiver or staff may be unaware of or unable to provide what the individual with AD needs, and this can result in the individual's frustration, anger, and ultimately disturbing behavior. The unmet need could be basic, such as discomfort, lack of privacy, embarrassment, an underlying medical condition, boredom, sensory deprivation, or poor vision as a result of wrong prescription eyeglasses (Cohen-Mansfield 2001).

Social Learning Approach

The social learning approach suggests that the response behavior reinforces the initial negative behavior. For instance, the ABC approach, despite providing a consequence believed to extinguish the behavior, may in fact serve to encourage the dysfunctional behavior because it gains attention, which may be the purpose on its own.

Wandering
The act by a person with dementia of walking, riding, or driving off unsupervised, leading to a potentially dangerous situation.

WANDERING

Wandering is common in all dementias, including AD. Administrators need to be concerned about wandering because it can cause harm or even death and thus significant problems for the nursing home, personal care facility, or daycare facility. **Wandering** is the unmindful movement "on foot or by other means [that results] when certain cognitive losses and environmental circumstances intersect, causing [a] person to become lost in an unsupervised and potentially unsafe setting" (Silverstein,

Flaherty, and Tobin 2002). Individuals with AD-related dementia who walk around the halls or gardens of a personal care, nursing home, or daycare facility are not wandering; rather, they are merely pacing, perhaps due to agitation, and not in an unsafe environment in which they can get lost.

According to the Alzheimer's Association (2012) more than 60 percent of individuals with AD will wander off and get lost (referred to as eloping). Many LTC residents wander repeatedly. Forty-five percent of elopements from nursing homes, daycares, and personal care homes occur in the first 48 hours after admission (Green 2005), and administrators need to be mindful of this statistic and respond appropriately. To maintain a satisfactory level of security, individuals with dementia or AD should be assumed to be a wandering/elopement risk. The risk factors for wandering are somewhat related to the preclinical and mild stages of AD. Someone in the severe stage of AD is unlikely to be capable of ambulating to the point of wandering, but the possibility should be a consideration.

Other wandering risk factors include lack of social interaction, anxiety, unmet physical needs, agitation, boredom, excess energy, noise, crowds, and lifelong patterns (e.g., perhaps the resident was employed as a delivery person). Although wandering can occur at any hour and in any season, it is most prevalent in late afternoon or early evening; in spring or summer; and on the first warm day after a long cold or rainy spell. Because most wanderers walk and take small steps at a slow speed and have a greater step-to-step variability, the wanderer generally travels one mile or less from the starting point and is found not far from the point last seen (PLS). When given the opportunity, a small percentage of wanderers will drive; hail a cab; take a bus, train, or subway; and even hitchhike, depending on whether they resided in a rural or urban area.

It is incumbent on the administrator to develop policies and procedures to address wandering and getting lost either inside or outside the facility. These policies and procedures should be specific and should include what immediate actions should be taken, how a search (inside or outside the facility) should be conducted, and what happens if the individual is not found. The policy may even include provisions for volunteers to report in an emergency situation to assist in finding a wanderer.

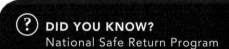

? DID YOU KNOW?
National Safe Return Program

The Alzheimer's Association offers membership to its National Safe Return Program for a small fee. The program was enacted by the US Congress in 1982 and operates 24 hours a day, 365 days a year. Members of this program receive educational information on wandering; jewelry, wallet inserts, and other paraphernalia that will help identify the person as a wanderer; and forms that, when completed and returned, provide searchers with identifying information, medication listings, and special instructions critical to finding an individual who wandered away. The information on these forms can be shared with the authorities with a simple phone call or a keystroke to further facilitate a search. Enrolling in this service is a small investment in limiting a facility's liability in the event of an elopement.

Factors to Consider Regarding Wanderers

Following are questions that the administrators and staff should consider when admitting a person who wanders:

◆ What type of dementia does the individual have? Behaviorally, it is less challenging to cope with AD patients than individuals with frontotemporal dementia because the latter have difficulty with or may be unable to inhibit their behavior and thus periodically create a disturbance.

◆ At what stage of the individual's illness does the facility become unable to provide care? Perhaps in a daycare, the administrator may not be able to manage a chronic wanderer who has frontotemporal dementia and thus tends to become agitated or aggressive.

◆ What specialized training has the staff received to care for this individual?

◆ What protocols, environmental modifications, and specialized staff training have been implemented to safely care for this individual if he wanders?

◆ What is this individual's current level of physical acuity, and are the facility and staff equipped to address it?

A critical consideration in dealing with wanderers is exit control—the location of the exit door, the type of foot traffic on the other side of the door, and the management of people allowed to enter and exit a secured unit. The attractiveness of the exit door, the signage on it, and even the hardware attached to it are issues with wanderers. Thus, it is advised to camouflage exits to limit wanderers' curiosity. Locking devices and alarms are financial considerations as they can be expensive; however, they are necessary to safeguard residents at risk for wandering.

To provide a safe pacing environment, LTC facilities may consider creating paths—either inside or outside (or both)—designed as a circle or figure eight. The paths may be further enhanced by featuring window-shopping opportunities—areas with a hutch and a bench that allow the resident to take a break, sit, and rummage through drawers in which safe, approved items are placed. Another accommodation to pacers is placing a pedometer on a constant walker, with his permission, to track the daily number of steps or miles he logs; monitoring the data would prevent exhaustion, dehydration, or a similar negative scenario. When implementing ideas such as these, the administrator needs to consider the type of environmental controls desired, the level of staff training required, the availability of consultation support for difficult Alzheimer's clients, and the appropriate staff-to-patient ratio.

Sundowning

Sundowning is a symptom that is exhibited by approximately 20 percent of individuals with Alzheimer's or other dementias and refers to an increasingly confused, anxious, and agitated state that occurs in early evening or into the night. Although the cause is unknown, it is aggravated by fatigue, low lighting, and visible shadows. The administrator should be familiar with nonpharmacological interventions for sundowning, including well-lit rooms (until bedtime) and purposeful activities that keep the individual occupied and engaged. If necessary, the physician or psychiatrist can also prescribe pharmacological interventions. Because melatonin levels decrease with age and may be reduced by 50 percent in individuals with AD, a melatonin supplement is another option (Tabloski 2010).

Sundowning
A symptom exhibited by some people with Alzheimer's or other dementias characterized by confusion, anxiety, and agitation in the early evening or into the night.

Difficult Communication

The administrator needs to be mindful of the mild to extreme difficulty experienced in communicating with those who have AD and other dementias. Aphasia, as defined earlier, is a disorder that robs a person of the ability to communicate, including receiving or sending messages or both (Green 2005). Staff members require training on the various types of aphasia and on effectively communicating with those who

♦ forget what they are talking about in the middle of a point and get frustrated in the process,

♦ go back to speaking in their native language,

♦ stick to the same words because they cannot find the appropriate terminology,

♦ use neologisms to describe common things,

♦ have difficulty organizing words logically,

♦ use offensive language, and

♦ prefer to point rather than talk.

These difficulties vary in severity depending on the AD stage and type of dementia. To ease some of these difficulties, staff should practice the following tactics:

1. Face the person and remain calm.
2. Attempt to identify the feelings or emotions rather than the words to understand what the person is attempting to communicate.
3. Check for hearing or vision problems that might hinder communication.

4. Use the person's full name with title (e.g., Mrs., Mr., Sister, Dr.).
5. Speak slowly, using simple words and omitting conjunctions, as they can complicate the message.
6. Ask one question at a time, and allow ample time for the response.
7. Include the person in the conversation if he is in the room, and refrain from talking about him as if he is not there.
8. Be patient.
9. Use gestures and pictures of objects or actions (e.g., an image of someone drinking coffee).

Staff who can effectively communicate with clients and residents typically have a better relationship with these individuals and experience fewer dysfunctional behaviors (Williams et al. 2009).

PHARMACOLOGICAL TREATMENT

The pharmacological management of the cognitive symptoms of AD consists of the cholinesterase inhibitors—Aricept (donepezil), Exelon (rivastigmine), Razadyne (galantamine), and Cognex (tacrine, no longer used)—and Namenda (menmantine), a non-cholinesterase inhibitor. Cholinesterase inhibitors are usually beneficial when administered during the early stages. The non-cholinesterase inhibitor Namenda has been effective in the later stages when combined with Aricept. The pharmacological approach has proven to be successful 50 percent of the time, modestly slowing the progression of cognitive impairment and reducing difficult behaviors and some psychiatric symptoms in patients (Hallberg and Norberg 2005).

This improvement translates into an individual with AD who is somewhat capable of self-care, which can reduce staff workload. Although administrators need not be experts in medications, it is to their advantage to understand that drugs, while helpful, can create problems if not prescribed correctly. Pharmacists should be consulted in difficult cases. A pharmacist can analyze over-the-counter and prescription medications to determine whether they are appropriate and whether they contribute to an underlying problem. Due to normal age-related changes, the elderly are more susceptible to side effects, which when not recognized can increase staff workload and negatively affect the clients' and residents' quality of life.

No magic pills can solve the problems that arise from AD, and administrators and staff should consider non-pharmacological approaches, as described in this chapter, before adding pharmacological options. Medications should never be used to treat family or staff anxiety, nor should they be used as chemical restraints.

A LOOK AHEAD

New and seasoned administrators must stay current with the ever-changing discoveries in the field of dementia, specifically AD. They must be prepared to provide effective services to the existing population, and understand insurance and governmental standards to meet and maintain their facility's certifications. Administrators and staff must work efficiently and avoid providing services deemed ineffective or obsolete. Likewise, they should be constantly aware of and knowledgeable about new discoveries in AD treatment, including new medications, diagnostic innovations, and creative interventions that improve care. Being current with trends helps facilities expand their potential customer base and thus increase profitability.

This chapter provides a broad overview of Alzheimer's disease and its management in LTC facilities. Future administrators should conduct further study into this important topic to enable them to effectively provide quality care to this population.

FOR DISCUSSION

1. Why is it important for an administrator to have an understanding of Alzheimer's disease?

2. Should staff do everything for the client, knowing the activities may be completed faster than if the client performs them? Why or why not?

3. Explain the negative outcomes of wandering in any facility.

4. Can too much programming cause behavioral problems?

5. Briefly describe the chronic care model.

CASE STUDY: PROGRESSING FROM MILD TO SEVERE STAGES OF ALZHEIMER'S

Seventy-five-year-old Mrs. Fox was referred to the facility for an assessment. She was cooperative for the interview and initially tried to answer all the questions, but many times she gave up rather quickly. Her affect was flat, and she denied experiencing visual or auditory hallucinations. She was able to maintain her attention and made fair eye contact. She stated that she would sometimes cry and that her memory was "not bad." She reported a good appetite, stated she had no trouble sleeping, and denied any feelings of depression. She did appear to have a hearing impairment and noted that her vision was fine. She continued to attend church services and was able to say the Rosary. She indicated that she was not feeling well and would like to feel better.

Mrs. Fox has multiple physical problems for which she is presently receiving medical treatment. She has been diagnosed with a dementia (Alzheimer's type). She has periods of suspiciousness and believes that people are removing things from her room. She often sits in her room in various stages of unsuitable dress at inappropriate times. Staff reports that she has been confused for about a year but has been significantly impaired for the past two months.

Mrs. Fox shows a significant problem with recent memory, and her remote memory is also impaired. She is now beginning to wander, and the symptoms of aphasia, apraxia, and agnosia are becoming more evident. Her suspiciousness may be the result of her frustration over things she cannot find or cannot explain. In other words, she is using various defense mechanisms to make sense of her erratic, unpredictable world. She lacks insight into her impaired memory and other symptoms. She showed no improvement after taking Aricept, the prescribed medication for her Alzheimer's disease; instead, she showed both cognitive decline and progression of the disease. When Aricept was discontinued, there was a rapid decline in her cognitive scores. Assessing individuals for depression when cognitive impairment is present is difficult, but she appears to be depressed. As noted, she admitted to sometimes crying. She also needs medication to induce sleep, and according to staff she has appeared sad for the last two weeks.

Mrs. Fox's prognosis is poor, but several interventions can improve her quality of life. The wandering, confused behavior, and memory problems will only worsen as she enters the severe stage, where sitting and lying down will replace wandering as she succumbs to the disease.

CASE STUDY QUESTIONS

1. In what stage of AD is Mrs. Fox, and what symptoms support your response?

2. What behavior will indicate that Mrs. Fox is entering the severe stage of Alzheimer's disease?

3. If staff were to attempt to involve Mrs. Fox in many activities and make significant demands on her to clean her room and bathe herself, how might this affect her behavior?

CHAPTER 6

Hospice, Palliative, and End-of-Life Care

Judith Jopling Sayre, PhD, and Reetu Grewal, MD

LEARNING OBJECTIVES

After studying this chapter, you should be able to

➤ define the key terms essential to understanding the delivery of care at the end of life in a variety of settings, including inpatient and long-term care environments;

➤ understand the theoretical and philosophical foundations of today's practice of hospice and palliative care;

➤ understand the history of the hospice movement, its growth and development in the United States, and its relevance to residents of long-term care facilities;

➤ understand key medical issues related to end-of-life care, including interdisciplinary pain and symptom management;

➤ understand the importance of such key issues as advance directives to end-of-life care;

➤ be able to discuss the ethical, spiritual, and social issues involved in the delivery of hospice care; and

➤ understand the economic issues of hospice and palliative care relative to the inpatient and long-term care environments.

INTRODUCTION

End-of-life care, as practiced in the growing field of hospice and palliative medicine, is a relatively new specialization in US healthcare, but it is of increasing importance as the country's population ages in greater numbers. The goals of hospice and palliative medicine are to provide comfort to the dying, offer relief from suffering not only to the patient but also to her caregivers, and instill the acceptance of death as a natural part of life (NHPCO 2012). This philosophy contradicts the traditional model of medicine, the primary goal of which is to cure disease and which views death as a failure. Once viewed with skepticism by the medical community, hospice and palliative medicine are now recognized (in large part due to a grassroots effort by the public) and are quickly emerging as prominent components of US healthcare.

The field of hospice and palliative medicine presents unique challenges and opportunities for healthcare administrators, including the great variety of locations in which this care could take place, the economic impact of end-of-life care, and the multitude of medical, social, and spiritual issues that affect such care.

THEORETICAL AND CONCEPTUAL FOUNDATIONS

Hospice care addresses the physical, psychological, social, and emotional issues of patients and families when a patient is facing the end of her life. It is based on centuries-old principles and grounded in a holistic philosophy.

HOSPICE PHILOSOPHY

In contrast to the traditional curative model of care, **hospice** provides support and comprehensive care for the dying and focuses on maintaining quality of life by relieving the patient's physical, emotional, or spiritual suffering (NHPCO 2012). Hospice care may be delivered in the hospital, in specialized hospice inpatient facilities, in LTC facilities, or in the home. Hospice care is provided primarily through a Medicare benefit, and patients qualify on the basis of disease-specific criteria, which in general indicate that the person has six months or less left to live.

Hospice today is an integral part of palliative medicine. An emerging specialty, palliative medicine extends the principles of hospice "upstream" in the disease process and thus benefits a wider population at an earlier point in the disease process (Ferris 2005). Any patient with a life-limiting illness, regardless of how far along her disease has progressed, qualifies for **palliative medicine**. This broader view of palliative medicine accepts that some curative therapies may be appropriate even though the patient has been diagnosed with a fatal disease. For example, an individual in the middle stages of Alzheimer's disease would not yet qualify for hospice care but may still have troubling symptoms that would benefit from medical attention. This person would be a candidate for palliative medicine.

End-of-life care
Care provided to patients approaching the end of life that is focused on pain relief, comfort, respect for the patient's decisions, support for the family, and interventions to help psychological and spiritual needs.

Hospice
Treatment that provides support and comprehensive care for the dying and focuses on maintaining quality of life by relieving the patient's physical, emotional, or spiritual suffering.

Palliative medicine
The comprehensive, multidisciplinary care of patients with life-limiting illness. Palliative care extends the principles of hospice but begins at an earlier point in the disease process, and accepts that some curative therapies may be appropriate even though the patient has been diagnosed with a fatal disease.

Dame Cicely Saunders, founder of the first modern hospice facility, defined the centrality of the dying patient to hospice goals: "You matter because you are you. You matter to the last moment of your life, and we will do all we can, not only to help you die peacefully, but also to live until you die" (Clark 2006). According to Florence Wald, former dean of the Yale University School of Nursing and often credited with the spread of the hospice movement in the United States, "As more and more people—families of hospice patients and hospice volunteers—are exposed to this new model of how to approach end-of-life care, we are taking what was essentially a hidden scene—death, an unknown—and making it a reality. We are showing people that there are meaningful ways to cope with this very difficult situation" (Yale University 2008).

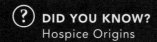

(?) DID YOU KNOW?
Hospice Origins

Archeological evidence from human prehistoric sites suggests that early humans frequently cared for injured family and group members. Healed skeletal fractures and evidence of advanced arthritis, for instance, indicate that some individuals received long periods of support and nursing care. Many religious beliefs, including early Christianity, also emphasized a religious and community responsibility to care for the sick and dying. By the fourth century, as pilgrims began journeying across Europe, monks in monasteries along pilgrimage routes began caring for individuals who needed shelter, became ill, or faced death on their journey (Golding 1981). It was then that the word *hospice* originated, from the Latin *hospes*, meaning host or guest.

HISTORY OF THE HOSPICE MOVEMENT

The idea of hospice as a site dedicated to the care of the dying was first applied in 1842 by Jeanne Garnier, the founder of the Dames de Claire in Lyon, France. As the nineteenth century drew to a close, hospitals were increasingly focused on new cures and procedures, not on care for the dying. The modern concept of hospice is credited to Dame Cicely Saunders, a British physician who, in 1967, established St. Christopher's Hospice (2011) in London. Inspired by a dying patient, Dame Saunders started a program that included both inpatient and home care for the terminally ill. Dame Saunders began developing the hospice concept when she lectured at the Yale University School of Nursing in 1965. Her philosophy of "We do not have to cure to heal" found a receptive audience. Florence Wald, dean of the school at the time, founded Connecticut Hospice in 1974. The first hospice organization in the United States, it was modeled after St. Christopher's Hospice.

A more holistic approach to the dying process was introduced to the public in 1969 by the publication of *On Death and Dying*, by Dr. Elisabeth Kübler-Ross. This best-selling work destigmatized the discussion of death and established the now well-known **five stages of grief** model for coping with death. By the late 1970s the federal government, through the Health Care Financing Administration (HCFA; now the Centers for Medicare & Medicaid Services, or CMS), began to test programs at hospices throughout the United States. These early programs were followed by the

Five stages of grief
A five-stage psychological model, first proposed by Dr. Elisabeth Kübler-Ross (1969) in *On Death and Dying*, that describes five emotional stages—denial and isolation, anger, bargaining, depression, and acceptance—that many people experience as they deal with the knowledge of their approaching death.

creation of the Medicare Hospice Benefit in 1984 as part of the Tax Equity and Fiscal Responsibility Act. Individual states were also granted permission to include hospice benefits under Medicaid. Today, many insurance companies also offer a hospice benefit, although Medicare still covers the majority of hospice care.

The National Hospice and Palliative Care Organization (NHPCO), established in 1978, has helped promote public education about hospice and palliative care and encouraged the development of palliative medicine (Yale University 2008; NHPCO 2012). In 2006, more than 4,500 hospice programs were in operation, and approximately 36 percent of all patient deaths in the United States occurred under hospice care (NHPCO 2007).

CORE ISSUES IN HOSPICE AND PALLIATIVE CARE

Hospice and palliative care utilizes an interdisciplinary approach to dealing with core patient issues, including medical and psychosocial issues at the end of life.

KEY MEDICAL CONDITIONS

Most people immediately think "cancer" in relation to patients in hospice or palliative care, but such care is appropriate for many other illnesses as well. Any ailment considered life limiting, including the end stage of many chronic diseases, qualifies for hospice or palliative care. Examples of noncancer diseases include Alzheimer's-type dementia; end-stage emphysema; ALS, or Lou Gehrig's disease; chronic kidney disease that requires dialysis; end-stage AIDS; and end-stage congestive heart failure. In fact, 59.9 percent of patients admitted to hospice in 2009 had a noncancer diagnosis (Yale University 2008; NHPCO 2012). In recent history, the majority of hospice deaths were due to chronic illness rather than cancer (Miñino et al. 2007).

Pain

Pain management
Comprehensive assessment of and plan for a patient's total pain, including physical, psychological, and spiritual pain.

Regardless of which illness brings a patient to seek hospice, pain is one of the most common symptoms treated by hospice and palliative care providers. Traditional healthcare practice uses a Likert pain scale that ranges from 0 to 10, with 0 being no pain and 10 representing excruciating pain such as childbirth (Likert 1932). Unfortunately, this scale can be misleading; the number on the scale that represents unbearable pain may differ significantly between patients. For example, one patient may feel that a pain level of 5 is not tolerable, but another patient with the same condition may feel that a level of 8 is not tolerable.

Another common problem in **pain management** is that physicians often are reluctant to prescribe adequate medication to relieve pain out of fear that their patient could become addicted, that the patient may sell pain medications for money, or that their medical license may be revoked for overprescribing narcotics. In the palliative care model, providers continue to use the traditional pain scale, but pain is also viewed as a highly personal experience unique to the individual. Only the person who is suffering can define his pain level, and, regardless of the number given on the scale, only he can say whether the pain is tolerable. Additionally, hospice and palliative medicine researchers approach pain from a multidimensional perspective, recognizing that a patient's pain could be a manifestation of emotional or spiritual distress; they have developed tools to measure the many factors that affect a patient's pain level (Melzack 1975). This concept, known as **total pain** and developed by Dame Saunders (1979), recognizes that a person's suffering is due not only to physical pain but also to spiritual, psychological, and social distress.

> ***Total pain***
> A concept developed by Dame Cicely Saunders that recognizes that a patient's pain has more than just a physical component, and also includes suffering due to spiritual, psychological, and social aspects.

This new paradigm of pain management also supports the use of narcotic pain medications without the fear of promoting addiction. In 2001, a California jury found a physician guilty of elder abuse for not adequately treating a terminally ill patient's pain (Tucker 2004). This verdict indicates that treating pain adequately is not only a moral and ethical issue for providers but a legal one as well. The American Pain Society has taken a strong stance advocating appropriate pain treatment for the dying, emphasizing that pain management is essential to quality patient care (American Pain Society Task Force 2006). Studies indicate that individuals who receive hospice care, including those in LTC facilities, have better control of their pain than those who do not use hospice care (Miller et al. 2009; Follwell et al. 2009).

Other Symptoms

In addition to pain, close attention is paid to other commonly occurring physical symptoms in end-of-life care, including fatigue, nausea, constipation, loss of appetite, insomnia, shortness of breath or air hunger, itching, and hiccups. Nonphysical symptoms, such as anxiety, depression, agitation, and delirium, can be equally distressing to the patient and caregiver and thus are treated with equal importance. Other dimensions of care include spiritual distress, which is discussed later, and social issues such as the patient's inability to participate in social gatherings because of illness.

It is easy to see how feelings of isolation and abandonment may develop in an individual who is no longer able to meet her friends at the weekly bingo game because she feels too ill to participate or someone who is afraid to visit with loved ones because he fears that disclosure of his impending death will upset the family. Hospice and palliative medicine provide a holistic approach to the patient's suffering in that both address the medical and nonmedical issues with equal importance and consider these factors to be interrelated in the way they affect the patient's quality of life (Delgado-Guay et al. 2009).

> ⚠ **CRITICAL CONCEPT**
> New Approaches to Hospice and Palliative Care: Optimizing Therapy

Hospice and palliative care teams often participate in discussions of the benefits and burdens of medications and interventions, keeping in mind the patient's life expectancy and goals of care (Holmes et al. 2006). An example of the inherent dilemma is the use of statins, a class of medication used to lower cholesterol. Although statins have many preventive benefits, such as lowering the risk of heart attack and stroke, their administration may no longer be beneficial for a person who has widespread cancer, who has less than six months to live, and whose goal of care is to remain as comfortable as possible. The medicine presents the burden on the patient of having to swallow another pill and exacts additional cost to the patient and to the healthcare system. When the patient is more likely to die from a cancer-related complication than a heart attack or stroke, the benefit of the statin is lessened. Thus, hospice and palliative medicine providers often are tasked with a thorough review of the patient's medication list, with the goal of removing nonessential medications during end-of-life care.

While many medications and therapies are discontinued when a patient enters hospice or palliative care, at times new medications and therapies are started. Pain and other symptoms often can be managed appropriately with currently available medications, but for those symptoms not well controlled by available treatments, new medications continue to be developed (Abrahm 2011). Other advances include new chemotherapy agents that may not cure the cancer but may shrink the tumor and thus provide symptom relief. Hospice and palliative patients also are benefiting from more frequent use of palliative radiation treatments to help slow tumor growth and reduce pain.

As the utilization of hospice and palliative medicine grows, the types and number of therapies will continue to grow as well. These new treatments are rarely cost effective, but the cost of hospice and palliative care is often much lower than the cost of traditional medicine because hospice and palliative care discontinue therapies not directly aimed at patient comfort. With the advent of newer and often more expensive therapies, administrators will need to be good stewards of healthcare by performing a cost-benefit analysis to determine whether the benefit gained by a patient from a particular therapy is worth the cost to the facility.

INTERDISCIPLINARY APPROACH TO HOSPICE MANAGEMENT

Hospice patients require a multitude of services, such as attention to their disease process and associated symptoms, spiritual and emotional support, assistance with navigating increasingly complex healthcare systems, and support for family members. The depth and breadth of services needed to address these issues and the recognition that no single professional can adequately deliver all of them dictate a team approach be used in treatment.

The team approach to healthcare is not a new one, but it has been reorganized within the realm of hospice and palliative medicine. The traditional model of the interdisciplinary healthcare team involves a top-down approach. Usually a physician is at the head of the team and directs patient care through the medical chart, the main form of communication in a traditional medical setting. Medical consultants, nurses, social workers, administrators, and other clinical personnel generally obtain information and communicate to one another via orders and notes that are recorded in the chart. Unfortunately, interpersonal communication is often lacking with the traditional medical team model.

The interdisciplinary approach used by most hospice and palliative care teams differs in that all members' input is considered on an equal footing regardless of role, and face-to-face communication about patients is the norm. This approach is the key to hospice management, where physicians and nurses work side by side with social workers and chaplains to deliver comprehensive and appropriate care.

Other members of the team may include administrators, pharmacists, physical therapists, and certified nursing assistants. Volunteers also play an essential role on the interdisciplinary team; many hospice programs offer a training course for community volunteers to introduce them to the hospice philosophy and to acquaint them with the unique challenges they may face while caring for a very ill patient. Volunteers talk and visit with patients, providing caregiving family members an opportunity to step away for a time. Some volunteers even offer comforting music and pet therapy. In addition, the insights and observations provided by volunteers about a patient and the family dynamic are invaluable to the hospice interdisciplinary team.

Medicare considers the interdisciplinary approach so important that, as of December 2008, CMS (2008c) requires hospice organizations, in order to maintain certification, to conduct interdisciplinary team rounds and to establish and constantly adjust the plan of care for each patient. These rounds occur weekly, and all members of the multidisciplinary team are required to attend. Each team member offers insight about the patient's treatment plan and the concerns brought up by the individual and his caregivers. The problems are then solved together by the team. Inclusion of the patient and caregivers when formulating and adjusting the plan of care is a mandatory part of the CMS regulation. These weekly team meetings occur for hospice teams in inpatient hospice facilities, LTC facilities, and home care settings and can provide valuable information to administrators, who often sit on the hospice review committee. If a question arises about whether a patient continues to qualify for hospice on recertification, documentation from weekly team meetings provides the essential information regarding that patient's ongoing needs, treatment plan, and health status. This information represents an accurate description of the client and her case for those who may not be directly involved in her care.

COMMUNICATION

As the average life span increases and advances in healthcare continue to emerge at a rapid pace, patients and families often have unrealistic expectations of cure. Denial of death has been a prominent feature in Western society, and the fear of death (thanatophobia) makes discussions about end-of-life care awkward for healthcare consumers and professionals alike. Unfortunately, these discussions may not occur until the dying process is under way, by which time efforts to honor a person's wishes concerning her end-of-life care are difficult to fulfill. Studies indicate that appropriate discussions with physicians and caregivers about end-of-life care are associated with less aggressive medical care, earlier hospice referrals, improved quality of life for the dying, and better caregiver adjustment in bereavement (Wright et al. 2008).

With the increasing public awareness of hospice and palliative medicine, medical educators have begun focusing on such key communication skills as delivering bad news and conducting family conferences (Larson and Tobin 2000). Three main areas of communication are addressed here: (1) communication with the patient and caregivers, (2) communication within the multidisciplinary team, and (3) communication with other healthcare providers.

The dying process is an extremely personal matter that must be handled with the utmost caring and compassion. Healthcare professionals involved in hospice and palliative medicine need to understand the terminal illness itself so that they can effectively manage the patient's physical, emotional, and spiritual distress. This understanding comes from frequent and ongoing dialogue among the individual, the family and other caregivers, and healthcare professionals about goals of care and treatment plans. Another area of communication is teaching the patient and caregivers what to expect as the dying process occurs. This knowledge helps alleviate fears of the unknown. Additionally, hospice and palliative medicine providers facilitate communication between the terminally ill patient and his loved ones, which allows strengthening or healing of relationships before death occurs.

Medical conditions can change rapidly during the dying process, so everyone involved in the care must be aware of what is going on. For the administrator, regular communication with care teams is important. Knowledge about patients' conditions helps the administrator make decisions about appropriate utilization of resources. Administrators also need to be sensitive to burnout, a common problem in this often emotionally challenging work environment. Open communication among staff members is the best insurance against work-related stress. In addition, communication between the hospice physician and the patient's primary care physician (or supervising LTC physician) is critically important to carrying out the treatment plan. For example, nonhospice providers may be unaware of advances made in pain and symptom management and thus benefit from updated information from the hospice physician. When a medical condition becomes more complex, sometimes hospice and palliative care professionals must call on the expertise of other consultants outside of the hospice organization. Consultants may include wound care nurses, who manage severe wounds, and podiatrists, who manage ingrown toenails. These conditions can greatly detract from the patient's quality of life. Be aware, however, that consultants are often reluctant to provide care to hospice patients because of concerns that their service may not be reimbursed and because of the prevailing attitude that "nothing can be done" for individuals in hospice. Administrators play a key role as advocates in the local community for such resources. They should communicate with local physicians and care providers about the needs of their patients. They can arrange payment agreements between the consultants and the hospice and discuss the structure for reimbursement, which is often an obstacle for outside consultant care. Additionally, they should promote the positive attitude that hospice and palliative medicine are about enhancing the patient's quality of life despite his limited life expectancy.

> ⓘ **CRITICAL CONCEPT**
> The Dimensions Model and Its Application to End-of-Life Care
>
> Just as the dimensions of care model (see Chapter 1) has been shown to be a useful construct in understanding and promoting quality within the LTC environment, it also provides insight into compassionate end-of-life care. During this time, the patient and family benefit greatly from an administration that facilitates the delivery of new medical technologies, flexible residential services, and a variety of home and community-based services. For example, hospice today is no longer based on a "no further treatment" model. Instead, palliative medicine now benefits from a variety of new pain and symptom relief modalities, such as wound care, new pharmaceutical therapies, and therapeutic radiation.
>
> Modern hospice delivery systems are more flexible than in the past, allowing patients to move more freely from an inpatient setting back to a less restrictive residential environment as symptoms are brought under control. This flexibility is facilitated by hospice home services, including volunteer providers, that can assist dying individuals whether at home or at an LTC facility.

ECONOMIC CONSIDERATIONS

With America's rapidly aging population, the economic impact of end-of-life care has become a major political and healthcare concern.

Medicare Conditions of Participation

To qualify for the Medicare Hospice Benefit, the hospice patient must be eligible for Medicare Part A and must have a physician's statement that he has a terminal condition with a life expectancy of six months or less. Given the medical complexity and individual circumstances surrounding a terminal illness, determining the exact life expectancy of a person is virtually impossible. An individual diagnosed with a terminal illness could live longer than the anticipated six months. Because of this unpredictability, the Medicare Hospice Benefit stipulates two initial 90-day recertification periods, followed by an unlimited number of 60-day periods. At the end of these recertification periods, a physician must again state that in her professional opinion the individual's life expectancy is six months or less. The person may choose to revoke or re-enroll in the Medicare Hospice Benefit at any time.

Any hospice that receives certification, and therefore can bill Medicare for services, must adhere to the rules and regulations set forth by CMS. In hospice care, these rules are known as Conditions of Participation (CoPs). The CoPs cover all aspects of hospice care—from admission criteria to recertification to documentation of services—and establish the minimum standards for patient health and safety. When hospice was first made available in the early 1980s, the HCFA published a set of CoPs, which were in effect for more than 20 years. In June 2008, CMS released an updated version of the CoPs, which took effect in December 2008 (Randall 2008). Important changes to the CoPs have occurred in all major areas (CMS 2008b). Patient and family involvement in the development of a plan of care is one area that received much attention in the new CoPs. Specifically, once the person is enrolled in a Medicare-certified hospice program, she must receive a copy of the rights and responsibilities both verbally and in writing. These rights and responsibilities include receiving important information regarding pain and symptom management, participating in the development of the treatment plan, and refusing care. Additionally, within 48 hours of electing hospice care, the patient must receive an initial nursing assessment, which determines immediate needs for care so that they can be met. Within five days of the patient's enrollment in hospice, the multidisciplinary team must complete a full assessment, including physical, psychosocial, and spiritual needs; offer bereavement counseling; and develop a drug profile. This information is then used to create an individualized plan of care, and it must be updated at least every 15 days by the team with input from the patient and his family.

These time frames, as well as the areas of bereavement counseling and drug profiles, are new to the CoPs. That is not to say that bereavement counseling and drug profiles are not given at present, but the specific documentation requirements on these issues have increased.

For example, bereavement counseling is an important part of hospice care, and it is often administered both formally and informally by all members of the multidisciplinary team. Hospice members now must document bereavement counseling at their initial and all subsequent visits. In terms of the drug profile, Medicare requires documentation of not only the list of medications being used but also the rationale for their use, the potential for drug interactions, and any required laboratory monitoring as a result of a medication. Increasing the involvement of pharmacists in the work of the multidisciplinary team is important in reviewing patients' medication list. While this task is feasible in the inpatient hospice setting, it can be potentially challenging in the home care and LTC environments due to the difficulties of coordinating meetings among patients and families, pharmacists, and other hospice staff members.

Another area included in the updated CoPs is Quality Assessment and Practice Improvement, or QAPI. This section mandates that hospice organizations track outcomes data, such as organizational processes of care and patient care indicators, and design and implement methods to achieve improvement in treatment outcomes and quality-of-life indicators. These performance improvement projects became mandatory in February 2009. Ultimately, the responsibility for executing these projects falls on the governing body of the hospice, including its administrators.

Cost Analysis

According to the NHPCO's National Data Set from 2006, the Medicare Hospice Benefit pays for approximately 84 percent of hospice care. The rest is paid through private insurance (8 percent); Medicaid hospice (5.3 percent); uncompensated or charity care (1.7 percent), which includes almost all pediatric hospice care, as few hospice benefits exist for children; and self-pay or other payer (0.7 percent).

The Affordable Care Act, passed in March 2010, included changes to the payment structure of hospice care, a proposed decrease in reimbursements for hospice care, new quality reporting standards, increases in research and education on pain management, and a provision for terminally ill children to qualify for hospice care through Medicaid (Health Care and Education Reconciliation Act 2010). As of this writing, the impact of this legislation on hospice care in the United States has yet to be seen.

Approximately 40 percent of all Medicare costs occur in the last month of life (CMS 2008b). A large study conducted at Duke University Medical Center in 2007 showed that on average, patients electing hospice care at the end of life resulted in lower—by $2,309 per patient—Medicare costs in the last year of life (Taylor et al. 2007). Cost-saving benefits per day were seen for up to 233 days of care for cancer patients and up to 154 days for noncancer patients. Once these numbers of days were eclipsed, the cost of care under the Medicare Hospice Benefit began to exceed that of nonhospice care. Another study, published in 2009, found that adult cancer patients who had discussions with their physicians regarding end-of-life care were more likely to receive hospice care and less likely to undergo costly interventions, such as hospital admission and intensive care stays, in their last week of life than patients who did not have such conversations (Zhang et al. 2009). The cost of end-of-life care for those who had discussions with their physicians was about 35 percent lower than the cost incurred by those who did not have these conversations—$1,876 versus $2,917.

Hospital-based palliative care teams are also expected to reduce overall healthcare costs. Palliative care teams help facilitate end-of-life discussions on such topics as the benefits and burdens of therapies, the patient's goals of care, and earlier referrals to hospice—all of which can contribute to decreased length of stays, discontinuation of costly therapies, and prevention of future hospitalizations. In addition to improvements in quality of life, cost savings gained by using palliative care within the acute hospital setting were validated in a large study in California. The 2007 California Pacific Medical Center study showed that after having a palliative care team visit, the average hospitalization costs decreased by about 33 percent and the average length of stay decreased by about 30 percent (Ciemins et al. 2007). Overall, patients who received consults from the palliative care team had 14.5 percent lower daily costs compared to patients with similar conditions who were not seen by the team. Furthermore, a 2002–2004 study evaluating cost of hospital stays across eight hospitals found that utilization of hospital-based palliative care teams was associated with significant cost savings (Morrison et al. 2008).

LOCATIONS

Hospice care can be provided at several physical locations. The patient's private home is the primary setting, followed by nursing homes, skilled nursing facilities, other hospice units, and assisted living facilities. According to NHPCO (2007), 42 percent of hospice deaths occurred in a patient's private home, followed by 22.8 percent at a nursing facility, 19.2 percent at an inpatient hospice unit, 10.5 percent at an acute inpatient hospital, and 5.5 percent at an assisted living facility.

Medicare reimbursement for hospice care is directly associated with location of care; for example, the rate of reimbursement for routine home hospice is significantly lower than that for hospice care provided at an inpatient facility. Individuals who receive hospice care at a private home are visited by a hospice nurse at least once a week and may receive some help with bathing and grooming from hospice aides. Aside from brief periods of crisis or continuous care, home services do not provide 24-hour care. The majority of hospice care typically comes from family or friends or providers from privately hired home health agencies.

In the United States, about 25 percent of all hospice deaths between the years 1989 and 2001 occurred in an LTC facility (Center for Gerontology and Health Care Research 2005). However, this number does not include patients who were transferred to an acute inpatient hospital in the days or hours prior to their death. Individuals who are enrolled in a hospice program while residing in an LTC setting receive better pain management (Delgado-Guay 2009) and are less likely to be hospitalized at the end of their life (Gozalo and Miller 2007). Many LTC residents are unaware that they may receive hospice care while in the facility, and reluctance of healthcare workers to initiate conversations regarding end-of-life care promotes the underutilization of hospice care in such facilities (Casarett et al. 2005). LTC facilities that provide hospice care for their residents must have a contractual agreement with a Medicare-approved hospice provider. The facility is still responsible for providing care to the patient; however, all hospice-related treatments are the responsibility of the hospice organization. For example, a resident who suffers from end-stage lung cancer would continue to receive all of his regular care from the LTC staff. Additionally, he would receive visits from a hospice nurse and physician, who would adjust the medications and treatments for his lung cancer and provide any durable medical equipment such as oxygen tanks or a nebulizer machine, and he would be offered the services of chaplains and volunteers just as those home-based patients would.

Providing hospice care in an LTC facility is not without challenges. Confusion often arises about who is "in charge" of the patient's care—the hospice team or the LTC team. A hospice physician may write an order for a medication, but the LTC staff members are the ones who actually administer the medicine. Studies have found that LTC patients under hospice care are often undertreated in both pain and non-pain symptoms (Rodriguez et al. 2010; Oliver, Porock, and Zweig 2005). Furthermore, using hospice care in an LTC setting offers some economic disadvantages. Under the current Medicare Hospice Benefit, payment for routine home care provided in a home setting is no different than that in an LTC setting. The routine home care rate, which is paid to the hospice agency, does not include payment for room and board, so if a client elects hospice care while residing in an LTC facility, she becomes responsible for paying room and board and the facility receives a lower reimbursement rate for its services. For many patients covered by the Medicare Hospice Benefit, using the skilled nursing facility benefit is more cost-effective than paying out of pocket for room and board. A survey of nursing home administrators found that lack of education regarding hospice care, nursing staff shortages, and financial issues were the biggest barriers to using hospice services in their facilities (Rice et al. 2004). More research, education, and efforts directed toward improved communication between hospice and facility staff are needed to ameliorate this situation.

More than one in every five hospice agencies has an inpatient hospice unit (NHPCO 2007). Inpatient hospice units are often used when a person's symptoms cannot be adequately managed at the home or the LTC facility. A move to an inpatient hospice unit also provides brief periods of caregiver respite or allows medications to be rapidly adjusted to attain adequate symptom relief before the individual is discharged to her home. Inpatient hospice facilities also are used either when the person (or his family) chooses to not die at home or when the caregivers are uncomfortable with providing end-of-life care at the home.

Palliative medicine is typically used by interdisciplinary teams in the acute inpatient hospital setting. The team consults with the dying individual, whose goals may be to transition from primarily curative to comfort-based care. Some hospitals also have a palliative care unit within the facility for individuals who are actively dying but are too unstable to or cannot transfer to an inpatient hospice facility or the home. These units are often managed by the palliative care team and are staffed by specially trained nurses and other ancillary caregivers, who provide all comfort measures, including attention to pain and symptom management. Often, these units are located in an area of the hospital away from the noise and activity of the regular units, and any treatments not aimed at providing comfort, such as lab draws and taking vital signs, are discontinued so that the patient and her family can experience a peaceful atmosphere. According to data from the American Hospital Association and the Dartmouth Atlas of Healthcare, about 50 percent of hospitals with more than 50 beds have a palliative care team, although the scope of services provided varies among hospitals (Goldsmith et al. 2008).

ETHICAL ISSUES IN HOSPICE AND PALLIATIVE CARE

Professional caregivers are obligated to practice ethical healthcare; they must not only provide good-quality healthcare but also do what is right for the dying individual. With the growth in advanced medical technologies, myriad new treatment options and healthcare approaches are available. In hospice and palliative medicine, ethics plays an increasingly important role as the options for end-of-life care multiply. The terminally ill may not be able to communicate their wishes as they enter the dying process, and if previously they did not clearly communicate their wishes in an **advance directive**, their loved ones may find making such decisions on their behalf particularly difficult. Families are asking not only what can be done but also what should be done. With myriad treatment options facing families at the end of a patient's life, the simple **DNR (do not resuscitate) order** may be inadequate. Patients and their families may find that a more complete advance directive can convey the patient's specific wishes regarding such treatment options as tube feeding or continuation of artificial ventilation. As part of an advance directive, the patient may designate someone as his **healthcare surrogate** to help make complex decisions in the event that the patient is no longer capable.

Ethical dilemmas may arise when members of the multidisciplinary team have differing ideas about values and responsibilities than those of the patient and family or when no consensus can be reached on what is right or good for the patient. Consulting

---

Advance directive
Information provided to a healthcare provider that details an incapacitated individual's wishes for medical care.

DNR (do not resuscitate) order
Instructions, usually written by a physician after discussion with a patient, telling other healthcare providers not to try to restart a patient's heart through cardiopulmonary resuscitation or other treatments if the patient's heart were to stop beating.

Healthcare surrogate
The person designated by a patient to make healthcare decisions for the patient in the event that he is no longer able to make decisions. If no one has been designated by the patient, by default the next of kin is the healthcare surrogate.

an ethics team can help resolve ethical dilemmas. These ethics experts can provide an objective review of the case and talk to conflicted staff, the patient, and family members about their views on the issue. After working through a case, the ethics team makes recommendations, which are documented in the patient's chart.

Most hospitals have an ethics team, and hospice organizations are beginning to follow suit. Members of an ethics team can include physicians, nurses, social workers, chaplains, administrative staff, and board members as well as legal and healthcare professionals from the community. Most ethics teams meet at regularly scheduled times or on an as-needed basis, and generally a member of the ethics committee is available on call for issues that arise outside of normal business hours.

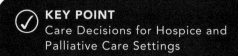

KEY POINT
Care Decisions for Hospice and Palliative Care Settings

Questions such as "How aggressive should Mother's care be?" or "Should we consider artificial nutrition?" arise frequently in the hospice and palliative medicine setting. For some people, making these decisions is straightforward, but for many others it is a complex process that can be emotionally challenging. When trying to resolve these conflicts, the basic principles of bioethics and the person's values, including cultural, religious, and spiritual beliefs, must be considered.

Two ethical dilemmas unique to hospice and palliative medicine are physician-assisted death and palliative sedation. Physician-assisted death, which includes physician-assisted suicide and physician-assisted euthanasia, involves prescribing lethal doses of medication to the terminally ill to hasten death. In physician-assisted suicide, the dying individual is responsible for deciding if and when the medication is used and for administering the medication, whereas in physician-assisted euthanasia, the physician administers the medication. In the United States, physician-assisted death is currently legal only in the states of Oregon, Washington, and Montana (O'Reilly 2010). Palliative sedation can legally be provided in the last few days of life for severe physical symptoms that do not respond to the typical doses of medications (American Academy of Hospice and Palliative Medicine 2006). These symptoms can include pain, agitation, difficulty breathing, and tremors; and although they may have been controllable earlier in the illness, symptoms may acutely worsen in the days just prior to death. Palliative sedation is recommended when all other options for treating the patient's suffering have been exhausted. In palliative sedation, sedating medications are administered to keep the patient in a state of unconsciousness while other symptom-control medications are continued. Palliative sedation operates on the principle of double effect, which acknowledges that the primary goal of palliative sedation is to alleviate suffering and not to hasten death. While a patient's life expectancy may be inadvertently shortened by the administration of palliative sedation, this is not the intent of the intervention. Maintaining open clear communication about palliative sedation is important in obtaining informed consent and ensuring that the individual and/or family members understand the risks and benefits of the procedure and that it is in accordance with their wishes. In some hospice and palliative care units, providers must obtain an ethics consult before initiating palliative sedation.

CURRENT ISSUE
Multicultural Issues in Hospice and Palliative Care

Hospice and palliative care are rapidly growing specialties and are gaining recognition. In 2009, according to the Yale Medical Group (2011), hospice programs served approximately 1.56 million people in the United States. However, among minority groups, use of end-of-life services is less common.

National data indicate that blacks and Hispanics with heart disease, cancer, diabetes mellitus, and kidney diseases do not receive the same quality of care and level of hospice assistance as do whites with the same diagnoses. Studies have suggested that culturally specific resistance to hospice principles may exist, especially among African Americans; this research indicates that greater diversity in hospice teams would make hospice care more acceptable to minority populations (Crawley 2005; Yancu, Farmer, and Leahman 2009). The disparities in access to healthcare on the basis of racial, ethnic, and socioeconomic factors have been well documented, but the racial and ethnic disparities in using hospice services have received little analysis. However, epidemiological studies indicate significant racial and ethnic differences in cause of death, with blacks and Hispanics receiving less optimal care (Cohen 2008). The comparatively few studies concerning racial and ethnic differences in hospice care may partially reflect the focus on the individual and the relative newness of the field of hospice and palliative medicine. However, those studies that have been conducted reveal significant disparities in such areas as pain and symptom management and increased use of restraints, especially among black and Hispanic nursing home residents (Green et al. 2003; Cohen 2008), making strategy development to deal with such inequities an urgent priority.

These findings are supported by increasing demographic data gathered from epidemiological studies that reveal evidence of bias and discrimination in critical end-of-life care. High-quality end-of-life care provided by hospice teams must ultimately focus on the patient and her family to reflect the patient's cultural background and personal preferences, values, and goals.

Spirituality and Religion

Perhaps no other field in medicine is more uniquely suited to address a person's spiritual needs than hospice and palliative medicine. Each religion has beliefs, rites, and rituals that are performed during the dying process or after death. The definition of spirituality, however, goes beyond the realm of religion.

The Association of American Medical Colleges Task Force (1999) offers the following definition of spirituality:

> Spirituality is recognized as a factor that contributes to health in many persons. The concept of spirituality is found in all cultures and societies. It is expressed in an individual's search for meaning through participation in religion, and/or belief in God, family, naturalism, rationalism, humanism, and the arts. All these factors can influence how patients and health care professionals perceive health and illness and how they interact with one another.

In most healthcare settings, chaplains are tasked with obtaining a patient's spiritual history and addressing her spiritual needs. Chaplains differ from traditional faith leaders in that they minister to patients of all spiritual beliefs, both religious and nonreligious. They provide support to patients by relating their experience with illness to patients' spirituality. Chaplains continue to fulfill this important role in the hospice setting and are in fact a requisite part of the hospice team, but other members of the team are expected to help in this role as well. Multiple studies have shown that patients would like their physicians to show interest in the patient's religious beliefs (King and Bushwick 1994; MacLean et al. 2003). Because spirituality can serve as an important means of coping for the dying and their loved ones, all professionals who deal with end-of-life care should be familiar with taking a spiritual history. The spiritual history can give important insight into a person's beliefs and helps the multidisciplinary team better relate to his experience.

Training and Retraining of Professionals

Despite having roots that date back many centuries, hospice and palliative medicine are still considered relatively new fields in the United States. Not until 2006 did the American Board of Medical Specialties acknowledge these disciplines as unique subspecialties.

Any physician trained in family medicine, internal medicine, obstetrics and gynecology, pediatrics, emergency medicine, physical and rehabilitation medicine, psychiatry, neurology, radiology, surgery, or anesthesia can complete fellowship training and become board certified in hospice and palliative medicine. As the importance of hospice and palliative medicine continues to be recognized, a major effort by the medical community is under way to incorporate these principles in the training programs of healthcare providers. In 2001, the Hospice/Home Care Working Group released a statement following its national consensus conference encouraging education for medical trainees in the realm of palliative care and home visits (Billings et al. 2001). Many professional schools now offer introductory lectures and elective courses or tracks within a required course that teach hospice and palliative medicine principles.

For administrators, the Center to Advance Palliative Care (CAPC) offers conferences and materials to help launch and sustain a palliative care program in the hospital setting. The CAPC (2012) and the Robert Wood Johnson Foundation formed the Palliative Care Leadership Center, a collaborative effort to help all members of the multidisciplinary team learn from successful palliative care programs via a yearlong mentoring program and an intensive two-day training course. Other resources for administrators in this emerging field include websites such as Health Resources Online (2011), which offers updates in Medicare and Medicaid services, marketing strategies, and a monthly newsletter called *Hospice Letter*. The NHPCO also offers information and resources aimed at educating all members of the multidisciplinary team, including administrators.

A Look Ahead

The old (those aged 65 or older) and the very old (those aged 85 and beyond) are the fastest growing segment of many industrialized societies, including the United States. Current projections indicate that by 2030, almost 70 million people—20 percent of the entire US population—will be older than age 65 (US Census Bureau 2008). The oldest members of the baby boom cohort reached age 65 in 2010 and began to join the population of older people who suffer from chronic, progressive, and terminal illnesses (Morrison and Meier 2004; Lang and Quill 2004). During the last years of their lives, many of these individuals, faced with diminishing independence, chronic pain, and psychological distress, will need significantly increased family and medical support (Higginson 1999). Technology has begun to greatly improve the activity levels and health of those in their sixties and even seventies, but the extension of longevity will inevitably pose dramatic implications for the delivery of quality, compassionate, and individualized end-of-life care. The need for such services also will affect the economies of many industrialized nations. Currently, much of each individual's lifetime healthcare spending is concentrated at the end of life (Zhang et al. 2009). The cost savings and improvements in a dying person's quality of life as a result of hospice and palliative care are reasons that utilization of these services is expected to increase.

The benefits of hospice and palliative medicine are now increasingly recognized, but numerous barriers to such care still exist. In addition to the previously discussed limitations of the Medicare Hospice Benefit, barriers include the traditional focus of Western medicine on the curative model of healthcare; lack of research leading to an evidence-based approach for palliative medicine; and physician discomfort with issues surrounding end-of-life care, including communicating with patients about the need for hospice or palliative care. The sheer demographics of a rapidly growing elderly population, combined with an increased acceptance of hospice and palliative medicine, already have begun to present unique challenges and opportunities for healthcare administrators.

Quality medical care in a hospice setting is challenged by a number of significant medical issues, especially pain management and symptom control. Healthcare administrators must understand the fundamental differences between pain management in a traditional setting and pain control in the palliative medicine paradigm, wherein the focus is on each patient's pain threshold and adequate medication for full relief. Because hospice patients qualify for the Medicare Hospice Benefit on the basis of disease-specific criteria and life expectancy prognosis, administrators must familiarize themselves with the rules and regulations set forth by CMS. The ethical issues in hospice and palliative care, especially as they coincide with the growth of advanced medical technologies, also can pose challenges. The entire multidisciplinary team must understand the essential bioethical principles involved and be able to communicate with the patient and the family about the patient's cultural, religious, and spiritual values.

Unlike in the top-down model of a traditional interdisciplinary healthcare team, the coordination among the multiple specialties needed in hospice care results in increased equality among team members and in more face-to-face communication. The inherent nature of the hospice team and its rapid evolution require administrators to be especially proactive in ensuring that all team members are given opportunities for ongoing professional training. Several organizations, such as the American Academy of Hospice and Palliative Medicine and the Center to Advance Palliative Care, offer conferences and materials to help administrators develop and maintain strong multidisciplinary palliative teams.

FOR DISCUSSION

1. Explain the relationship of hospice and palliative care. How are these two concepts, which are related to end-of-life care, similar and different?

2. What is the key distinction between the hospice philosophy and the traditional model of medicine?

3. What were the respective impacts of Dame Cicely Saunders, a British physician, and Dr. Elisabeth Kübler-Ross, a Swiss psychiatrist, on the establishment of the modern hospice movement?

4. Pain management is a key medical issue in palliative medicine and hospice care. Briefly discuss how the hospice paradigm of pain management differs from pain management approaches in a more traditional practice setting.

5. To qualify for the Medicare Hospice Benefit, a dying person must have a physician's statement that he has a terminal condition with a specifically limited life expectancy. What is this expectancy? What recourse is available for the patient who lives longer than the original expectations?

6. The provision of hospice care may come with many ethical dilemmas. Discuss the impact of new medical technologies on the delivery of quality hospice care.

7. Describe the hospice multidisciplinary team approach to care delivery. How does it differ from that found in the traditional medical inpatient setting?

8. Name some of the available resources for hospice and palliative care team members, including administrators, for training and retraining opportunities.

9. Name some of the demographic factors that influence the rapid growth of palliative medicine as a medical specialty and the need for increasing availability of inpatient and in-the-home hospice care provision.

CASE STUDY: PALLIATIVE CARE CHOICES

Mrs. Guevara is a 78-year-old who has been suffering from memory loss for several years. She currently resides in a skilled nursing facility as she is unable to care for herself. Her husband passed away last year, and her adult daughter, Karen, lives out of state. Sometimes Mrs. Guevara gets lonely and feels frustrated by her lack of independence. Despite taking medication for Alzheimer's disease, her condition has been steadily progressing. She gets confused easily and sometimes accuses the staff of stealing her belongings. In addition, she has developed bladder incontinence and difficulties maintaining her balance. Her appetite has decreased, and she tires easily. She often falls asleep while talking to Karen on the phone.

One night, Mrs. Guevara forgot to call for assistance and collapsed in the bathroom. She moaned quietly in pain, and a nurse later found her still lying on the floor.

Mrs. Guevara was taken to the facility's emergency department. When Karen received this news, she came immediately to the hospital. Karen demanded that "everything be done" to help her mother. Mrs. Guevara was admitted to the hospital and received intravenous (IV) fluids for dehydration and antibiotics for a urinary tract infection, and the orthopedic surgeon evaluated her for a broken wrist. An already confused Mrs. Guevara, now in an unfamiliar environment, became agitated alone in her room that night. She pulled out her IV line and tried to climb out of bed. In her attempt, she fell out of bed and hit her head. A CT scan of her head revealed a small bleed into her brain. Several days later, Mrs. Guevara's urinary tract infection had resolved through treatment. However, she appeared more confused than she had been upon admission, and she was having trouble swallowing her food. She underwent an evaluation by a speech therapist, who determined that every time she swallowed, she aspirated and a small amount of food went into her lungs. Karen asked about a feeding tube and how to care for her mother when she was discharged. The hospital physician called the palliative care team to meet with Mrs. Guevara and Karen to discuss her current and future healthcare issues. Mrs. Guevara was too confused to participate in the decision-making process, and because she did not complete an advance directive, the team relied on Karen to make decisions on behalf of her mother.

The palliative care team reviewed the natural course of Alzheimer's disease with Karen and informed her that what was happening to her mother is not uncommon. Often, when patients with Alzheimer's disease undergo an acute setback, their dementia and related complications can progress much faster. Together, Karen and the palliative care team tried to figure out what Mrs. Guevara's wishes would be. They discussed the benefits and burdens of artificial nutrition as well as the probability that any minor illness in the future would be distressing to Mrs. Guevara. The palliative care team notified Karen that at the current state of illness, her mother would qualify for hospice care, and they proceeded to review the philosophy of hospice care. After meeting with the palliative care team and taking into consideration her mother's values, Karen decided that her mother would not want a feeding tube but would want to return to her skilled nursing facility with help from the local hospice provider in managing her comfort. The next day Mrs. Guevara was discharged from the hospital.

CASE STUDY QUESTIONS

1. What issues need to be considered initially regarding Mrs. Guevara's care?

2. What issues will Mrs. Guevara face once her health status changes, and how should they be addressed?

3. How can hospice help Mrs. Guevara and Karen?

4. What hospice services could be provided to Mrs. Guevara while she is residing in a skilled nursing facility?

Diversity and the Delivery of Long-Term Care Services

Carol Molinari, PhD, and Mary Helen McSweeney-Feld, PhD

LEARNING OBJECTIVES

After studying this chapter, you should be able to

➤ identify the long-term health needs of elders by ethnicity/race, gender, and sexual orientation;

➤ discuss health disparities of diverse elders;

➤ discuss how ethnicity, race, gender, and sexual orientation affect diverse elders' preferences for residential or home and community-based long-term care services; and

➤ discuss how cultural competency among long-term care providers and staff is critical to delivering residential or home and community-based long-term care services.

INTRODUCTION

The continued growth of the senior population in the United States is commensurate with the increase in the ethnic and racial diversity of this population. In 2005, 20 percent of elders in the United States were considered part of a minority group—African Americans, Asians, Hispanics, and Pacific Islanders; however, by 2050 these minorities are projected to account for half of the senior population (Vincent and Velkoff 2010). The general health of seniors is improving, but studies have found that minority elders are less likely to receive routine medical care and that this care is of poorer quality than that received by white elders (Baldwin 2003). In 2002, the Institute of Medicine issued a report, titled *Unequal Treatment: Confronting Racial and Ethnic Disparities in Health Care,* that confirms race/gender/socioeconomic-based inequities exist in medical screening, treatment, and outcomes across common chronic diseases such as cancer, diabetes, heart disease, and HIV/AIDS (Smedley, Stith, and Nelson 2003; Gehlert et al. 2008). Given these disparities, diverse elders' health and functionality are lower, which then increases the likelihood that these seniors will need LTC.

Consequently, LTC managers and providers must understand the health and cultural needs and preferences of this emerging majority of diverse elders to ensure that residential or home and community-based services (HCBS) are better equipped and prepared for this population. Culturally competent LTC can help mitigate some of the disparities noted in the Institute of Medicine's report. This chapter provides an overview of the cultural needs and health disparities among diverse elders and shares information that will assist managers and providers of residential or home and community-based services to deliver culturally competent LTC.

WHAT IS DIVERSITY?

Diversity

The variation in cultural, personal, and lifestyle attributes of individuals, including ethnicity, race, age, sexual orientation, and socioeconomic status.

Diversity is the variation in cultural, personal, and lifestyle attributes that can be observed among a group of individuals. A diverse group, for example, could include men and women of all ages, racial and ethnic backgrounds, sexual orientations, income and educational levels, religious affiliations, political views, marital status, and physical and mental capacities (Betancourt et al. 2005). This chapter focuses on the diversity in gender/sex, ethnicity/race, and sexual orientation of the elderly population.

For our purposes, the term "diverse elders" is used throughout the chapter to refer to seniors who represent minority groups.

HISTORY OF RESEARCH ON DIVERSE ELDERS

In 1971, diverse elders were recognized as an area of gerontology. Concomitantly, the National Caucus and Center on the Black Aged was established. Afterward, the National Association for Hispanic Elderly, National Indian Council on Aging, and National Asian Pacific Center on Aging were formed, spurring research on elder populations of color.

> **⚠ CRITICAL CONCEPT**
> Defining Diversity
>
> To better frame this discussion, a brief definition of the following terms is necessary:
>
> - *Gender* is the "socially constructed roles, behaviors, activities, and attributes that a given society considers appropriate for men and women." *Sex*, on the other hand, is "the biological and physiological characteristics that define men and women" (WHO 2011).
> - *Race* is the classification that binds a group that shares inherent physical characteristics, such as skin and hair color, facial shape, and even height (Relethford 1990). Ethnicity, on the other hand, is a cultural identity, including ways of dressing and speaking, that an individual adopts for a number of reasons, such as to fit in with his social environment.
> - *Sexual orientation* is a person's romantic inclination toward those of the same sex (homosexuality), different or opposite sex (heterosexuality), or both sexes (bisexuality).

The US Census Bureau is the primary source of information for such research. To address the problems of misclassification of data about nonwhite groups (which led to the undercounting of minority groups), in 1997 the Census Bureau expanded the race category list to include the following:

- American Indian or Alaska Native
- Asian
- Black or African American
- Native Hawaiian or other Pacific Islander
- White
- Some other race

People who complete the census may now check off one or more races and may write in their racial identity. For ethnicity (see the definition given in the Critical Concept box), the categories are Hispanic or Latino and Not Hispanic or Latino, and people who identify as this ethnicity could be of any race; "in the federal statistical system ethnic origin is considered to be a separate concept from race" (US Census Bureau).

National studies of minority populations from the 1970s and 1980s suffered from small, nonrepresentative samples and were often restricted to comparisons of blacks and whites. However, research methodology has improved since that time, and studies that examine broad minority categories and incorporate race with gender have emerged. Population data demonstrate shifts in the proportion of diverse seniors 65 years were older. Based on census data from 2008, 13 percent of seniors in 2010 were racial minorities, but that percentage is expected to increase to 23 percent of seniors by 2050 as minority children today reach old age. Hispanic elders are expected to increase from 7 percent in 2010 to almost 20 percent in 2050 and as such account for much of the growth in racial and ethnic elders (see Exhibit 7.1). Despite the growth in the number of diverse elders, this population is likely to encounter oppression and discrimination (Torres and Moga 2002).

Exhibit 7.1

Projected Minority Distribution of Seniors in 2010 and 2050

RACE	2010 % of 65+	2050 % of 65+
All races	100.00%	100.00%
White alone	86.82%	76.86%
Black alone	8.50%	11.92%
Asian alone	0.58%	8.52%
AIAN alone*	3.31%	1.04%
NHPI alone**	0.10%	0.25%
Two+ races	0.69%	1.42%
ETHNICITY		
Non-Hispanic	92.90%	80.12%
Hispanic all races	7.10%	19.78%
Hispanic white	6.67%	18.39%
Hispanic nonwhite	0.44%	1.39%

*   AIAN = American Indian and Alaska Native
** NHPI = Native Hawaiian and other Pacific Islander

SOURCE: US Census Bureau (2008b).

LONG-TERM HEALTH NEEDS OF ELDERS BY GENDER, ETHNICITY, AND SEXUAL ORIENTATION

The over-65 population in the United States is not homogeneous. Disparities in health status within this population can best be understood through an examination of the characteristics of the group by gender, ethnicity, and sexual orientation.

OLDER WOMEN

The aging society is mainly composed of females. In the United States, women represent 58 percent of the aged 65 to 74 population and 77 percent of the over-85 group (Federal Interagency Forum 2008). Women's patterns of underemployment; family caregiving; and low wages, pensions, and Social Security benefits contribute to making them more vulnerable than men to poverty and chronic illness later in life (Moen and Chermack 2005). These economic concerns are major determinants in elder women's level of life satisfaction and quality of life (Choi 2001).

Despite these obstacles, older women have proven to be resilient. They are skilled at multitasking and at forming and sustaining friendships and social supports, and such abilities may be attributed to their experiences as caregivers for children and, in many cases, parents and other older adults. As women's educational attainment and employment opportunities increase all over the world, women in the future will have more economic resources that could enable them to age in their communities.

Poverty and Chronic Illness

Marriage can protect women against poverty in old age. Less than 5 percent of older married women face poverty, compared with 17 percent of unmarried older women (Federal Interagency Forum 2008). Despite the higher rate of longevity among older women in all industrialized and nearly all developing countries, they experience higher rates of illness, physician visits, and prescription drug use associated with acute and chronic illnesses (Moen and Chermack 2005).

Older women's poorer economic status increases their health risks. Compared to their wealthy counterparts, poor elderly women tend to live alone, have inadequate diets, have limited access to health and wellness information, and have fewer regular dentists and physician visits. Older men are more likely to have life-threatening chronic diseases, such as heart disease, cancer, and stroke, and thus are prone to die earlier. However, older women are more likely to experience disabling effects of multiple chronic problems related to age. For example, autoimmune diseases, such as thyroid disease and arthritis, affect more women than men (55 percent and 43 percent, respectively) (Federal Interagency Forum 2008). Such chronic health conditions can interfere with daily functioning (i.e., activities of daily living [ADLs] and instrumental activities of daily living [IADLs]), requiring the person to seek regular medical and social services.

Older women are less likely than older men to engage in leisure physical activity, such as dancing. While women tend to engage in walking, yard work, or household chores as a way to keep active, overall, women's inactivity increases with age. In a Medicare Beneficiary Survey, 32 percent of elder women reported they were unable to perform any functional activities (e.g., stoop, reach over head, write, walk two to three blocks, lift ten pounds) (Federal Interagency Forum 2008). Among the very old (85 or older), 65 percent of women, compared to 50 percent of men, were identified as likely to need to enter a nursing home.

LTC Preferences

Older women represent 71.2 percent of nursing home residents and 64 percent of home care consumers (Jones et al. 2009; Caffrey et al. 2011). Because of their lower socioeconomic status, they make up 70 percent of Medicaid beneficiaries aged 65 to 84 and 80 percent of those aged 85 or older (Hooyman and Kiyak 2011). In a study, a group of disabled women aged 65 and older were asked to name the ideal LTC setting for a range of healthcare needs, such as help with ADLs, IADLs, and dementia-related issues (Wolf, Kasper, and Shore 2008). Sixty-six percent of respondents preferred to be taken care of in their private home if they needed ADL or IADL assistance. For a scenario involving dementia, half of the respondents agreed that the nursing home was their best option. This study indicates that older women perceive that certain LTC settings are best for certain physical and mental needs; this perception drives their preferences.

OLDER AFRICAN AMERICANS

Among older African Americans, the prevalence of chronic disease is twice as high as among whites. Heart disease rates, for example, are decreasing among white males but increasing among black males. Furthermore, mortality rates for heart disease, stroke, and cancer are higher for African Americans and occur at a younger age than for non-Hispanic whites. African Americans also experience higher rates of type 2 diabetes and are twice as likely to die from complications from diabetes as whites (McDonald et al. 2004; Wen, Cagney, and Christakis 2005).

African Americans have a shorter life span than whites, with a longer period of declining functional ability and disability. Older blacks are twice as likely to be incapacitated as are white elders (Angel and Angel 2006). Marital status affects the health of African Americans. The proportion of married African Americans is lower than any other racial minority. Among African-American elders, 56 percent of men and 24 percent of women are married, compared to 75 percent of white elder men and 42 percent of white elder women (Administration on Aging 2009).

Although African Americans are less likely than whites to enter nursing homes, they do so more than other racial minority groups. African Americans who live in nursing homes are more limited in their daily living activities than their white counterparts. And they are less likely to be discharged, because of their disabilities or impairments (Administration on Aging 2009).

OLDER HISPANICS OR LATINOS

Hispanics or Latinos are the largest ethnic minority and the fastest growing population in the United States. The term "Latino" refers to people born in or who have direct ancestors from Mexico, Puerto Rico, Cuba, and countries in Central and South America. This ethnic group shares a common language (Spanish) but is diverse in terms of geographic location, income, education, and cultural heritage.

Cubans make up the largest number of elder Latinos, and Mexicans represent the smallest. More than any other minority group, Latinos have retained their native language. Among Latino elders, about 33 percent speak only Spanish and 70 percent never completed high school (compared to a 30 percent nongraduation rate for elders of all races) (Munet-Vilaro 2004).

Older Latinos have lower mortality rates than non-Latino whites for certain disease conditions, such as heart disease, cancer, or stroke (Wallace and Villa 2003). One exception is that among Mexicans, disease rates increase as their length of stay in the United States increases. The reason may be that Mexicans are more likely to acquire type 2 (adult onset) diabetes than whites (Wallace and Villa 2003).

Mexicans, Puerto Ricans, and Dominicans develop chronic and disabling diseases early in life, which could lead to ADL limitations later on and thus the need for ADL assistance (Aranda 2006).

Health differences among Latinos may be observed by sex. Latina women are at increased risk for hypertension and related heart disease (Borrell, Dallo, and White 2006), and they are more likely than Latino men to have chronic diseases. Mortality from cervical and uterine cancers is higher among Latina women than white women. Also, older Latina women experience more depression than older white women. To better understand these health differences among elderly Latinas, consider this recent research finding of a study by Shuster and colleagues (2009): More than half of the Latina women who participated in the study were sedentary and did not exercise regularly. This is an important finding because physical function is the key determinant of independent living and thus LTC needs.

OLDER NATIVE AMERICANS

Native Americans or First Nations refer to indigenous American people, including Alaskan natives. This racial minority is a diverse population marked by about 300 native languages and myriad cultural traditions. Sixty percent to 70 percent of Native Americans live

KEY POINT
Diverse Elder Services

Historically, other minority elder groups relied on residential or home and community-based LTC services less often than did white elders due to the availability of caregivers in their immediate families. However, with growth in educational levels of successive immigrant generations and downturns in the world economy, caregivers now balance work responsibilities with caregiving time. This trend signals two implications for the field:

1. More frail elders will seek LTC care in the future.

2. LTC organizations, administrators, and caregivers and other professionals need to provide culturally competent services.

in urban areas rather than on reservations, and about 7 percent of the Native American population is 65 years or older.

Life expectancy has increased dramatically for younger Native Americans, which may be attributed to the acute care services provided by the Indian Health Service. Three times as many Native Americans as non-Native Americans die before age 45, but from age 65 mortality rates for this population are comparable to non-Native Americans (John 2004). Specifically, up to age 75, Native Americans have higher mortality rates than whites; between ages 75 and 85, however, the mortality rates plummet and become lower than the rates for whites (John 2004). At this age, the chronic disease rates go up, creating a demand for LTC. This trend poses a concern for the Indian Health Service because it is focused on providing acute care, not chronic care.

Native Americans have the poorest health of all Americans, which may correlate with the poverty prevalent in this population. Elder Native Americans experience high rates of diabetes, hypertension, heart disease, stroke, influenza, accidents, and obesity-related diseases (Kaufman 2002). Compounding the issue, they rarely see physicians, and they harbor mistrust of non-Native American healthcare professionals. Their hospitalization rates are high, while their outpatient visits are low (John 2004).

Elder Native Americans aged 65 to 74 typically have some form of functional impairment, particularly mobility limitations. Given these disabilities, they lack access to many LTC services and, in self-reports, rate their health lowest among all racial groups.

OLDER ASIANS/PACIFIC ISLANDERS

The Asian/Pacific Islander (API) racial group is itself highly diverse, including a large number of distinct cultural groups that speak a multitude of different languages (US Census Bureau 2007). Adding to this diversity is the ongoing immigration to the United States of elder Asian Americans, whose children and grandchildren are also immigrants. About 60 percent of these elders do not speak English, and most practice traditions and values that differ from those in the West. The language limitation and cultural practices serve as barriers to accessing healthcare and LTC services.

Since 1970, APIs have represented 43 percent of the older immigrant population in this country (Min and Moon 2006). Older APIs are the second fastest growing minority group in the United States, and they have great longevity. The longer they live, however, the more they face the potential for physical and/or mental impairment that renders them functionally dependent and thus in need of LTC services. Historically, APIs used nursing homes far less frequently than other minority groups (McCormick et al. 1996); however, the Japanese preferred nursing home care for their elders suffering from dementia more than whites did for their elders with the same problems (whites preferred home and community-based services) (McCormick et al. 2002). A study of Japanese elders in Seattle found that LTC preferences reflect different generations' perceptions of racism and threat (McCormick et al. 1996). Conversely, a study of Korean elders in Chicago found a shift in preference toward greater acceptance and use of residential as well as home and community-based LTC services (Shin 2008). This finding was corroborated by Min and Moon's research (2006), which showed that Korean elders chose nursing homes after a stroke.

ELDERS' SEXUAL ORIENTATION

When examining the concept of aging families, the issues of gay, lesbian, bisexual, or transgender (GLBT) elders should be included. Consider that one in four same-sex relationships includes a partner who is aged 55 or older (Lambert 2005). The elderly are made to feel invisible in a youth-oriented society, and this invisibility is more extensive among GLBT elders.

Elder GLBT Research

Few studies have been conducted to examine the intersections of race/ethnicity, culture, social class, and sexual orientation in old age. Furthermore, neither the US census nor the Centers for Disease Control and Prevention's National Health Survey collects information on sexual orientation or gender identity (Lourde 2009). Consequently, the exact number of GLB elders is not known, although estimates put this population in the 1 million to 3 million range (based on the assumption that 3 percent to 8 percent of the general population are GLB). The number of transgender elders is completely unknown.

Some researchers argue that the aging experience of gay men and lesbians is different due to their sexual orientation and identity (Butler 2006; Barranti and Cohen 2000). A 2006 MetLife survey of 1,100 self-identified GLBT adults aged 40 to 61 reported that their greatest concern about aging was discrimination due to their sexual orientation. Not until 2003 did the US Supreme Court rule the sodomy laws used as a basis for arresting homosexuals in some states to be unconstitutional.

GLBT elders have the same concerns as other elders in terms of accessing health-care, budgeting limited or nonexistent income, and finding living arrangements.

Feeling of Isolation and Discrimination

GLBT elders must fight societal hostility and discrimination associated with their sexual orientation. Such situations have contributed to GLBT elders' feelings of isolation from the rest of society. As a result, many GLBT elders have tried to pass as heterosexual to minimize the antagonism, and they continue to pursue this strategy when they seek health and LTC services. Still other GLBT elders have resorted to staying closeted. Coming out, or revealing one's sexual orientation to family and friends, is difficult, and it is even more difficult for minorities and for working-class men (Hooyman and Kiyak 2011). The closeting strategy continues in the LTC setting, as some GLBT elders fear discriminatory treatment from their providers. This secrecy, in turn, prevents the providers from responding to these elders' special needs and thus reinforces the perception that the providers and the services they offer are not hospitable (Lourde 2009).

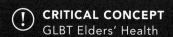

CRITICAL CONCEPT
GLBT Elders' Health

Being closeted or living in isolation can be harmful to a GLBT elder's health:

1. Secrecy could lead to depression and other physical and mental health problems (Lourde 2009).
2. Fearing discrimination, GLBT elders are five times less likely than straight seniors to visit the doctor (Chambers 2004).
3. Older gay men who do not share their sexual orientation with their physicians and other caregivers risk receiving misdiagnoses. For example, early signs of HIV/AIDS such as skin discolorations could be mistaken as normal signs of aging.
4. Older lesbians who do not disclose their sexual orientation may not be screened for early stages of breast cancer or other diseases. According to the Institute of Medi-cine report mentioned earlier, "lesbians were at heightened risk of cervical cancer, Alzheimer's, fibromyalgia, arthritis, heart disease, and hypertension" (Smedley, Stith, and Nelson 2003). Additionally, older lesbians have been overlooked in re-search on women's health.
5. The majority of lesbians and gays have been part of a couple, even a family, at some time in life. In old age, however, they tend to be single and have no children, unlike their heterosexual counterparts (Kurdek 2005). This adds to their feeling of being alone and having no support system.

Lack of Finances

Another area of difficulty for GLBT elders involves finances. Unlike straight elderly couples, GLBT elders in a relationship frequently do not receive marital benefits. For example, the death of a homosexual partner may leave the remaining partner without survivor benefits. If they were not legally married, the survivor is not entitled to Social Security benefits, widow/widower's pension, and other assets left by the deceased. Compounding this problem is that GLBT elders are less likely to have private health insurance (outside of Medicare) than straight seniors are (Lourde 2009).

All of these factors contribute to GLBT elders' greater need for residential long-term care: fewer financial resources coupled with inadequate medical care, isolation, and no children to care for them.

DISPARITIES IN HEALTHCARE AMONG DIVERSE ELDERS

As mentioned earlier, research has found that minority elders receive less routine medical care and lower quality of care than white elders. For example, elder African Americans are 62 percent less likely to receive anticoagulants after a transient ischemic attack than white elders. Similarly, elder Mexicans receive 36 percent fewer prescriptions after myocardial infarction (Smedley, Stith, and Nelson 2003; Betancourt et al. 2005). The differences in morbidity are presented in Exhibit 7.2, and the differences in mortality are shown in Exhibit 7.3 (Byrd, Fletcher, and Menifield 2007).

Several aspects of the US health system influence these disparities among minority elder groups, including GLBT elders (Byrd, Fletcher, and Menifield 2007):

- Attitudes of healthcare providers
- How patients understand and seek healthcare
- How healthcare providers offer services
- The organizational system

Cultural competency is a critical element in addressing these disparities. It must be developed at the individual and organizational level over an extended period of time.

		EXHIBIT 7.2
African Americans	1.5 times more likely to have a stroke	Disease Morbidity: Diverse Elder Population Versus Whites
	1.5 times more likely to have hypertension	
	2.5 times more likely to have diabetes	
Native Americans	2 times more likely to have diabetes	
Hispanics or Latinos	2 times more likely to have diabetes	

SOURCE: Data from Smedley, Stith, and Nelson (2003) and Baldwin (2003).

Exhibit 7.3
Disease Mortality:
Diverse Elder
Population Versus
Whites

African Americans	50% more likely to die of stroke
	20% more likely to die of heart disease
	30% more likely to die of cancer
	30% more likely to have diabetes-related amputation
Hispanics or Latinos	50% more likely to die from diabetes-related complications

SOURCE: Data from Smedley, Stith, and Nelson (2003) and Baldwin (2003).

Cultural competency
The ability of individuals or organizations to understand the global view of clients from diverse cultures and adapt their practices to ensure their effectiveness.

CULTURAL COMPETENCY

Cultural competency is a system of care that is responsive to cultural needs and preferences of diverse populations. The focus of cultural competency is to develop a complete understanding of a person's racial, ethnic, and cultural background and social identity and how these elements affect the person's attitudes and feeling about health and healthcare. With this knowledge, the provider can design and implement interventions that are respectful and sensitive to the individual's beliefs, traditions, and practices. Cultural competency also extends to considerations of language and other communication systems, such as translation services available to those (e.g., clients and family members) whose native language may not be English. In a melting-pot society, cultural competency covers the respectful treatment of people, regardless of age, race/ethnicity, disability, gender, or sexual preference.

In December 2000, the US Department of Health and Human Services published CLAS (culturally and linguistically appropriate services) standards that could be used by all types of healthcare organizations. The 14 CLAS standards are intended to achieve the following (Office of Minority Health 2001):

♦ They provide a common understanding and consistent definitions of culturally and linguistically appropriate services in healthcare.

♦ They offer a practical framework for the implementation of services and organizational structures that can help healthcare organizations and providers be responsive to the cultural and linguistic issues presented by diverse populations.

The need for cultural competency training for leaders of healthcare organizations and its connection to quality outcomes for patient care are emphasized in healthcare management research (Dreaschslin and Hobby 2008; Curtis and Dreaschslin 2008). Because of the profound extent to which a person's gender, race/ethnicity, sexual orientation, and cultural background can influence perceptions of health and quality of care, many medical schools and training programs have integrated cultural competency into their curricula (Chen 2009).

A Look Ahead

As the elder population becomes more diverse, the challenge for LTC providers and administrators is to provide culturally competent care along the LTC continuum. The Centers for Medicare & Medicaid Services, The Joint Commission, and other health-care organizations have introduced measures and guidelines for assessing LTC facilities' translation services (or their availability) for elders whose native language is not English. Because culture is a highly influential factor in the clients' health beliefs, behaviors, and health itself, delivering culturally appropriate and competent LTC is critical. Those who can overcome this challenge are poised to become the quality leaders in long-term care.

As historical trends in international migration show, diversity and cultural competency training in LTC are global issues. Many European Union countries are facing economic and societal challenges due to the influx of immigrants from non-European nations, and these problems will be exacerbated as the elders in these family units age in place. Emerging economies faced with conditions of famine and political unrest will face shortages of caregivers for their elders who remain in tribal villages and homelands. Developing global cultural competency standards to effectively address these caregiver-shortage problems will be an ongoing need.

Issues related to many groups of elders have yet to be studied. For example, studies of the needs of GLBT elders are limited, and research on black and Latino elders has primarily focused on African Americans and Puerto Ricans and has overlooked elder immigrants from Africa, Central America, and South America. As immigrants continue to move throughout the global economy, healthcare leaders need to assess and evaluate the health needs of diverse elders and develop culturally competent approaches to help them successfully age in their communities.

For Discussion

1. Define the social constructs related to diversity: gender, ethnicity, race, and sexual orientation.

2. Explain the demographic trend associated with the emerging majority of diverse elders.

3. Explain how elder women's longevity is increasing their LTC needs.

4. Why do diverse women face more obstacles in aging than their white counterparts?

5. Discuss health disparities affecting African-American elders.

6. Discuss health disparities affecting Hispanic elders.

7. The high incidence of chronic disease affects many diverse elders. Pick two groups of diverse elders, and discuss how their illnesses affect their LTC needs.

8. Why do GLBT elders have trouble being accepted as residents in LTC facilities?

9. How does language affect diverse elders' ability to obtain services for the aging?

10. For what diverse elder groups are poverty and lack of access to healthcare services a major issue?

11. What role do culturally competent providers play in reducing health disparities among diverse elders?

12. Discuss LTC preferences among diverse elders that are likely to affect residential or home and community-based LTC services.

CASE STUDY: CULTURAL COMPETENCY COUNTS AT GALTIER HEALTH CENTER

Galtier Health Center is a nursing home located in St. Paul, Minnesota, a state whose Hmong population is second only to that in California (Tate 2009). The Hmong comprises people who originated from or have ancestors in mountain villages in Vietnam, Laos, China, Burma, and Thailand. Since 1992, Galtier has been providing LTC services to the Hmong community. This focus has led Galtier to develop several innovative approaches to delivering culturally competent long-term care.

First, Galtier partners with Hmong groups, leaders, businesses, organizations, and other interested parties in the community. In this way, Galtier is able to educate the community about skilled nursing and promote the services it offers and the benefits that a Hmong family can realize by sending their elderly to Galtier's facility. This outreach is critical, especially because in the Hmong language the term "nursing home" is nonexistent.

Second, Galtier actively recruits staff from the Hmong community. Galtier has many native Hmong speakers on staff, enabling the facility to communicate well with its patients and their families about their healthcare needs and preferences. In this way, the care or treatment is culturally and medically competent. For example, if an elderly man develops an illness, the Galtier staff will not just administer the required medications to alleviate pain and discomfort but will also approach the illness holistically, because the Hmong believe that an ailment has physical and spiritual aspects. A healer may be called in, and this person will work with the staff and the physician to develop treatments and therapies that combine Hmong traditions with Western medicine.

Third, Galtier works with its Hmong community partners through its Southeast Asian Committee, whose membership includes Galtier's staff and leadership and community members. Additionally, Galtier has established a Hmong Resident Council. The committee and the council ensure that the Hmong residents at Galtier are given a voice. In this way, Galtier can respond to these residents' concerns, make changes according to their suggestions, and incorporate or adopt cultural practices and preferences (e.g., making rice a dietary staple; bringing in a shaman or healer) into daily operations and care delivery.

Galtier's close association with the Hmong community it serves ensures that the nursing home remains respectful of the Hmong people and their cultural traditions, achieves active participation from the Hmong residents and the larger community, and improves the Hmong elders' quality of life.

CASE STUDY QUESTIONS

1. Name several internal and external conditions needed for an LTC organization to replicate Galtier's culturally competent approach.

2. Discuss three key strategies used to ensure a culturally competent LTC environment.

3. Identify two ways you would evaluate a nursing home's cultural competency and sensitivity.

4. Explain how Galtier integrates the Hmong residents' cultural preferences in its daily operations and LTC delivery.

Management Issues

In recent years, healthcare providers have seen many changes in the population size and characteristics of people needing long-term care services. Individuals seeking long-term care services have also seen changes in the variety of settings and care, and in their forms of delivery. Added to these developments are changes in the external environment such as new technologies for the provision of healthcare services, new regulations, and new criteria for care management and reimbursement of healthcare services.

Part III of this book focuses on the management issues that arise from these dimensions of the long-term care service delivery system. These chapters discuss changes in the design and management of long-term care facilities and services, human resources issues, developments in laws and regulations, ethical considerations facing long-term care service providers, and changes in reimbursement for services. An overview of issues that will continue to affect service design and delivery of long-term care concludes this section, providing students and long-term care professionals with opportunities to develop new approaches and solutions.

CHAPTER 8

Management and Leadership in Long-Term Care Settings

Suzanne Discenza, PhD

After reading this chapter, you should be able to

➤ differentiate the special nuances of managing and leading in long-term care organizations as opposed to other healthcare settings;

➤ understand the effects of leadership style and attitudes on organizational culture and on managing and motivating individuals within long-term care settings;

➤ apply management techniques relative to staff recruitment, hiring, retention, mentoring, and motivation;

➤ form, facilitate, and empower effective interdisciplinary teams and quality circles in long-term care settings; and

➤ engage internal and external stakeholders in strategic planning processes and innovation initiatives within long-term care settings.

WHAT IS MANAGEMENT?

Management is management is management, and it is essentially the same in all settings, including LTC settings. Or is it?

Certainly, one can argue that a basic definition of management can be applied to all organizations in which individuals are engaged in the production of goods and services and in which a hierarchy of workers exists, whereby some are supervised by others. For example, Samuel Certo and S. Trevis Certo (2009, 8) offer this definition of management: "the process of reaching organizational goals by working with and through people and other organizational resources." Rose Dunn (2010, 13), writing specifically about healthcare settings, asserts that "the type of organization in which you work does not matter; managerial functions are the same for a commercial or industrial enterprise, not-for-profit or for-profit organization, professional association, government agency, and hospital or other healthcare facility." This definition needs to be taken at least one step further for LTC settings: Management should protect and address the special needs of the vulnerable individuals who depend on the organization's care. To do less may negate the important differences in managing the resources for dealing with frail and vulnerable human beings—particularly managing the dedicated individuals who are charged with caring for these clients.

FUNCTIONS OF MANAGEMENT IN LTC SETTINGS

Management textbooks ascribe to varying frameworks for understanding management functions—the work performed within an organization. Beaufort Longest and Kurt Darr (2008, 238–45), however, provide a comprehensive framework for six "functions that are fulfilled in the management process," with specific application to healthcare settings. Following is a brief description of each of these functions (as defined by Longest and Darr) along with examples of activities related to one issue that is common in many LTC settings—pressure ulcers.

♦   *Planning:* the process of charting a course of action for the future, including its mission and desired objectives.

   Example: Plan the quality indicators that the facility wants to address in the immediate future related to a reduction in pressure ulcers among LTC residents.

♦   *Organizing:* the developmental efforts and activities of management in achieving the organization's mission and objectives through orderly use of resources.

   Example: Form a skin integrity team to assess skin integrity and presence or absence of pressure ulcers for each resident on a weekly basis.

◆ *Staffing* (also called human resource management): the wide range of activities, programs, and policies related to acquisition, retention and maintenance, and separation of human resources.

Example: Hire physical and occupational therapists who have knowledge of proper positioning of residents in beds and wheelchairs; also, hire wound care nurses or other specialists to treat pressure ulcers.

◆ *Directing:* the system for initiating action in the organization through leading, motivating, and communicating with those whom managers direct.

Example: Set up reporting systems for staff to ensure that policies and procedures for reducing residents' pressure ulcers are communicated and followed and to empower all employees and reward them as appropriate.

◆ *Controlling:* the regulation of activities and performance of an organization through measuring and correcting the activities of people and things to ensure objectives are accomplished.

Example: Track the reduction in pressure ulcers among residents and the severity of ulcers when occurrences arise; also, correct staff members who do not follow the turning schedules for bed-bound residents or the standing schedules for wheelchair-bound individuals.

◆ *Decision making:* intertwined with all other functions of management, the element of problem solving and choosing among alternatives.

Example: Decide which set of pressure-reducing mattresses or wheelchair systems to purchase within budgetary constraints.

THE MANAGEMENT HIERARCHY

Governing Body

Governance in many organizations is defined narrowly in terms of the governing board's oversight of the organization's operations. Some expand the scope of governance to include administration activities. The **governing body**, frequently referred to as the board of directors, is defined by John Pratt (2010, 358) as "the policy-making arm of the organization" and has legal and fiduciary responsibility for how the organization functions. Its responsibilities include developing the mission and vision statements and the operational policies of the organization, monitoring the organization's programs and financial performance, hiring and evaluating the CEO, and providing financial and human resources.

Governing body
The oversight and policymaking arm of the organization, with legal and fiduciary responsibility for how the organization functions; frequently referred to as the board of directors.

Longest and Darr (2008, 61) contend that critical shifts in the current healthcare environment have had a "profound effect" on governing bodies, whereby "members can no longer be chosen as a way to honor them or because they might make financial contributions. The pressures and need for [governing bodies] to be effective will increase, and this means recruiting people who understand health [in this case, LTC] services, are prepared in business matters, and have backgrounds that are relevant to the [health services organization]."

Administration and the Management Team

Administration

Those employees who manage the day-to-day operations of the organization and who carry out the policies of the governing body; also known as the management team.

Administration, on the other hand, is "made up of those employees of the organization who manage the day-to-day operations of the organization" and "carry out the policies of the governing body" (Pratt 2010, 358). In LTC organizations the senior management team typically includes the chief executive officer (often, the licensed nursing home administrator [NHA]), the medical director (or the chief medical officer [CMO]), the director of nursing services (DON), the chief operating officer, the chief financial officer, and perhaps the director of rehabilitation. These officers may work from corporate offices to provide oversight for their counterparts in individual facilities. Each facility operates under a management team whose duties include executing the six functions of management and directing the activities in their specific departments. Following is a brief description of the key leadership positions in LTC facilities:

◆   All states require skilled nursing facilities to have a licensed administrator—typically, a licensed NHA; requirements for assisted living facility administrator licensure vary from state to state. These administrators must pass an examination demonstrating their competencies in such areas as patient care, financial management, human resources management, marketing, laws, and regulatory codes.

◆   One administrative position that is under increasing scrutiny is the assistant administrator (AA), sometimes referred to as the administrator in training (AIT). In addition to assisting the administrator with a plethora of management duties, the AA or AIT provides on-the-job training and mentoring for new graduates of health administration programs. Due to severe reimbursement cutbacks in Medicaid, Medicare, and other funding for LTC, many organizations have all but eliminated the AA and AIT positions. In an urgent response to this situation, Susan Gilster and Jennifer Dalessandro (2010, 11) made the following argument during their presentation at the American College of Health Care Administrators annual conference:

More than 7,000 administrators will leave their position this year alone, and the pool of incoming candidates has diminished. The roles and responsibilities of an administrator can be overwhelming.

Frustrations arise from the inability to manage it all, and be an effective leader. This session will make the case for assistant administrators and outline how having a person in such a role is advantageous for the organization's quality of care, satisfaction levels, and profitability.

◆ The CMO is required by Medicare regulations to ensure coordination and appropriateness of medical services. The CMO is also responsible for maintaining quality of care in the facility and for credentialing independent physicians who provide services to residents. Furthermore, the CMO oversees the medical care provided by home health agencies and other home-based services.

◆ The DON often serves as the chief clinical officer. Supervision of the direct patient care staff, pharmacy, and lab is typically under the DON's purview.

Section I of the Appendix shows a simple organizational chart of a typical nursing facility.

Strategic Planning

At some point during the planning function, the governing body or management team, along with key internal and external stakeholders (such as community members), engage in **strategic planning**. Connie Evashwick and James Riedel (2004, 105) define strategic planning as "the process of determining the organization's goals, measurable objectives, and direction for the immediate future, as well as reaffirming the organization's mission and long-range vision." Short-term strategic planning generally involves goal setting for the coming year, while long-term planning typically establishes aims for the next two to three years. Good plans provide criteria for decision making, align all stakeholders on important issues, and develop in an ongoing, nonlinear fashion. Despite the fact that many LTC organizations are less diligent with strategic planning due to limited "internal resources to devote to 'planning' rather than daily operations," Evashwick and Riedel (2004, 106) insist that "in the future, as the field of long-term care becomes more complex, and more competitive, strategic planning will be imperative."

A widely debated topic is who should be involved in strategic planning in LTC organizations. Intentional inclusion of a diverse array of participants is now considered key to a successful process. The governing body and management team should drive the larger goals of the plan, but representation and input from all departments and employees (e.g., first-line care staff, housekeeping, food service, admissions, accounting, medical records), clients or residents and their families, and community stakeholders should be solicited

Strategic planning
The long-term planning process by key stakeholders in which the organization's goals, measurable objectives, and direction for the immediate future are determined.

throughout the planning process. For example, if one strategic goal is to move the skilled nursing facility toward a more resident-centered model, the development of the objectives should, at a minimum, include residents, their families, all direct care staff, food service and housekeeping employees, the medical staff (because physicians will no longer be the ultimate decision makers), and the management team. Strategic planning for adult day centers, on the other hand, may need to include clients and their families, staff members, service providers who see clients at the centers (e.g., home health workers, social workers, traveling podiatrists, and dentists), and members of neighborhood associations.

The act of strategic planning is an orderly process. First, it establishes or reaffirms the organization's mission (i.e., what it does, what purpose it serves) and vision (i.e., where it wants to go) statements. Second, it analyzes the organization's stakeholders and customers, its internal resources, and the external market, including the competition and regulatory constraints. Of particular importance during the internal organization review is the participation of staff in a SWOT (strengths, weaknesses, opportunities, and threats) analysis. Such brainstorming efforts, as well as development of specific goals and objectives that affect individual departments, allow buy-in and commitment of staff at all levels of the facility. Last, it develops broader goals, short-term objectives, and a specific plan of action, which delineates the responsible parties and timetables for completion.

It is a short-sighted organization that does not take steps to communicate the strategic plan to first-line managers and to integrate the plan into all aspects of day-to-day operations. The planning team must continue to evaluate the impact of implementing the plan, making adjustments as needed to ensure that the plan remains relevant as conditions change inside and outside the organization.

LEADERSHIP VERSUS MANAGEMENT OF LTC FACILITIES

Leadership has been a more elusive concept to define than **management**, although most experts agree that leadership is an essential element of the organizational climate. Rose Dunn (2010, 481) states, "Leadership plays an important role in organizational life and ultimately makes the difference between an effective and an ineffective organization. . . Leadership is a process by which people are imaginatively directed, guided, and influenced to select and attain goals." Dunn emphasizes the voluntary nature of this process, whereby followers want to engage in the activities that the leader espouses.

DIFFERENTIATION OF ROLES

Two proverbial questions asked during discussions of leadership roles within an organization are (1) What is the difference between leadership and management? and (2) Are good managers necessarily good leaders?

The answer to the first question may be best illustrated by contrasting what managers do with what leaders do. Managers are involved in maintaining the day-

Leadership
The process by which people are voluntarily and "imaginatively" guided (Dunn 2010) and influenced in choosing and attaining the goals of the organization.

Management
In long-term care entities, this is the process of reaching organizational goals by working with people and other resources to protect and address the special needs of the vulnerable individuals depending on the organization's care.

to-day operations of the organization (i.e., the status quo), while leaders are considered the visionaries of the organization, constantly challenging existing paradigms, embracing change, and moving the organization forward into the future. An example in the LTC setting is that management makes sure that staff logs daily entries into clients' paper medical charts, that care plans and physicians' orders are followed, and that all lab and radiology reports are filed in the appropriate sections. The leaders in the same LTC facility, on the other hand, pursue the adoption of portable electronic medical record devices to streamline operations and to help the organization meet HIPAA (Health Insurance Portability and Accountability Act) mandates.

The answer to the second question, whether good managers are necessarily good leaders, is provided by Dunn (2010, 482), who unequivocally states that although these terms "are often used interchangeably, they are not synonymous. A person who has formal positional authority may use formal legitimate authority and power to get things done; on the other hand, an individual who has no position of formal authority may use the leadership influence but is not the manager." In the LTC setting, an example is the NHA who directs the staff to expedite breakfast by getting all the residents into the dining room by 6:30 am. The NHA's order may be followed, but staff members resent it because they feel it is unnecessary to rush and are aware that residents do not wish to eat breakfast or to get out of bed so early. In other words, the employees involuntarily comply with the manager's directive, but they do not view her as a leader who knows how to provide resident-centered care. As Dunn (2007, 435) contends, "a manager can do a reasonably good job of managing without being a leader. From the view of organizational effectiveness, however, it is desirable for the manager to also be the leader."

LEADERSHIP STYLES, ATTITUDES, AND COMPETENCIES

In the past few decades, various styles of leadership have emerged, including the following:

◆ *Autocratic or directive style.* The leader gives specific instructions and closely monitors employees; the leader exercises single-handed decision making.

◆ *Laissez-faire or hands-off style.* The leader provides little or no direction, giving employees the freedom to make their own decisions and solve their own problems.

◆ *Democratic or participative style.* The leader involves employees in decision making and problem solving and emphasizes cooperative teamwork throughout the organization, although the leader retains the final say.

In recognition of the fact that no one leadership style may be effective with all workers at all times under all circumstances, but rather should change with the particular situation, the current thinking is that good leaders should adopt a situational leadership style. Moreover, the two leadership styles cited most recently in leadership literature—transformational leadership and adaptive leadership—have moved center stage. These styles are based on the idea that leaders can move their organizations forward by listening to their followers and adapting to the realities of a rapidly changing economic and social environment. Certainly, no industry has experienced more rapid change in recent years than the LTC industry.

Transformational leaders inspire their workers with a shared vision of the future. Adaptive leaders, on the other hand, not only embrace change but also rely on a style in which "participants ha[ve] to be drawn together to discern a new pathway" when the solution to an issue or a problem is essentially unknown (Roberts 2007).

The relevance of any leadership style is that it generally reflects the attitude of the leader toward her workers. The majority of the literature on managers' and leaders' attitudes and actions cites Douglas McGregor's Theory X and Theory Y (McGregor 1960) to describe the general assumptions made by managers about workers. According to Theory X, managers and leaders hold negative assumptions about workers, believing in their inherent dislike of work and indifference to organizational goals. For example, a nursing home administrator may think that a certified nurse assistant (CNA) or a nurse is "only in it for the money," does not care about the residents, and will only do the minimal amount of work expected in his job. As a result, the administrator may use a directive leadership style to ensure that the facility's objectives are met.

On the other hand, according to Theory Y, managers and leaders hold positive assumptions about employees, believing that most workers want to take responsibility for their work and want to help achieve organizational goals. For example, the administrator who operates under this assumption thinks that the CNA or activity staff member personally enjoys making a positive difference in the lives of the residents and works hard in the process. In this case, the administrator assumes a participative leadership style to engage her employees in decision making and to give due consideration to their ideas. Furthermore, a Theory Y management team may adopt a laissez-faire style to allow for increased discretion and innovation.

A third model, Theory Z, applies to motivating employees. Although proposed by William Reddin in 1977, this theory has drawn renewed attention recently because it more easily aligns with contemporary theories of situational leadership. It recognizes that "leaders must change their styles according to the situation" and to the "competence and commitment of each worker or group" (Singh 2005, 430). In LTC facilities, Theory Z translates to giving more direction to less skilled workers, such as kitchen workers or housekeeping staff, and more opportunities for direct care employees, such as nurses and CNAs, to become involved in restorative feeding programs.

While it is important to adopt the appropriate leadership styles and attitudes to accomplish organizational goals, it is equally important to understand which qualities and competencies enable good leadership. Leadership expert Warren Bennis (2003) proposed

> ## ⚠ CRITICAL CONCEPT
> ### LTC Leadership and Emotional Intelligence
>
> Daniel Goleman (2004), a scholar on **emotional intelligence,** has found that a direct relationship exists between emotional intelligence and measurable business results. He names the five qualities of an emotionally intelligent leader: self-awareness, self-regulation, motivation, empathy, and social skill (see the Appendix). In LTC settings, most workers want to see these qualities in their leaders. Specifically, they want to serve under managers who are motivated by more than their paycheck or the prestige of their position, who display empathy and sensitivity for the condition of their staff and clients, and who know how to monitor and temper their own emotional responses so as not to alienate others.

six traits a good leader must have: integrity, dedication, magnanimity, humility, openness, and creativity (see Section II of the Appendix for more on these attributes).

MENTORING

One of the most effective experiences through which to learn leadership skills is mentoring. Mentoring is a process whereby an experienced leader (for our purposes, a seasoned LTC manager) partners with a novice manager (the protégé) to impart personal and professional knowledge and insight. Following are some mentoring techniques that could be adopted by LTC administrators (Bell 2002):

Emotional intelligence
The personal attributes of great leaders that involve "qualities of the heart" (Goleman 2004), such as empathy and self-awareness.

- ◆ Create a safe haven for trust and risk taking.

- ◆ Develop the art of listening, and ask effective questions.

- ◆ Give advice while minimizing resistance.

- ◆ Use the power of storytelling.

- ◆ Balance guidance with freedom.

SETTING AND LIVING BY THE ORGANIZATIONAL CULTURE

As defined by Samuel Certo and S. Trevis Certo (2009, 443), **organizational culture** is "a set of shared values that organization members have regarding the functioning and

Organizational culture
A set of shared values, norms, and rituals that organization members have regarding the functioning and character of their organization.

existence of their organization." Evolving slowly over time, and significantly affected by the leadership style of an organization's managers, this culture "has dimensions such as organizational rituals, special language, norms, and habits." While frequently not verbalized, the culture may manifest itself in company mottos or slogans that try to capture the essence of how the organization hopes to do business. For example, one company providing therapeutic services to home health agencies, assisted living facilities, and nursing homes in Colorado promoted its motto "success through teamwork" as an important aspect of its organizational culture. Such manifestations engender workers' pride. An excellent resource for LTC administrators and managers is Susan Gilster's book *Changing Culture, Changing Care*. Gilster (2005, 19) notes, "We have lost our way. Many in long-term care have forgotten what they were designed to do—to serve others by providing compassionate care for the older adults who can no longer be cared for in their homes. . . . It is time to refocus and to reestablish service as our primary function." The model presented in Gilster's book includes seven "S.E.R.V.I.C.E." components: *s*ervice, *e*ducation, *r*espect, *v*ision, *i*nclusion, *c*ommunication, and *e*nrichment.

RECRUITMENT, HIRING, AND RETENTION

Staffing, according to Rose Dunn (2010, 359), "is the managerial function concerned with the procurement and maintenance of human resources to fulfill the institution's goals." More important, according to Dunn, "Once goals are determined, departments are set up, and duties and task relationships are established, people must be placed to give life to what would otherwise be an empty structure." This could not be truer than for LTC facilities, where fragile individuals come for all kinds of assistance.

A needs assessment—a forecast of the number, types, and competencies of workers needed—must be undertaken in healthcare settings before recruitment begins. Douglas Singh (2005, 458) approaches staffing levels from the standpoint of either total number of staff members (or full-time equivalents) or skill mix (which Singh defines as "the ratio of staff members with a particular skill type [e.g., RNs versus CNAs] to the total staff in a unit"). Two primary factors determine the levels of staff and skill mix needed: the volume factor (e.g., number of patients) and the weighting factor (i.e., intensity of resources used).

One common example of staffing decisions made in LTC facilities involves the ratio of nursing staff to residents. The University of Minnesota (2011) website "NH Regulations Plus" provides one of the most complete analyses of nurse staffing ratios in the United States. Because federal standards are minimal, most staffing regulations in the country are enacted at the state level, resulting in huge variances in requirements; 18 states have no numerical ratios for nurse staffing. One frequently used model involves merely following a specification of total nurse staff (including the nursing spectrum from registered nurses to CNAs) ratio, which ranges from 1.5 total hours per resident per day in Louisiana to 3.0 hours per resident per day in California and Vermont. Some states require ratios for different levels of care (e.g., skilled nursing versus assisted living facility or intermediate care facility, and still others specify the ratios per shift (e.g., days, nights, swing).

After staffing determinations are made, recruitment, selection, and hiring may begin. Recruitment may involve consideration of either interested internal candidates (existing employees) or external applicants. Advertising, screening, interviewing, and background checks are typical elements of the recruitment, selection, and hiring processes.

Suitable LTC employees—from frontline workers to managers—are typically not motivated by high salaries or prestige; thus, it is imperative that administrators understand why applicants are seeking to fill such a demanding position, what qualities to look for in these candidates, and how to retain these people once they are employed. "Settling" for able bodies with minimum qualifications (or hiring the first person who applies) is tempting for administrators, particularly in light of pervasive staffing shortages in the LTC industry. However, that approach does not pay off in the long run. A strategic manager perseveres to find suitable individuals. The following questions may help in this regard:

- ◆ Is the candidate passionate about working with elderly, disabled, and vulnerable individuals and about helping to improve these clients' quality of life?

- ◆ Can the candidate interact comfortably with these individuals and demonstrate a respectful, compassionate, and positive attitude?

- ◆ Is the candidate a good listener and a good communicator? Is he willing to provide client-centered care?

? DID YOU KNOW?
What Attracts LTC Workers to the Field?

LTC recruiting involves determining how to appeal to suitable applicants. Following are common elements of the workplace that attract LTC employees:

- Workers in home health agencies are attracted to jobs that provide autonomy and freedom of movement. These employees like to be able to set their own schedules and hours to see patients in their home or care setting.

- Workers in hospices are attracted to a setting that is dedicated to providing palliative or comfort care as well as facilitating end-of-life and spiritually oriented experiences.

- Workers in assisted living or continuing care retirement communities are attracted to the rich histories and stories of people and the opportunity to interact with the elderly or disabled in enjoyable activities and events.

- Workers in nursing homes are attracted to serving society's most vulnerable individuals.

As Singh (2005, 456) emphasizes, "success in attracting and retaining employees tends to be self-sustaining; organizations with a satisfied and well-qualified staff are able to attract capable and enthusiastic people." At all levels of the organization, workers want to feel valued, to be rewarded (minimally through verbal praise) for their efforts, and to feel respected as a contributing part of the care team. They need to feel that management cares foremost about the residents and employees and that financial results are a consequence of good care rather than the driving force of the facility's operation. In this way LTC organizations not only attract but also retain good workers.

◆ Does the candidate understand the need to protect the clients' privacy, autonomy, and desire for confidentiality?

These questions should be followed up by checking the candidate's qualifications, credentials, work history, criminal background, references, and other relevant information. Additionally, the administrator must assess the person's fit with the organization's culture, mission, value system, and existing employees.

Attenuating Turnover and Discipline

Particular attention should be paid to increasing employee job satisfaction and to reducing job burnout. These goals can be achieved by decreasing work stressors caused by the job's high emotional and physical demands. The ultimate aim of managers in their retention efforts is to reduce high employee turnover, which is defined as "the proportion of job exits or quits from a facility in a year" (Buchbinder and Buchbinder 2007, 242). As noted by Connie Evashwick and James Riedel (2004, 66), "Unusually high turnover, either in the entire organization or in a single department, usually points to a management problem."

A study by Christopher Donoghue and Nicholas Castle (2009) points to the relationship between NHAs' leadership style and turnover rates for registered nurses, licensed practical nurses (LPNs), and nursing assistants. Findings indicate that for all three positions, the consensus manager style (the NHA solicits input from staff) correlates with the lowest level of staff turnover, while the shareholder manager style (the NHA does not solicit input or provide information) correlates with the highest turnover level (Donoghue and Castle 2009). The results of this study can guide NHAs' efforts to better engage their employees in decision making, improve staff performance and satisfaction, and enhance the quality of care.

Additionally, reducing turnover depends on the organization's ability to decrease work stress and burnout, especially for CNAs, who are engaged in low-paying, often unappreciated work. Minimizing the CNA's shift extensions, double shifts, and excessive overtime (caused by sick and other call-ins) can be achieved through planning to use contract or "pool" nursing services when the need arises, an option that is less expensive in the long run than constantly replacing staff. In fact, fewer staff call-ins (often related to stress on the job) occur when such a plan is in place. Honoring break schedules, holding team-building activities (such as sharing a late-shift snack or an after-hours bowling event), and creating incentives that reward good work (e.g., paid time off or gift cards) further improve staff retention. Rotating tasks within departments allows for cross-training and helps break up stressful, monotonous routines. (The next section discusses this topic further.)

Despite the best efforts to have sound management practices in place, managers occasionally encounter discipline issues—when employees "fail to abide by established rules and standards even after having been informed of them" (Dunn 2010, 566)—that can threaten morale, teamwork, and the facility's overall reputation. Take, for instance, a home health aide (HHA) who notes on her timesheet that she provided one hour of care (e.g., bathing, dressing, changing bandages for a recently discharged surgical patient) but brags to another HHA that she actually only spent 20 minutes in the client's home. Once informed, the manager must address this infraction immediately to (1) send a message to other HHAs that such cheating is not acceptable and cannot be tolerated by the agency and (2) avoid the perception that the agency provides less-than-adequate care. A negative reputation may eventually reach the client and the physician, who in turn will not make further referrals to the agency.

Progressive discipline—increasing penalties for repeat infractions—is generally considered standard practice in most LTC facilities. In the case of the timesheet-cheating HHA, she may first receive a verbal warning; for the next infraction, her pay may be docked and she may receive counseling and a written warning. A further offense could result in termination.

In cases where the offense is not intentional but rather the result of careless oversight (such as failure to answer a call light in a nursing home), the manager should "first assume no malice"—an idea based on the Hippocratic Oath that creates a win-win climate. By first assuming that the employee intended no harm, the manager is giving the employee ample opportunities to redeem himself. Use of heavy-handed discipline, especially when other techniques may be more effective, is the surest way to lose the interest, dedication, and service of sensitive and patient-centered employees—the types of people that LTC facilities should seek to attract.

EMPOWERMENT AND MOTIVATION

Empowering employees at all levels and motivating them to help the organization carry out its mission and goals are two sides of the same coin. **Empowerment**, according to Rose Dunn (2010, 420), "permits individuals within a work team to make certain decisions about their work assignments, schedules, and other related items." The savvy manager is able to empower his workers by not only providing the appropriate resources to achieve job tasks but also delegating authority so that the workers can use their independent judgment and make decisions without close supervision. To operate under an empowerment framework requires assurance of adequate job skill sets and basic trust that the workers will meet expectations. Susan Gilster (2005, 32) describes how the value of empowerment translates to LTC facilities:

> Staff needs to be given the freedom to take action and make the necessary decisions for the residents. Do not belittle or scold staff for a poor decision. If you do, they will not make decisions on their own again, and the organization will not grow. . . . Teach and guide them to make a better decision in the future. . . . Most of the time when leaders trust in others and give staff a chance, they will exceed expectations.

Empowerment
Permitting people working within teams to exercise their own independent judgment and to make decisions regarding their work activities.

Motivation
The process by which organizational leaders arouse and energize the inner needs or drives of individuals working within the organization to promote organizational goals.

Motivation, on the other hand, "is the process affecting the inner needs or drives that arouse, move, energize, direct, and sustain human behavior" (Gilster 2005, 445). Virtually all textbooks on management offer theories for motivating the workforce, but which strategies have the greatest impact on engaging employees? Research reveals at least three responses to this question:

◆ *Not all employees are motivated by the same set of strategies.* In fact, each individual is motivated by a different combination of strategies reflecting her unique experiences and personal characteristics. While one employee may be motivated by public recognition in the LTC newsletter or during a staff meeting, another worker may respond best to opportunities for advancement and increasing job responsibilities. Of course, some employees are most motivated by tangible rewards, such as a pay raise, a bonus, or free tickets to a sporting event. Consequently, a manager must get to know her employees and then tailor the rewards according to each individual.

◆ *Most workers are motivated by a combination of intrinsic and extrinsic incentives.* Extrinsic incentives are often tangible rewards, such as money, promotions, praise, and flexible schedules, provided by LTC managers with the intent of increasing productivity. Intrinsic rewards are typically intangible and are felt internally by the employee because they appeal to his value system; they may include interesting and meaningful work, shared goal setting and decision making, or a culture of caring. The latter is particularly important in LTC settings, as personal satisfaction often comes with a sense of "making a difference" in the lives of others.

◆ *LTC workers need the opportunity to reenergize or revitalize to remain motivated.* Edward Hallowell (2005) and Nancy Shanks (2007) discuss the problems that develop when employees work on "overloaded circuits." Burnout leads to a decline in motivation, underperformance, and decreased productivity. Management must ensure that staff members are allowed regular breaks while on the job and that they are given real vacation time without fear of being called back in because of staffing shortages. The ability to take periodic stress days, which could be drawn from the worker's pool of sick days, is especially needed in LTC facilities (particularly nursing homes and hospice) because of the emotionally draining nature of working with frail, high-needs individuals experiencing daily life-and-death struggles. On-site wellness, relaxation, and exercise programs for workers provide further opportunities for reenergizing.

FACILITATING INNOVATION

Two initiatives that have received a large amount of attention in the area of innovation are electronic medical records (EMRs) in nursing care facilities in response to HIPAA mandates and resident-centered culture change in response to increased demands from aging baby boomers for improved quality of life. Yet in light of staffing shortages and tremendous financial pressures, little encouragement and few, if any, resources have been given to individual managers or frontline staff to foster innovation in improving the daily lives of either residents or caregivers.

Susan Gilster (2005, 59) refers to a visioning process in LTC facilities that involves "thinking, reflecting, and brainstorming, in which all [management and direct care staff] are given the opportunity to dream about what will be created" to improve the lives of residents and their families. Noting that this process moves a group toward a common destination through uniting and exciting them, Gilster provides examples of innovative solutions in such areas as individualizing resident care, activity programming, making resident rooms and common areas more homelike, and being more accommodating to families. For example, residents should be allowed to sleep later each day and then enjoy a continental breakfast, if they so desire. This shift in practice results not only in satisfied residents and families but also, though it may seem contradictory, time saved and increased staff satisfaction. Dealing all day long with the negative behavior of a resident who did not get the amount of rest he wants and needs is far more problematic and time consuming for staff than just allowing the resident to sleep late and providing an individual breakfast from the kitchen. Whether referred to as innovation or visioning, this process is part of the culture change movement described in greater detail in Chapter 9.

Finally, community partners (including vendors, other healthcare institutions, other not-for-profit agencies serving the aging and the disabled or chronically ill, financial institutions, and the central business group) may be asked to help the LTC facility come up with innovative ideas and initiatives to improve services for both residents and caregivers. This strategy might be especially helpful for managers of home and community-based services who interact directly with external organizations.

FORMING AND FACILITATING INTERDISCIPLINARY TEAMS

A team consists of a group of individuals who influence one another toward the accomplishment of shared objectives. In LTC facilities, teams may be formed on a permanent basis, such as with departmental or functional teams (e.g., nursing unit, dietary, safety), or on a temporary or ad hoc basis, such as with quality improvement (e.g., skin care, falls prevention) or individual patient care teams. Ad hoc teams are typically cross-functional and bring together individuals with expertise on a particular

Interdisciplinary team
A group of individuals from different disciplines/areas of expertise within the long-term care setting who influence one another toward shared objectives to meet the needs of individual residents or groups of residents with related issues.

Conflict resolution
Negotiation by the manager where compromise is the desired outcome in an LTC setting in which opposing goals between any combination of residents, families, and/or employees become counterproductive.

issue or with knowledge of the needs of an individual resident. Team size may or may not be an important consideration. A patient care team may consist of all staff members involved with providing care and other services, the resident, and his family. Other teams may consist of all staff members within a certain department. All teams must be neither so large that the size impedes the completion of project goals nor so small that the group is too exclusive. Teams of three to seven members are often considered most efficient. Literature on **interdisciplinary teams** reveals the common elements of teams, including the following:

◆ Member empowerment to encourage innovation

◆ Authority to make decisions and accountability for outcomes

◆ Support from administration, including time to meet, resource provision, and rewards for performance

◆ Effective leadership and member commitment

◆ Mutual respect, effective communication, and **conflict resolution**

Exhibit 8.1 lists some advantages and disadvantages of using teams in LTC facilities. The list in the exhibit is purposefully not exhaustive. For instance, Dunn (2010, 467) argues that establishing teams "places authority in the hands of those closest to the product or service to make decisions that will affect that product or service." Whether providing services at the client's home or in a nursing home, for example, the CNA or HHA is the individual who provides the bulk of hands-on care, is most familiar with the client's needs and desires, and first notes any changes in the client's physical or emotional status.

EXHIBIT 8.1
Advantages and Disadvantages of Teams in LTC Organizations

Benefits/Advantages	Challenges/Disadvantages
Improved coordination of care	Conflict between team members
Improved quality of care	Costs of staff time spent in meetings
Greater job satisfaction of workers	"Free riders" not sharing the work
Greater resident satisfaction	Poor communication
Increased productivity	Unclear goals and poor leadership
Decreased staff turnover and costs	Lack of management support

SOURCE: Dunn (2007); Buchbinder and Thompson (2007); Mickan (2005).

Inclusiveness and Accountability

The LTC manager must play a significant role in two other elements of effective teams: **inclusiveness** (i.e., each member feels valued) and **accountability** (i.e., each member is responsible for team objectives and following through on them). To foster inclusiveness, the manager must engender a sense of shared purpose among the team members, encouraging them to make a significant difference in pursuit of the organization's mission. Equally important to team engagement is how employees are treated throughout the process (Gilster 2005, 76–77):

> Employees actually want most to be respected, heard, included and to be part of the decision-making team. . . . Inclusion enhances their interest and participation and gives them a sense of ownership in the operations and facility achievement. It gives them something to work for. There seems little that staff will not try as long as they are part of the discussion and understand the reason to do so.

Curtis McLaughlin and Arnold Kaluzny (2006) address the importance of team composition to a sense of inclusion by all of its members. They warn, for example, about heading quality improvement teams with physicians (or nursing directors), whose status and demeanor may intimidate some subordinates, preventing them from speaking up for fear of being wrong or looking foolish. Team leaders must have the ability to relate well with all team members, to promote open and honest dialogue, and to respect and recognize each member's contributions. In the LTC facility, the team leader might be an experienced CNA or a respected staff LPN who is involved in hands-on patient care. Who better to lead a patient care conference than the direct care team who works with the resident?

Teams also need to be accountable for their performance. John Pratt's (2004, 52) emphasis on outcome-oriented accountability may be applied to teams:

> Providers of long-term care services should have a high degree of accountability, both to those using their services and to those paying for the services. To attain that accountability, the system should focus on outcomes, not on process, as is largely the case with the current system. To begin with, the system should be designed to gauge results, particularly as they affect quality of life.

Thus, the manager must not only provide the team with appropriate resources to accomplish its objectives but also help the team focus on outcomes. The team must establish clear timelines for completing specific tasks or steps in the process and clear assignment of individual responsibility for completing each task. Even more important, the LTC manager must make sure that the team's recommendations are carried out. Few experiences are more demoralizing for team members than to have the results of their hard work shelved by management to await a better or more financially lucrative time to roll

Inclusiveness
Making sure each member of the organization's team feels valued as an important contributing member.

Accountability
The importance of the employee or team meeting established objectives as well as follow-through on the part of management in carrying out the team's recommendations.

out the ideas. In-service training or debriefing of participating staff should be scheduled immediately to allow implementation to begin. This, more than almost any other activity, will affirm and excite the team to take on further tasks.

The following section discusses the work of two LTC teams: patient care teams and quality teams.

Effective Case Management

Douglas Singh (2005, 597) describes case management as "a centralized coordinating function in which the special needs of older adults [arguably, any resident requiring care] are identified and a trained professional (or team) determines which services would be most appropriate, determines eligibility for those services, makes referrals, arranges for financing, and coordinates and monitors delivery of care to ensure that clients are receiving the prescribed services." While a specific case manager may be assigned to each resident of an LTC facility, it is the patient's or resident's care team that should ensure that all aspects of case management are executed appropriately and correctly, from the time of admission to discharge. In skilled nursing facilities, long-term residential care, and many assisted living facilities, periodic (at least monthly) meetings are held for each resident, with attendance by all individuals involved with the individual's care. This team may include staff members from the nursing, dietary, rehabilitation, social services, activities, medical records, and finance departments and may occasionally include representatives from housekeeping or environmental services departments, if needed. Because they are often the team members most familiar with a given resident, CNA representation is imperative. In resident-centered care facilities, the attendance of the resident and her support system (e.g., family, close friends) is paramount. Only with this comprehensive representation on the team will individualized care for each resident be guaranteed.

Typically required for facility-based settings, effective case management is now the norm for many home and community-based services organizations. Home health care agencies frequently set up care conferences either in the home (allowing attendance of clients, their families, and other caregivers) or with the care team in the agency itself. Health status, care progress, and need for ongoing services are often discussed. Adult day centers provide case management, using care teams to address the individual needs of the client and her family, such as diet, activities, medical/therapy services, and emotional support. Hospice case management addresses spiritual and emotional support for the client and family as well as end-of-life physical, social, and medical support for the client.

Quality teams, also referred to as quality circles, are charged with **continuous quality improvement (CQI)**—the ongoing critical examination of resident care processes within LTC facilities. Rose Dunn (2010, 303) notes that the team is "assigned a project to assess or is asked to identify problems, isolate the causes, and develop practical solutions for more effective methods to ensure that the work is accomplished error free the first

Continuous quality improvement (CQI)
The ongoing critical examination of resident care processes within long-term care facilities through which team members identify problems, isolate the causes, and develop practical solutions for more effective methods.

time." Connie Evashwick and James Riedel (2004) further emphasize the importance of positively influencing costs as well as client care. Quality teams differ from facility to facility depending on the resident mix, the types of problems encountered, and the financial resources or constraints of the organization. In nursing facilities, typical quality teams may address skin integrity or wound care, wheelchair positioning, mattress surfaces for pressure ulcer prevention, weight loss, dietary issues related to swallowing problems, or falls prevention. In assisted living facilities, quality teams may address financial management needs, memory support, exercise and activity programs to maintain physical functionality, or other ways to assist the resident in maintaining independence. As is characteristic of CQI, such needs and supports are addressed on an ongoing basis to reflect changes in patient, resident, or family status.

A Look Ahead

The all-too-common cliché in LTC management and leadership is that nobody really knows what the future holds. Yet despite the limitations of the unknown, we must recognize the need to adjust to the rapidly changing, crisis-like environment of healthcare and LTC administration and that the way to stay nimble is through transformational and adaptive leadership. We can also see that a culture change in long-term care is upon us, as our aging society demands care and services that far surpass the dismal institutionalization to which the frail, elderly, and other vulnerable individuals have been traditionally subjected. Recent recognition of this need for culture change in government regulations will further drive this movement forward.

Still other changes in the LTC industry will be embraced as a matter of organizational survival. For instance, adoption of EMRs will be widespread despite their significant expense; this technology will provide uniformity, efficiency, and rapid transfer of client information. Various stakeholders, including the local community, will demand the LTC organization's participation or leadership in corporate social responsibility activities that give back, such as greening initiatives (e.g., recycling of wastes, use of environmentally responsible products) or local volunteerism. All of these changes will require that LTC organizations have in place managers and leaders who are forward thinking, innovative, resilient, and adaptable. In short, they must be open to and excited by these possibilities.

For Discussion

1. Describe the organization and roles of the governing body and administrative team in a long-term care facility near your home or one that you have visited. How does the administrative structure compare to that of a hospital?

2. Identify the external and internal strengths, weaknesses, opportunities, and threats faced by an LTC facility in which you work or have volunteered or with which you are familiar. Does this facility have a strategic plan and goals? Do administrators communicate this information to their staff and the public? How? (Or, if not, why not?)

3. Are good leaders necessarily good managers? Why or why not? Provide support and examples for your position.

4. In this era of rapid change in healthcare, which leadership style is most conducive to moving long-term care organizations toward being more aware of the needs of their residents and their communities? Discuss two leadership qualities that you feel such leaders must possess.

5. What steps should a good manager take to retain employees? How does leadership contribute to retaining good workers?

6. Discuss strategies that may be effective in motivating or reenergizing employees in high-stress LTC settings. Give specific examples for specific types of workers (e.g., nurses, CNAs, housekeeping staff).

7. List some advantages and disadvantages of using interdisciplinary teams to accomplish much of the work in LTC settings. Discuss ways in which managers can effectively form a team and provide the team with the support it needs to accomplish its goals.

8. How might good managers and leaders foster both innovation and accountability among team members? Provide specific examples and suggestions.

9. Describe the importance of quality teams in LTC facilities. From your experiences or from your reading and research, discuss one such team in an LTC facility (e.g., falls prevention team). What problem did this team address, and what were the team's objectives? What solutions did the team develop, and were they adopted?

CASE STUDY: A TALE OF TWO NURSING HOME ADMINISTRATORS

Facility A was run by an autocratic nursing home administrator (NHA) who preferred to lead her employees in an atmosphere of fear and intimidation. Any individuals who ignored or challenged her directions were either fired on the spot or targeted to be ushered through a rapid succession of disciplinary steps often leading to their termination. Turnover was high, but the NHA did manage to keep "happy" employees willing to follow her lead. She practiced measured favoritism by giving certain staff members financial incentives, offering better work schedules, and leaving them free from harassment. Employees were pitted against each other by being encouraged to turn each other in for not following the rules, although the NHA gave plenty of lip service to teamwork. Employees were also told to keep costs down above all else, and they were rewarded for not recommending costly rehabilitation services, better wheelchair seating or bed surfaces, or extra food or liquid snacks that would increase the food services budget.

As soon as the facility's management was alerted to an impending state survey, the NHA immediately assigned a manager and a team of employees to a nursing wing/hallway, storage area, service (e.g., medical records, kitchen), or common area (e.g., dining room, activities room) to ensure that those areas would meet all state standards when inspected, despite the fact that those areas were disregarded during the rest of the year. The NHA ordered staff to scrutinize the medical records for missing or incriminating material and to alter them accordingly. Leaky faucets were quickly repaired, equipment was sterilized and/or checked for malfunction, resident bathrooms were scrubbed, and residents were dressed and groomed with uncharacteristic care. Staffing (which was often deficient) was increased, and regular routines (e.g., therapy, care conferences, quality team meetings) were temporarily suspended to allow all staff members to participate in the all-out effort to look good for the surveyors. A "guard" was posted in the front window to warn of arriving surveyors, and a few members of senior management were ready to greet and delay the surveyors so that other managers and their teams could complete a final cleanup.

Facility B was run by an NHA who used a democratic-style leadership approach, believed strongly in teamwork, and served as chief facilitator of resources for the ongoing work of teams throughout the facility. Excellent performance and innovative practices, which increased care quality and overall satisfaction, were immediately rewarded with team recognition, special celebrations (e.g., ten-minute popcorn breaks, tea parties), and opportunities for career advancement. The organizational culture was resident centered, (with a motto of "residents first"), and everyone worked toward the mission of providing high-quality care. Teams were encouraged to look for ways to improve the safety, well-being, and comfort of their charges. Employees at all levels were empowered to lead teams or offer suggestions, resulting in happy workers and low turnover. Client and employee satisfaction were thus high, resulting in an average daily census near 100 percent and a waiting list for potential admissions.

Unlike the situation at Facility A, the ongoing emphasis on excellence and teamwork by the NHA in Facility B eliminated the need for particular changes in routine when the facility was informed of an upcoming survey. The facility and all pertinent records were already in tip-top shape, staff were prepared and empowered, and residents were happily engaged in their everyday activities. When the state surveyors arrived, no last-minute special efforts were needed; it was business as usual, with strong evidence of ongoing judicious management and leadership.

The results of both surveys were as expected. Facility A did not "fail" the survey, but it was given 11 deficiencies of varying severity in both patient care and facility cleanliness and maintenance. The rumor was that the staff sabotaged the efforts, resulting in a major deficiency given for the alteration of medical records. Characteristically, the NHA was punitive toward the staff whose areas received deficiencies, and little was done to correct previous poor practices. Facility B was deficiency-free in the area of resident care, but it was given one minor deficiency for a loose ceiling tile in the kitchen, a defect that was corrected before the surveyors left the building. The NHA rewarded all staff, residents, and their families with a huge celebratory party that same week and gave special recognition to teams involved in areas that received commendation from the surveyors.

CASE STUDY QUESTIONS

1. What management and leadership principles were used by the NHA at Facility B? How did they differ from those used by the NHA at Facility A?

2. Did the leadership styles of the NHAs significantly affect the surveys' outcomes? Why or why not?

3. Based on your readings and/or experiences with LTC facilities, what management or leadership practices might be employed by an NHA to achieve successful patient care outcomes and resident and staff satisfaction?

APPENDIX: MANAGEMENT AND LEADERSHIP BASIC PRINCIPLES

I. Organizational Chart

Exhibit 8.2 shows a simple chain-of-command (or chain-of-responsibility) chart within a typical nursing facility.

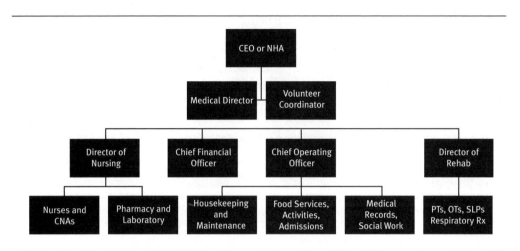

EXHIBIT 8.2
Organizational
Chart of a
Nursing Home

II. Qualities of Leadership

Following are excerpts from Warren Bennis's "Personal Qualities of Leadership," from the book *On Becoming a Leader* (2003):

• Integrity means alignment of words and actions with inner values. It means sticking to these values even when an alternative path may be easier or more advantageous.

• Dedication means spending whatever time and energy on a task is required to get the job done, rather than giving it whatever time you have available.

• A magnanimous person gives credit where it is due. It also means being gracious in defeat and allowing others who are defeated to retain their dignity.

• Humility means recognizing that you are not inherently superior to others and consequently that they are not inferior to you.

• Openness means being able to listen to ideas that are outside one's current mental models, being able to suspend judgment until after one has heard someone else's ideas.

• Creativity means thinking differently, being able to get outside the box and take a new and different viewpoint on things.

In another article published by the Leader to Leader Institute, Bennis (1999) offers additional wisdom on attributes essential to leadership:

• Technical competence: grasp of one's field

• Conceptual skill: a facility for strategic thinking

- Track record: a history of achieving results

- People skills: ability to communicate, motivate, and delegate

- Taste: ability to identify and cultivate talent

- Judgment: making difficult decisions in a short time frame with imperfect data

- Character: the qualities that define who we are

Reproduced with the permission of Basic Books.

CHAPTER 9

The Design of Long-Term Care Environments

Jullet A. Davis, PhD; Christopher Johnson, PhD; and Reid Oetjen, PhD

LEARNING OBJECTIVES

After studying this chapter, you should be able to

➤ define the terms *sensory considerations, universal design, institutional design,* and *facilities management* as they are used in this chapter;

➤ understand the relevant regulations related to the physical environment of long-term care facilities;

➤ understand the management issues of the physical environment of residential care settings, including repair and preventive maintenance procedures;

➤ discuss the latest developments and movement in environmental design, including the Eden Alternative and the Green House Project; and

➤ understand the importance of disaster management, including creating a disaster plan to provide continuity of care to residents of residential care facilities in the event of an emergency.

INTRODUCTION

The enormous psychological, emotional, sociological, and physical well-being implications of a facility's environment are critical for all LTC administrators to address. A well-maintained environment improves the delivery of care and promotes resident-centered care. The buildings, grounds, and equipment all require regular attention and ongoing upkeep. The Code of Federal Regulations requires a facility to "be designed, constructed, equipped, and maintained to protect the health and safety of residents, personnel, and the public" (Allen 2007, 301). In addition, the physical design standards of LTC facilities are undergoing a revolution. It is no longer acceptable to build or design facilities using the medical model as a guide. A culture change focusing on resident-centered care is leading the revolution toward greater resident and client empowerment.

This chapter begins by outlining important considerations in designing or redesigning LTC facilities, particularly for residents with dementia. That section is followed by a review of the regulations surrounding the physical environment and the process of managing that environment. Next, the chapter addresses community-based designs. The chapter closes with a discussion of disaster management and provides related resources.

DESIGN OF LONG-TERM CARE FACILITIES

Healthcare facility design is a relatively new field that emerged in the early 1990s. A key theme in this area has been the need to transform healthcare settings into healing environments that improve resident outcomes through the use of evidence-based research. Research comes from a variety of fields, including evolutionary biology and neuroscience. Privacy, resident safety, and stress reduction are integral parts of this new philosophy of facility design.

Healthcare design specialists recognize the body-mind connection—that is, the physical environment has a strong impact on the psychological state of mind and, therefore, on physical health and well-being (Stewart-Pollack and Menconi 2005, 133). This connection is the result of two major influences: Robert Ader's science of psychoneuroimmunology and Roger Ulrich's **theory of supportive design**.

Robert Ader and Nicholas Cohen (1975) found that stress and anxiety can influence the function of the immune system, which, in turn, can inhibit the healing process. Consequently, environmental stressors, such as dim lighting, excessive noise, and brightly colored walls, can produce responses that hinder the healing process, especially for older persons. In 1995, Ulrich introduced the theory of supportive design, which encourages designers to promote wellness by creating "psychologically supportive" physical surroundings with three characteristics: (1) a sense of control over physical/social surroundings and access to privacy, (2) access to social support from family and friends, and (3) access to nature and other positive distractions in one's physical surroundings (Stewart-Pollack and Menconi 2005, 134). These concepts emphasize the importance of larger rooms to

Theory of supportive design

A theory formulated by Roger Ulrich (1995) that promotes wellness in long-term care by encouraging designers to incorporate psychologically supportive physical surroundings that encourage: (1) a sense of control over physical/social surroundings and access to privacy; (2) access to social support from family and friends; and (3) access to nature and other positive distractions in one's physical surroundings.

accommodate personal-space zones with greater privacy; the use of adjustable, comfortable seating; the incorporation of natural elements such as interior green spaces and windows with views of nature; and the presence of pets. Many of these themes are present in the philosophies of culture change, the Eden Alternative, and the Green House Project—all of which promote resident-focused approaches to providing long-term care. (These approaches were introduced in Chapter 3 and are discussed later in the chapter.)

SENSORY CONSIDERATIONS

As individuals age, their sensory needs and capabilities change. Many of these sensory needs require certain adjustments in the physical environment. Changes in vision and mobility are the two key sensory issues that require special attention. Federal statutes require facilities to be "well-lighted." To address vision needs, the facility may need to ensure that all residential areas have sufficient lighting, natural lighting, and lighting that decreases glare. To do this, the facility may consider replacing traditional fluorescent bulbs with T-5 or T-8 lamps, which simulate natural light and are energy efficient (Brawley 2006; Johnson 1998; Calkins 1988).

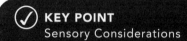

KEY POINT
Sensory Considerations

To address lighting needs, facilities should consider installing lighting that raises the level of illumination for residents and provides consistent and even light levels. Other suggestions include eliminating glare, using natural light when possible, and incorporating indirect lighting. Also, the facility should develop a lighting maintenance schedule so that these improvements continue to provide a safe environment (Brawley 2006, 64).

Related to vision needs, choosing the right colors is an important consideration. The key is to have high color contrast (Anderzhon et al. 2007; Brawley 2006). As the eyes age, the lenses thicken and become yellow, making distinguishing between colors difficult. Residents may find it challenging to differentiate floors from walls and may experience problems with depth perception. Therefore, using contrasting colors not only is aesthetically pleasing but also offers a level of safety for the resident. Some additional suggestions from the literature on lighting include raising the level of illumination, eliminating glare, providing access to natural daylight whenever possible, increasing luminance at task locations, and developing a lighting maintenance schedule to ensure proper maintenance of lighting (Brawley 2006, 64; Anderzhon, Fraley, and Green 2007; Brawley 2006; Johnson 1998; Calkins 1988).

Changes in residents' mobility can make certain environments risky. Several modifications must be made to minimize the safety risk for the residents and the liability of LTC providers. Many federal, state, and accrediting agency requirements are in place to ensure that facilities create safe environments. Following are some suggestions for preventing falls (Brawley 2006; Rollins 2000, 38; Johnson 1998; Calkins 1988):

- ◆ Repaint walls to create more contrast with floor surfaces.

- ◆ Do not oversimplify or make inappropriate modifications. A common error, for example, is installing grab bars without proper structural support.

- ◆ Use lighter-colored floor surfaces.

- ◆ Minimize changes in walking surfaces, and use slip-resistant covering when possible.

- ◆ Install more electrical outlets to minimize the use of extension cords.

Residents with Dementia

Residents with dementia experience special challenges with navigating the physical environment. John Zeisel and colleagues (2003, 697) discovered a positive correlation between "environmental design and agitation, aggression, depression, social withdrawal, and psychotic symptoms of residents with Alzheimer's disease." These residents may feel a greater sense of frustration and will perceive their environment as more stressful than would residents without dementia (Brawley 2006). Therefore, the physical environment should be designed to promote the highest level of functioning for residents with dementia. Zeisel and colleagues (2003) provide a literature review of studies that consider environmental features designed to improve outcomes for residents. Some of these strategies are presented in the nearby Critical Concept box.

LTC facilities may discover that these designing or remodeling suggestions will lead to improved quality of life for residents with dementia. These modifications are not limited to new or remodeled structures; they can also be implemented in older buildings. For example, residents with dementia have better outcomes when they have a private rather than a shared bedroom (Brawley 2006). It is worthwhile for the administrator to attempt to employ innovations in the physical environment to improve outcomes for all residents.

Universal design
A resident-centered approach to the design of the environment that focuses on the needs of the users regardless of functional impairments or disabilities.

Universal Design

According to the Institute for Human Centered Design, **universal design** is resident-centered design of the environment with the needs of the users in mind. It is not a single design element but rather a general orientation or framework that encompasses myriad design changes. Universal design is barrier-free, providing accessibility for all residents. Its focus is not simply on residents with functional impairments but also on those without disabilities; hence, this broad focus helps to limit the stigmatization associated with disability aids. Universal design is also known by the terms *inclusive design*, *design-for-all*, and *lifespan design*, and it is consistent with the principles of green design (Brawley 2006).

> **⚠ CRITICAL CONCEPT**
> Design Strategies for Dementia Patients
>
> Residents with dementia present unique challenges to LTC administrators. To address the needs of this population, facilities should consider using the following evidence-based design strategies:
>
> 1. Camouflaged exits reduce elopement attempts (note: the camouflage must meet Life Safety Code standards).
> 2. Private areas have proven to reduce aggression and agitation and to improve sleep.
> 3. Public or common areas that have an inviting (not institutional/hospital-like) décor encourage more socializing.
> 4. Walking paths equipped with devices to stimulate the senses and filled with activity opportunities lift clients' spirits and discourage the desire to leave the area; such design also engages the clients' visitors and loved ones.
> 5. Therapeutic garden access has shown to reduce elopement attempts and to improve sleep (Johnson 1998).
> 6. Thin carpet or tile with no specks, glare, or checkerboard designs should be used (Brawley 2006; Zeisel et al. 2003; Calkins 1988).
>
> These proven safety strategies lead to greater independence and fewer falls (Brawley 2006, 698).

INSTITUTIONAL DESIGN

According to the Centers for Medicare & Medicaid Services (CMS), LTC settings should be "homelike." However, older facilities—particularly nursing homes—are designed using the medical model, which is an institutional approach (Johnson 1998; Calkins 1988). The medical model approach is focused on meeting the needs of the staff. Thus, corridors are wide, privacy is nearly eliminated as residents are forced to share rooms, and the furniture and other fixtures are standardized (Joseph 2006). One of the reasons behind the continued use of institutional design methods is that most federal, state, and local regulations require that LTC facilities follow safety rules over homelike designs. A facility that wants to follow a design style that emphasizes safety along with homelike appeal sometimes has to seek a waiver. Given the importance of quality of life, facilities should address the regulatory hurdles to promote resident care on all levels. This section reviews a few new concepts in institutional design.

Overview

As noted earlier, the medical model promotes an institutional feel to LTC settings. Recent innovations in institutional designs promote greater resident freedom, autonomy, empowerment, self-reliance, independence, and comfort and overall give a more homelike feel to the facility. Having homelike and noninstitutional features, such as user-friendly flooring, good-quality lighting, and safety elements, throughout the space is the current trend. The design suggestions in this section are taken from designs implemented by actual LTC facilities across the country and are in accordance with the current gerontology architecture and interior design principles (Anderzhon, Fraley, and Green 2007; Brawley 2006; Zeisel et al. 2003; Calkins 1988).

Resident Room

Rooms are designed into clusters rather than grouped along corridors (Anderzhon, Fraley, and Green 2007). The cluster design allows for fewer residents on a given unit. The rooms are also single occupancy, which increases privacy and autonomy. If building single-occupancy rooms is not possible, then the facility may consider vertically splitting the room via the addition of a wall. This allows each resident to have some degree of privacy and eliminates the need for either occupant to enter the space of the other when entering or exiting the room. If space and funds are available, rooms can also be designed into suites. If a facility is unable to redesign the physical structure, it can take other steps to promote good outcomes, such as making furniture and fixtures flexible and customizable. For instance, the facility may allow a resident to bring her favorite chair, which would support a more homelike environment.

Nursing Station

Concomitant with the practical functions of nursing stations is their social role. John Peacock (1995) indicates that both staff and residents tend to congregate around the station, thus making it a meeting spot. The challenges for a new design are to encourage the social role of the nursing station and to minimize the negative aspects such as noise and the institutional look. Small changes can be made to the existing design to achieve both goals. For instance, the fortresslike counter can be removed and replaced by a dining room table and wall cabinets; this provides both workspace and a homelike gathering space. To combat the noise issue, Peacock (1995) suggests moving the nurse's station to a room. This allows staff to create a well-organized work location and allows for better noise control.

Shower Room

The design of a shower room should allow ease of use for both residents and staff. Some LTC facilities use a European design where the entire bathroom is essentially a large shower room (Brawley 2006). Facilities that are not able to redesign the shower room can make simple changes, such as installing more lighting for a brighter room, a fold-down shower seat or bench for safety and comfort, and removable shower chairs for better accessibility. The key to designing the shower room is flexibility: the greater the flexibility, the easier it is for staff to make needed adjustments to maximize resident comfort (Regnier 2002; Schwarz and Brent 1999; Calkins 1988).

Dining Room

Traditionally, nursing homes have used multiple tables in the dining room. Additionally, residents have few choices when it comes to the type of meals they eat and the time of day those meals are served. Recent innovations in resident dining employ fewer dining tables, more meal choices, and more flexible dining times. Some facilities have replaced the small four-seat tables with large tables (e.g., 8 to 12 seats) such as those found in many homes.

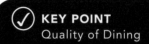

KEY POINT
Quality of Dining

One frequent source of complaints at LTC facilities is the quality of the food. Effective administrators understand that this is often one of the only areas over which a resident has control and thus incorporate strategies to improve the dining experience.

This minor change allows greater interaction among the residents. Another simple innovation is to set the table with silverware, napkins, plates, and glasses, much like many households do (Brawley 2006).

REGULATORY CONCERNS

LTC providers are among the most heavily regulated in the healthcare industry. This section reviews the relevant federal regulations related to the LTC physical environment and to its residents, staff, and visitors. The regulations discussed here focus on hazardous materials, building construction, fire protection, infection control, and resident comfort and protection.

AMERICANS WITH DISABILITIES ACT (ADA)

The **Americans with Disabilities Act** of 1990 is a federal law that established guidelines to ensure that all public and commercial buildings are accessible for persons with disabilities. The guidelines cover both the initial construction and future physical modifications to the facility. Violation of ADA rules can result in fines starting at $55,000 for first offenses

Americans with Disabilities Act
A federal law enacted in 1990 that establishes guidelines to ensure that all public and commercial buildings are accessible for persons with disabilities.

Life Safety Code
Established standards
that address items
that may cause fires or
other issues that would
affect resident safety.

and $110,000 for subsequent offenses (Department of Justice 2011). Many ADA-related lawsuits involve the violation of individual rights, but accessibility changes to the physical environment can also result in violation charges. For example, if a facility decides to create small corridors to achieve a homelike environment (a goal of culture change), it may find that it is in violation of ADA regulations (and also the **Life Safety Code**). Several notable cases against construction companies and other businesses include *United States v. Ellerbe Becket*, *United States v. Days Inns of America*, and *United States v. AMC Entertainment, Inc.* (A summary of these cases may be accessed at www.usdoj.gov/opa/pr/2000/June/369cr .htm.)

Title III of the ADA specifies that all new construction must be designed to be accessible by persons with disabilities. Likewise, renovations and other modifications to the facility must render the affected area accessible. In some cases, if an existing building has certain structural or architectural barriers, Title III requires the facility to remove the barrier. The rules do make allowances for undue hardship to the facility, such as when the cost of a compliance study is disproportionately larger than the cost of the renovations, but, as Peter Rauma (1992, 29) explains, "A display of 'good faith' may provide important defense in the event of a lawsuit. Certainly, the cost of a compliance study is a small price to pay compared to potential consequences of neglect or delay."

Administrators should seek legal advice from attorneys, architects, contractors, and other appropriate professionals when considering construction projects or renovations that might result in changes to ensure compliance with ADA rules. Professional advice is especially important when the facility is seeking to make modifications necessary to achieve culture change. The ADA rules may be found in the *Federal*

> ### ⚠ CRITICAL CONCEPT
> Complying with Federal Regulations
>
> The importance of complying with regulations cannot be overstated. Administrators must be well versed in all local, state, and federal regulations despite the fact that they are extensive, confusing, and ever changing. Ignorance is not a valid excuse for failing to comply with these regulations. CMS is the federal regulatory body for all LTC providers; however, CMS relies on codes written by the Americans with Disabilities Act, National Fire Protection Agency, and The Joint Commission, to name a few agencies. CMS requires that LTC facilities meet these codes by referencing them in the *Federal Register*.

Register (volume 56, number 144, July 26, 1991) as Final Rule Part III CFR 28, part 36. Compliance with the final rule is administered by the ADA's Architectural and Transportation Barriers Compliance Board, which is part of the US Department of Justice Civil Rights Division. The federal government may modify these rules in conjunction with the Council of American Building Officials and the American National Standards Institute in New York. Thus, periodically checking updates to this rule is important.

CENTERS FOR MEDICARE & MEDICAID SERVICES

Among the various regulatory agencies, the **Centers for Medicare & Medicaid Services (CMS)** is probably the most prominent. Section 483 of the Code of Federal Regulations lists the myriad rules CMS has established for long-term care facilities. These codes regulate numerous areas, including the physical environment, which is discussed in section 483.70. Covered items are discussed in general terms; however, specific mandates are detailed in the Life Safety Code of the National Fire Protection Association (NFPA). Administrators should regularly check the *Federal Register* for amendments to these documents to determine which edition of the Life Safety Code CMS requires facilities to comply with and when changes are proposed.

Centers for Medicare & Medicaid Services (CMS)
An agency of the Department of Health and Human Services responsible for regulating long-term care facilities.

OCCUPATIONAL SAFETY AND HEALTH ADMINISTRATION

Many of the guidelines from **Occupational Safety and Health Administration (OSHA)** relevant to LTC settings focus on staff safety. Not all of these guidelines are mandatory, but LTC providers may consider implementing them to ensure worker safety. For example, OSHA has established guidelines for ergonomics, exposure to blood and other infectious material, and decreasing slips, trips, and falls. The purpose of these guidelines is to reduce injury within the nursing home industry, which has some of the highest injury rates in the United States (Bureau of Labor Statistics 2006).

Occupational Safety and Health Administration (OSHA)
The federal agency charged with the enforcement of safety and health legislation; part of the Department of Labor.

NATIONAL FIRE PROTECTION AGENCY

For more than a century, the **National Fire Protection Agency (NFPA)** has been the leader in creating building safety guidelines. A nonprofit agency established in 1896, the NFPA publishes fire safety standards and codes and offers training throughout the world. Approximately every three years, the NFPA revises the Life Safety Code—standards that address items that may cause fires and other issues that have an impact on safety; the codes that govern long-term care facilities may be found in chapters 18, 19, 32, and 33. In addition to the actual codes, the NFPA also provides the *Life Safety Code Handbook*, an interpretive guide that is useful

National Fire Protection Agency (NFPA)
A nonprofit agency, established in 1896, whose mission is to reduce the burden of fire and other hazards on the quality of life by providing standards, codes, and training.

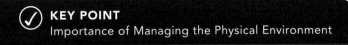

KEY POINT
Importance of Managing the Physical Environment

The importance of the physical environment or the physical plant is often overlooked by administrators. Without a properly operating plant, safe and effective care cannot be delivered to residents. Effective administrators ensure that an effective plan is in place to maintain the buildings, equipment, and related systems needed to provide a safe and high-quality experience to residents, staff, and visitors.

for LTC administrators who may be unclear about the meaning or application of a specific code. The key focus of the codes is on eliminating or minimizing the number of fire hazards. For LTC facilities, this means being vigilant about items that could be flammable, such as wall and ceiling finishes; issues that affect resident notification of a safety problem, such as alarm systems; and factors that affect residents' ability to leave an affected area, such as barriers to egress. The codes are extensive, and all LTC administrators must be acutely familiar with them to ensure facility compliance.

MANAGEMENT ISSUES OF THE PHYSICAL ENVIRONMENT

The LTC facility administrator is responsible for all aspects of the internal and external environment. A well-organized and properly maintained environment improves the ability of the facility to serve residents, staff, and visitors. "Optimized clinical care is an indirect outcome of [an] effective plant and environmental services" management program (Singh 2005, 362).

FACILITIES MANAGEMENT

Buildings, grounds, and equipment age at different rates. An effective facilities plan pays regular attention to all aspects of the physical plant. Scheduled maintenance, repairs, and replacements are necessary to avoid mechanical problems and facility obsolescence, which might result in a facility looking tired, old, and generally uninviting (Sasse 2007). Well-maintained buildings, equipment, and grounds convey an image of a robust, inviting facility to guests, residents, and facility staff.

MAINTENANCE

The facility maintenance department bears primary responsibility for monitoring all aspects of the plant. Regular assessments are crucial and should be conducted both informally and formally. An informal assessment may be conducted by simply walking around the grounds and buildings searching for existing and potential problems (Sasse 2007). Additional issues that maintenance should note are facility odors (both organic and inorganic), floor care, and other potential safety hazards (Dolan 2009). A formal assessment is accomplished more systematically through a structured method than by a random, haphazard approach. This structure includes a process for notifying the maintenance department of needed repairs and procedures for preventive checkups.

REPAIRS

Urgent and routine are the two general types of repairs (Singh 2005). Both require a system for alerting maintenance of the need for service. This system is especially important for urgent repairs, which may occur during times (e.g., evening, overnight) when no maintenance staff are available. Should any fixture, mechanical/electrical system, or other equipment cease to work or potentially threaten safety, the maintenance supervisor, administrator, nursing director, or other designee with sufficient authority must be contacted. If immediate attention is needed or the issue is beyond the staff's capability, the facility should be able to contact an outside firm that can correct the problem right away. Agreements with external vendors and repair contractors should be established before issues arise. The need for repairs is either discovered during maintenance's facility inspection or requested by staff throughout the day. Requesting a repair of either type employs a similar strategy: A work order is placed so that the repair can be scheduled and addressed in a timely manner.

PREVENTIVE MAINTENANCE

Preventive maintenance involves more than simply checking to see if everything is in good working order. A good preventive maintenance program includes tasks such as changing air conditioning and other filters, cleaning coils, tracking temperatures, testing sprinkler systems, and lubricating equipment. The basic rules of a good maintenance program include the following (Ratliff 1999):

- *Filing pertinent maintenance information.* Keep blueprints and other relevant information about the equipment in an organized, visible location.

- *Documenting the details of maintenance that is performed.* This log should be clear, indicating what repairs, parts replacement, and general upkeep have been performed on the buildings, grounds, and equipment.

In addition to these tasks, a preventive program should include weekly checks, revolving inspections, and ongoing upkeep (Singh 2005). Performing weekly checks ensures that equipment, especially emergency equipment, is functioning. During weekly checks, the fire alarm system can be tested.

Revolving inspections are conducted on a rotating schedule and involve a close examination of all areas of the facility. Depending on the size of the facility, the maintenance staff may take up to a week or longer to complete a full examination of the grounds, buildings, and equipment. Maintenance looks for issues that generally go unreported by others, such as the following (Singh 2005, 367):

♦   Leaky faucets

♦   Leaks at the bottom of toilets

♦   Windows that do not close or lock

♦   Doors that do not completely shut

♦   Missing ceiling and floor tiles

♦   Ventilation or exhaust problems in bathrooms, kitchen, laundry, and utility areas

♦   Scuffed walls in need of repainting or repair

♦   Curtains and other window coverings in disrepair

♦   Missing fire extinguishers

♦   Torn or buckled carpeting

♦   Nonfunctional patient call systems

♦   Burned-out or flickering light bulbs

♦   Signs of pest activity

♦   Cracks in the sidewalk or the parking lot pavement

Because of the wide array of issues that might be discovered during a revolving inspection, the LTC administrator must be fully involved in the process. Regular reports from the maintenance department are critical. The administrator should also engage in site checks to guarantee that maintenance has not missed a patient, staff, or visitor safety threat.

The final component of a preventive program is ongoing upkeep. As its name implies, ongoing upkeep focuses on the continuous activities to maintain the physical appearance of the facility. While wheelchair-scuffed walls may not be a safety issue, they make the facility less aesthetically appealing. The facility should have a plan in place to ensure that the building is physically attractive.

Preventive maintenance can save the facility from costly repairs and replacement. Using data from various sources, Wei Lin Koo and Tracy Van Hoy (2003) attempted to determine the costs and benefits derived from preventive maintenance. They discovered that investment in preventive maintenance leads to substantial returns on investment and can be up to a 500 percent return on investment.

HOUSEKEEPING

A critical role of the housekeeping department is to create a sanitary facility. Sanitary means both clean and safe. The housekeeping staff must use proper methods to minimize or eliminate the spread of disease and to appropriately store cleaning equipment and supplies. The products or chemicals used to sanitize and clean items must be approved by the Environmental Protection Agency (EPA). Furthermore, the cleaning and sanitizing process should follow the directions specified by the product's manufacturer or by a regulatory agency.

The housekeeping department is also responsible for odor control. Odors should not be covered up by using odor-eliminating sprays (Dillon 2005). Rather, an effective odor-control plan should entail daily and weekly cleaning schedules to ensure the proper disposal of odor-causing items. Although soiled linen may be the immediate cause of a new odor, "the housekeeping staff in nursing facilities must not handle either clean or soiled linens" (Singh 2005, 368). The task of removing soiled bed linen and other items used by residents should be assigned to the nursing assistants. Both OSHA and the Centers for Disease Control and Prevention (CDC) provide guidelines for the proper handling of soiled items. Odors can also come from carpeting, floor coverings, and other soft surfaces. Therefore, regular cleaning of these items is vital.

Another role of the housekeeping department is sanitation to control and combat the spread of infection. The prevalence of methicillin-resistant *Staphylococcus aureus* (MRSA) and other nosocomial infections in LTC settings is on the rise (Farr 2006). Thus, housekeeping must have access to the proper cleaning supplies. The EPA provides a list of registered antimicrobial cleaning supplies at www.epa.gov/oppad001/influenza-a-product-list.pdf. The administrator and the housekeeping supervisor both should be aware of the capabilities and limitations of these products. For example, concentrated bleach makes a good disinfectant when diluted, but an open container of bleach loses its effectiveness after 30 days. Product effectiveness is a critical consideration. Therefore, the housekeeping supervisor should periodically take cultures of surfaces throughout the facility to determine bacterial colony levels (Singh 2005).

LAUNDRY

The purpose of the laundry department in LTC settings is to wash all of the facility linens, including bedding, bath linens, and resident clothing. Laundry staff has the primary responsibility for collecting, sorting, washing, drying, and delivering laundry to the nursing units, and its personnel also play a key role in infection control because they are likely to come in contact with infected linen. Therefore, OSHA and the CDC have created guidelines for workers to follow when handling linens. According to the CDC, "although soiled linen may harbor large numbers of pathogenic microorganisms, the risk of actual disease transmission from soiled linen is negligible. Rather than rigid rules and regulations, common-sense hygienic practices for processing and storage of linen are recommended" (see www.cdc.gov/ncidod/dhqp/bp_laundry.html).

Following are specific recommendations from OSHA's bloodborne pathogens standards:

◆ LTC staff should bag soiled laundry inside the resident's room. The bag used for this purpose must be adequately sealed to prevent it from opening during transport.

◆ Gloves, gowns, and masks must be worn when handling or transporting soiled laundry regardless of whether it is bagged or not. To prevent the spread of disease, linens should not be shaken or handled in a way that would release contaminants into the environment, thereby making the transmission of disease likely.

◆ Laundry staff should follow appropriate hand-washing and hygiene practices after they have removed their gloves.

◆ LTC facilities should ensure that laundry is washed and dried in accordance with current infection control standards and procedures.

SAFETY AND SECURITY

Residents should feel both safe and secure. The facility is the residents' home, and as such it should protect residents from accidental and intentional harm, just as their own residences have done for them. The two types of safety are emotional and physical, and often, these types are intertwined. When residents feel physically safe, they also are likely to feel emotionally safe. Therefore, staff must maintain control over the physical environment to provide residents a feeling of emotional safety. Residents need to feel that the facility is properly secured and that intruders cannot enter. Thus, a system must be in place to ensure that staff members are aware of all visitors who enter the facility. Emotional safety also implies that employees are doing their jobs in a safe manner and providing safe care; poor quality of care is a threat to the residents' sense of emotional safety.

Emotional and physical safety is the responsibility of all staff, including those whose daily tasks do not entail direct patient care. For example, housekeeping needs to keep the floor free of debris and other hazards that can cause a resident to fall. Maintenance should place proper signage in appropriate locations throughout the facility. Signs, for the sighted and the blind, warn people (e.g., residents, staff, visitors) of dangerous, harmful, or infectious zones, such as chemical storage areas, stairs, or soiled linen rooms.

The facility's level of security affects residents' physical safety. Security includes protection of residents, staff, and visitors from physical harm and injury and protection of property (Singh 2005). Protection can be accomplished using a variety of measures, including security systems, security staff, unit lockdowns, appropriate lighting, police patrol, self-locking systems, door alarms, electronic surveillance systems in public areas, and surveillance systems in resident rooms (Acorn 2010). Each of these measures should be evaluated to determine if its relative merit outweighs the costs and the legal ramifications of its use. Prior to installing any security feature, the administrator should seek input from legal counsel and law enforcement officials.

In addition to resident protection, facility assets must be protected using established policies and procedures. Singh (2005, 374) suggests three types of security systems for these physical assets:

1. A system for ordering, receiving, storing, and maintaining inventory control of all supplies and materials
2. A system for tagging and inventory control for all movable capital assets
3. A key-control system that restricts access to various storage and office areas

The instrumental aspect of incorporating each system is proper documentation. Logs must be maintained that document incoming and outgoing items. During regular rounds, the maintenance department, in addition to monitoring for upkeep issues, should check the security devices to ensure proper functioning.

GREEN PRODUCTS

The number of environmentally safe cleaning and laundry supplies that can be used in the healthcare setting is steadily increasing. These products are environmentally friendly because they are nontoxic, noncombustible, noncorrosive, safe for aquatic life, and biodegradable; they have no chlorine, nonylphenol ethoxylates (NPE), ethylenediaminetetraacetic acid (EDTA), and nitrilotriacetic acid (NTA); and they are free of known carcinogens, have no reproductive hazards, and contain less than 1 percent volatile organic compounds (Dillon 2005). These characteristics thus make them safe for LTC residents and staff. LTC facilities interested in going green can download the *Green Guide for Health Care* at http://gghc.org/. This guide provides a list of environmentally friendly cleaning products and the recycled content of paper products.

INFECTION CONTROL

CMS requires LTC facilities to have in place an infection control program that prevents and monitors the development and transmission of disease. The infection control program is responsible for the following [483.65(a)(1-3)]:

1. Investigating, controlling, and preventing facility infections
2. Determining when and if resident isolation is necessary
3. Maintaining documentation of infection-related incidents and all corrective actions implemented

As noted earlier, the housekeeping department bears some of the responsibility for infection control. However, the facility must have a well-developed infection control program that addresses all aspects of infection control throughout the building and grounds.

CORRECTIVE ACTION

A corrective action plan is required by federal regulations to address deficiencies in the physical environment. As part of the quality assurance program, the corrective action plan should include a record of incidents and the corrective action steps in place. A comprehensive corrective action plan should contain the following elements: (1) how the corrective action will address any residents impacted by the deficiency; (2) the plan for identifying residents impacted or potentially impacted by the deficiency; (3) the safeguards employed to eliminate reoccurrence of the deficiency; and (4) how the facility will monitor the corrective action plan to ensure that the deficiency does not reoccur (Brown University, Center for Gerontology and Healthcare Research 2005).

COMMUNITY-BASED DESIGNS: AGING IN PLACE

The most direct definition of "aging in place" is living in the same community or home through the elder years. It involves creating an environment that supports the needs of the individual at all life stages. Numerous residential settings promote aging in place, such as continuing care retirement communities, but some individuals prefer to remain in their home. This section reviews ways in which a home can be modified to allow individuals to age in place.

Home Modifications

The first step in the decision to age in place is to determine if the current home can support the present and future needs of the elderly. Numerous websites provide assessment tools to determine the safety hazards in the average home. For example, the Senior Resource for Aging in Place presents an assessment tool that addresses some difficulties of seniors and offers a possible remedy for each; Exhibit 9.1 shows several examples from this tool, and the complete table may be found online (see www.seniorresource.com).

AARP also provides information on home modifications to meet aging-in-place needs. As would be expected, some of these suggestions include changing lighting, replacing doorknobs, lowering microwaves, installing an open-plan shower, and installing grab

EXHIBIT 9.1
Recommendations
for Seniors Who
Age in Place

Senior Difficulty	Possible Remedy
Balance and coordination problems	Bath seat in the tub or shower
Hearing impairment	Smoke detectors with strobe lights
Limited reach	Oven doors that swing to the side
Limited vision	Edge of counters a different color than the top
Poor hand and arm strength	Automatic garage door opener
Trouble bending	Elevated toilet or toilet seat
Trouble walking and climbing stairs	Threshold on door no higher than a quarter inch
Use of a wheelchair	Walk-in closet wide enough for wheelchair

SOURCE: Reprinted with permission from Senior*resource*.com.

bars. Safety is the focus of many aging-in-place modifications, but style and comfort are also important considerations. Some changes are minor (e.g., replacing light switches), while some are far more extensive (e.g., modifying the bathroom). Yet, they may all be necessary for the individuals to remain in their homes.

PHILOSOPHICAL EVOLUTION IN ENVIRONMENTAL DESIGN

CULTURE CHANGE

Culture change is the latest philosophical movement in the design of institutional settings such as long-term care. According to the Pioneer Network (see www.pioneernetwork.net/ CultureChange), culture change is "the national movement for the transformation of older adult services, based on person-directed values and practices where the voices of elders and those working with them are considered and respected. The core person-directed values are choice, dignity, respect, self-determination, and purposeful living."

Thus, culture change is not a singular task or event; rather, it is a series of tasks and environmental changes. This philosophy suggests a continuum of changes that a facility can implement along the culture change path. Nonetheless, the two necessary tasks associated with culture change are (1) resident-directed care and (2) staff empowerment (Rahman and Schnelle 2008). Culture change is a comprehensive process that leads to a change in staff attitudes and behaviors.

The research on the culture change movement is focused on two specific types of nursing home organizational designs—the Eden Alternative and the Green House Project. While these programs share similar philosophical underpinnings, they are unique.

Culture change
According to the Pioneer Network, "the national movement for the transformation of older adult services, based on person-directed values and practices where the voices of elders and those working with them are considered and respected. The core person-directed values are choice, dignity, respect, self-determination, and purposeful living."

Eden Alternative

A philosophy of providing long-term care services in an environment that promotes quality of life for all involved, as opposed to the traditional institutional model.

THE EDEN ALTERNATIVE

The **Eden Alternative** seeks to create an environment designed to reduce boredom, loneliness, and helplessness (Thomas 1996). This environment is achieved through decentralized management structures, team-delivered care, staff empowerment, resident participation in decision making, the inclusion of live plants into the design, and the encouragement of regular visits from animals and children (Barba, Tesh, and Courts 2002). The ten principles of the Eden Alternative are as follows (Eden Alternative 2009):

1. The three plagues of loneliness, helplessness, and boredom account for the bulk of suffering among our elders.
2. An elder-centered community commits to creating a human habitat where life revolves around close and continuing contact with plants, animals, and children. It is these relationships that provide the young and old alike with a pathway to a life worth living.
3. Loving companionship is the antidote to loneliness. Elders deserve easy access to human and animal companionship.
4. An elder-centered community creates opportunity to give as well as receive care. This is the antidote to helplessness.
5. An elder-centered community imbues daily life with variety and spontaneity by creating an environment in which unexpected and unpredictable interactions and happenings can take place. This is the antidote to boredom.
6. Meaningless activity corrodes the human spirit. The opportunity to do things that we find meaningful is essential to human health.
7. Medical treatment should be the servant of genuine human caring, never its master.
8. An elder-centered community honors its elders by de-emphasizing top-down bureaucratic authority, seeking instead to place the maximum possible decision-making authority into the hands of the elders or into the hands of those closest to them.
9. Creating an elder-centered community is a never-ending process. Human growth must never be separated from human life.
10. Wise leadership is the lifeblood of any struggle against the three plagues. For it, there can be no substitute.

Research on the effectiveness of the Eden Alternative found that implementing this type of design has resulted in improved outcomes for some elders. For instance, Brenda Bergman-Evans (2004) found that there were significant differences in levels of distress in terms of boredom and helplessness; however, there were not significant effects on loneliness.

However, other research found no major impacts on staff or residents from the implementation of this design (Singh 2005). One study found that some Eden homes have a negative effect on some residents (Denton et al. 1998). Thus, more research is needed before the true benefit of the Eden Alternative can be determined.

GREEN HOUSE PROJECT

Thomas (2003, 2004) suggested an evolution of the resident-centered approach, moving from the Eden Alternative to the **Green House Project**. The Green House Project is an innovative form of long-term care based on the social model of care that attempts to deinstitutionalize care and uses small ten-bed group homes for elders. It consists of "a complete reworking of the scale and physical environments of nursing homes, the organizational structure and staffing patterns, and the philosophy governing services" (Kane and Cutler 2008, 1). The main elements of the Green House Project include the following (Kane et al. 2005):

Green House Project
An innovative form of long-term care based on the social model of care that attempts to deinstitutionalize care and use small, ten-bed group homes for elders.

◆   Ten elders live in self-contained houses with private rooms and baths.

◆   Meals are cooked in the green house kitchen in the presence of CNA-level assistants called shahbazims.

◆   Shahbazims perform cooking, housekeeping, personal care, and laundry duties as well as facilitate elder development.

◆   Shahbazims do not report to nursing staff.

◆   All professionals (e.g., registered nurses, physicians, physical therapists) make up the clinical support teams that visit the green house.

◆   The emphasis is on quality of life for elders. (Quality of care is a given, but health and safety goals do not dominate the model.)

Additional features of the Green House Project include allowing residents to bring their own furniture and to choose their own room décor, wireless nurse-call systems, and medications stored in a locked cabinet in the resident's room (Singh 2005). It also encourages a closer relationship between the staff and the residents. This closeness is exemplified by elders and staff preparing meals, eating, cleaning, and doing laundry together. Research to date shows positive outcomes for residents living in a green house (Kane et al. 2007). For example, in a green house, residents reported having less bed rest, experiencing more activities, feeling less depressed, and improving in activities of daily living (Kane et al. 2007, 6).

OTHER INNOVATIVE DESIGNS

The Eden Alternative and the Green House Project are two prominent design models that have been gaining momentum, but other design initiatives are emerging. Providing an exhaustive list of these new designs is not practical, as numerous initiatives take place in single institutions. Each initiative attempts to implement various aspects of the culture change movement. Two themes that are repeated among facilities that have remodeled their physical environments are (1) smaller clusters of residents and (2) more resident choice and empowerment. Residents are given more freedom and control over the physical environment, emphasizing that the facility is now their home and not just the place where they receive care. The results are not overwhelmingly positive, but early reports do indicate some improved outcomes for residents living in these redesigned settings (Alden and Weisman 2004).

DISASTER MANAGEMENT

Disaster plan

A detailed written plan that includes procedures to meet all potential emergencies and disasters, such as fire, severe weather, and missing residents.

A **disaster plan**—a detailed written plan that includes procedures for responding to a natural or man-made catastrophe or mishap that has already occurred or is expected or likely to occur—is necessary for all LTC facilities. Staff members must be aware of this plan and must be sufficiently knowledgeable about their roles during a disaster. The need for a plan became especially clear during Hurricane Katrina, when several elderly individuals lost their lives due to the lack of knowledge concerning evacuations. As such, all staff must be trained on these procedures upon employment and engage in periodic reviews of these procedures. Each facility must conduct unannounced drills to determine staff responsiveness, knowledge, and ability to follow the plans and procedures should a true emergency arise. A comprehensive disaster plan should include the following considerations: (1) an evacuation plan that provides food, transportation, medical care as well as reentry to the facility after the event; (2) sheltering in a safe environment; (3) a specific plan for addressing the medical needs of the residents; (4) adequate staffing along with provisions for the staff's family members; and (5) a plan that is integrated with local emergency managers (Department of Health and Human Services 2006).

Nursing homes, and other LTC providers, should adapt the plans and procedures to meet the unique needs of their geographic region. The plan should also be a dynamic document, requiring the administrator and other responsible parties to perform regular reviews to ensure that the plan addresses the current characteristics of the buildings and grounds (Ross and Bing 2007; Seale 2010).

A LOOK AHEAD

The physical environment of LTC facilities has started to change. No longer is it acceptable to provide the institutional environment that is based on the medical model. Present and future users of long-term care (along with their families) are better educated about healthcare delivery and thus demand a homelike environment based on the social model. Design options for facilities, as well as modifications for existing structures, will continue to evolve as policymakers and laypeople become aware of the advantages of these changes in promoting quality outcomes for LTC residents.

FOR DISCUSSION

1. Briefly discuss the shift in design philosophy from the medical model to the social model.

2. What regulatory concerns should future administrators be aware of when considering adopting new design innovations for their facilities?

3. What are several sensory and safety considerations that administrators should consider when redesigning facilities? Discuss several challenges and find unique solutions to them on the Internet.

4. Describe both the Eden Alternative and the Green House Project. How are these approaches similar, and how are they different?

5. LeadingAge (www.leadingage.org) has created a prototype house, Leading Age Idea House, that shows how technology, universal design, and environmentally friendly construction can be harnessed to support independent, aging-in-place living. View the video at www.youtube.com/watch?v=Bs3mmFieWaA and describe your impressions of this house of the future.

CASE STUDY: REDESIGNING DILEMMA

Sally Smith recently took a position as the administrator of a suburban LTC facility in the southeastern United States. The facility has a large number of residents with dementia. The facility's board of directors told her that the residents' council asked if the dining room could be renovated to add more appeal, especially for visiting family members. Having a limited budget, Sally asked her interior decorator friend, Donald Desney, if he could help, given that he recently redesigned the living room and kitchen of her house. Donald decided to make the facility's dining room more dramatic and appealing to the Southern sensibilities of the residents. He replaced the dining room carpet with shiny, speckled linoleum. He picked a "Gone with the Wind" theme, using floral curtains, ruffled tablecloths, silk flowers on every table, a dark red color on the walls, and a large picture of Rhett Butler and Scarlett O'Hara painted on one of the walls.

Sally was pleased with Donald's redecorating ideas, and she was surprised that the residents were having problems. Many tripped and fell in their attempt to avoid walking on the speckled pattern on the floor. Many complained that they could not see their menu choices, and some with dementia became so agitated when they entered that they walked out without eating dinner. Sally was upset by these reactions. She thought to herself, "How could they not appreciate all the good work we put in to give them a new and improved dining space? They asked for this!"

CASE STUDY QUESTIONS

1. What should Sally have done before she redecorated the dining room, especially if she knew that a large number of residents have dementia?

2. What theories of supportive design were violated in this redesign?

3. What recommendations would you give Sally to encourage residents to return to eat in the new dining room?

CHAPTER 10

Strategic Marketing for Long-Term Care

Patricia R. Loubeau, DrPH

After studying this chapter, you should be able to

➤ understand the difference between marketing and selling to seniors and their families;

➤ understand how the senior market can be segmented for more effective marketing;

➤ develop options to target ethnic segments in the long-term care services market;

➤ understand the role of social media marketing in long-term care services; and

➤ examine some tips for marketing to seniors and learn how they are applied.

Strategic marketing
The process of developing a fit between an organization's goals and resources and changing market opportunities. It consists of the fundamental business planning tools of market research, a marketing plan, and its implementation.

Relationship marketing
A set of strategies that focus on the lifetime relationship with the customer rather than the individual transactions of the customer in order to increase profit. Relationship marketing captures customer share, or the share of the customer dollar, rather than the number of customers within the market share.

Selling orientation
An organization's primary focus on the needs of the seller rather than the buyer.

INTRODUCTION

Marketing has existed since commerce was invented, and even earlier, but only since the 1970s has it been an essential strategy for the healthcare industry. Prior to that time, reimbursement and lack of competition were such that the industry could survive nicely without the benefit of marketing. Today, everyone in the industry has an interest in healthcare marketing, whether it is marketing goods such as durable medical equipment, an idea such as the importance of a routine colonoscopy, or services such as home care or assisted living. Good **strategic marketing** is increasingly vital to a healthcare organization's financial success.

HEALTHCARE MARKETING: THE FOUNDATION

Many people have contributed to the collective knowledge about marketing. Philip Kotler provided the classic definition, which states that "marketing is a social process by which individuals and groups obtain what they need and want through creating, offering, and freely exchanging products and services of value with others" (Kotler and Keller 2006). A more recent philosophy that successful companies use is an extension of business marketing termed **relationship marketing**. This strategy takes marketing one step further to proactively build a bias or preference for an organization with the ultimate goal of a mutually satisfying long-term relationship. The basis for relationship marketing is a shift of the organization's thinking from a relationship made up of individual transactions to one of long-term customer loyalty. Inherent in this philosophy is the need for high-quality data that the marketer can use to track a customer's preferences, transaction history, and behavior over time. The goal is to move beyond satisfying the customer's immediate needs to establishing and maintaining a long relationship that is satisfying to both parties.

Historically, the concept of selling and that of relationship marketing have often been confused. The concepts are distinctly different. A company that adopts a selling philosophy or **selling orientation** focuses on creating sales transactions with little regard for building long-term relationships with customers. Selling assumes that customers must be coaxed into buying a service and that when they do they will probably like it. This is usually a poor assumption to make about a buyer.

An aggressive strategy, selling seeks to maximize sales volume while paying the least possible amount of attention to the customer's needs. It often requires a large-scale selling and promotion effort. The quality test of an organization with a selling philosophy is units of service or products sold. A selling strategy is often used where the supply of a product or service exceeds the demand. This strategy has, with less than desirable results, been practiced in some senior living communities when initial demand was overestimated and occupancy rates did not meet financial projections.

Marketing, on the other hand, is customer centered and seeks to make a profit by satisfying customer needs, wants, and desires more effectively and efficiently than competitors do. Marketing success is measured by a high-quality service plus a high level of awareness. Marketing aims to gain and retain customers over the long haul by establishing a meaningful long-term relationship.

Marketing and advertising are also frequently confused. Advertising, or more generally marketing communications of any type, is the last area to consider in developing the marketing mix (made up of product, price, promotion, and place). A product or service is designed to fulfill an unmet need or want, the most efficient and effective distribution system is designed, and the product or service is priced appropriately. Only then is the marketing communications plan designed to inform, persuade, or remind consumers about the product or service.

SEGMENTATION

Integral to the strategy of marketing is the idea of segmentation. **Market segmentation** is the opposite of mass marketing, or using the same marketing strategy for all demographics. The mass-market approach no longer works for the LTC industry. As a result, providers are adopting a marketing orientation that includes the use of segmentation.

Segmentation is breaking mass markets down into groups according to their buying habits and similar characteristics and targeting those customers most likely to use the product or service. The target market segment in LTC is no longer simply all individuals older than 65 years who qualify for Medicare or Medicaid. If an LTC service is to be successful, it must identify and promote itself as the best provider of attributes that are important to a particular market segment. Successful marketers know that a segmented market is more efficient to target than a broad, unfocused mass and that this technique wastes less money on low-probability contacts. Indeed, a marketing future for any healthcare organization may hinge on appealing to older demographics. The **marketing mix** can be tailored to appeal to the needs of a particular segment. A segmented market is also easier to research. Advertising strategy can pinpoint a refined market segment rather than use a "one size fits all" message that generally reaches nobody. In **market positioning**, marketers choose a segmentation that provides the organization with the maximal opportunity to achieve a leadership position in the marketplace.

Markets are rarely homogeneous, and the elder market is no exception. In fact, substantial heterogeneity and diversity characterize the older segment of the population. The elder market has diverse needs, lifestyles, and preferences. The most common mistake healthcare organizations make with age segmentation is to segment the elderly as anyone older than 65 years. While age may be a convenient and readily available criterion for defining the elder market, age alone is a poor predictor of behavior.

Markets are segmented along a variety of categories, including sociodemographic characteristics (e.g., age, gender, income), geography, psychography (e.g., attitudes, values, lifestyle), usage level of products or services (e.g., nonusers, ex-users, potential users), and cohort. Exhibit 10.1 illustrates the fundamental forces that shape differences in healthcare needs.

Market segmentation
Dividing a market into subsets in which each subset has characteristics in common.

Marketing mix
The product or service, price, promotion, and place or channels of distribution.

Market positioning
Choosing a market segmentation that provides the organization with the maximal opportunity to achieve a leadership position in the marketplace.

EXHIBIT 10.1

Motivating Factors
for Healthcare Use

Demographic Forces	Lifestyle Forces	Usage Behavior	Geographic	Cohort	Payer Status	Health Status
Age	Social class	First-time users	Zip code	1912–21	Medicare	Healthy
Income	Attitudes	Frequency of use	County	1922–27	Medicaid	Chronically ill
Gender	Values		State	1928–45	Self-pay	Acutely ill
Race/ethnicity	Interests				Private insurance	
Education	Activities					

SOURCE: Adapted from Fox and Jones (2009) and Elliott (2005).

An ideal market segment is of sufficient size, has the potential for growth, and most important, has a relatively underserved need. A marketer must ask, Does the segment have the potential to be profitable? A corollary issue to profitability is that the segment should be stable and long term. The market should also be actionable. In other words, an organization should have the capability and resources to develop effective programs to attract and serve a particular segment.

The overall eldercare market clearly meets these criteria. Seniors are a large and growing portion of the population who account for a disproportionate share of healthcare spending. They control a large proportion of the nation's discretionary income. In other words, they are economically sound enough for a marketer to profitably cultivate. They are also politically and economically powerful, reachable, and generally well insured. All these factors make them a highly desirable market segment. The marketing future of any healthcare organization may hinge on appealing to an older demographic. An organization that chooses to target a senior market segment should analyze both the targeted segment and its own capabilities to be sure it can match, and preferably exceed, competing offerings directed at the same segment. Similarly, the organization should examine its culture and mission to be sure it is consistent with the needs of this group.

In healthcare marketing, age segmentation is particularly relevant, and several strategies have emerged to attract this segment. An example is a medical group practice geared toward the elderly population. The practice might publish a brochure in 14-point type, use telephones with volume controls, offer specialized forms and devices to help seniors remember to take their medicine, and even designate one employee as a senior citizen representative who can help patients file insurance forms. The restrooms are adapted for the elderly with extra-wide doors, emergency call bells, extra lighting, and elevated toilet seats. The office is situated on a bus line, with adequate nearby parking and a well-lit, wheelchair-accessible entrance. The practice targets loyal users with newsletters, birthday cards, and health tips via e-mail to reinforce positive impressions and encourage continued loyalty.

EXAMPLES OF MARKET SEGMENTATION FOR SENIORS

Aultman Hospital in Canton, Ohio, is an acute care facility that has successfully segmented the senior market. The hospital's Prime Time Seniors Program includes a variety of services for patients aged 50 years or older. With 70,000 members, the program offers segmented consumers assistance filling out forms, discounts at area merchants, free parking, and invitations to educational, social, and travel programs. When members visit the hospital, they are welcome to free coffee and tea in the cafeteria and free notary services. Those who give blood four times a year receive a $25 gas card donated by a local merchant. The hospital website has a quiz called "Heart Aware" that takes about seven minutes to complete online. The quiz provides an immediate personal report that indicates an individual's overall risk of coronary artery disease along with ways to reduce development of disease. All these services are intended to establish an ongoing relationship with the senior marketplace (Aultman Hospital 2007).

The Senior Class program at Baystate Health, in Springfield, Massachusetts, offers tours, lectures, screenings, and other free services. Senior programs such as these are beneficial to organizations as they provide an excellent method to interact with the senior population and encourage them to be customers of their facilities.

The Osborn Retirement Community in affluent Rye, New York, has a tradition of gracious retirement living on its beautifully landscaped campus in Westchester County. Its residence includes independent living and assisted living facilities, skilled nursing care, short-term rehabilitation services, and dementia care. In 2007, to keep pace with and meet the needs of future residents, the organization surveyed local individuals about the factors that would be important when they considered a retirement community. Survey participants were also asked how (e.g., facility visit, in-home consultation, phone conversation, website, brochures, seminars) they would like to learn more about Osborn. Those who expressed a strong interest and demonstrated a current need for assistance were targeted immediately for a strong follow-up. Others with less pressing needs were followed up less aggressively. For each survey received, Osborn made a donation to the Alzheimer's Association. In addition to identifying potential residents, the survey helped Osborn identify service qualities for its particular market.

MARKETING TO DIFFERENT ETHNIC GROUPS

An assisted living facility cannot connect with all older consumers in large, broad, and diverse markets. Marketers sometimes pursue the same general segment as competing organizations and miss some potentially underserved and more lucrative segments. Focusing only on the largest segment may not be the best option, as competitive intensity can render that segment the least profitable (Berkowitz 2010). In recent years, organizations have paid greater attention to cultural and ethnic diversity. The face of the United States is changing. Latinos are the largest minority group, and many marketers have tailored their marketing strategies to meet the needs of this growing group.

Targeting ethnic segments in the assisted living arena is one way to effectively serve a distinct group of buyers with different needs and preferences. Freemont, California–based Aegis Gardens is an assisted living facility for the Bay Area's Korean population. Before breaking ground, the organization consulted a feng shui expert. The facility provides support for the Korean language and culture and serves Korean and Chinese food. The facility maintains an employee-to-resident ratio of nearly one to one, and staff members, who were recruited by consulting churches and local newspapers, are fluent in Mandarin and Cantonese. Resident activities include practicing Chinese calligraphy, making dumplings, participating in Chinese festivals, and playing mahjong. A popular resident activity is a simple form of Tai Chi that residents can do sitting in their chairs.

Segmentation by lifestyle is a common approach to the senior market. Others include social class, health status, income, and usage segmentation. Labels such as *healthy hermit*, *ailing outgoer*, *frail recluse*, and *healthy indulger* have been coined to classify various segments (Moschis and Mathur 1993). Additional classifications include those who are vitally active, those who suffer from health problems but have overcome or adapted to the problems, and those who are overwhelmed by their health issues.

Cohort
A group of people bound together in history by a set of events.

One of the newest ways to segment the market with significant strategic implications for healthcare organizations is by **cohort**. A cohort is a group of people bound together in history by a set of events. The current senior population is made up of three major cohorts. In the United States, those born between 1912 and 1921 were defined by unemployment and the Great Depression. Their thinking and planning are ruled by the idea of financial security. They are conservative spenders, and paying their bills for medical services or prescriptions is a central concern. These individuals place a priority on good bedside manner and are often accepting of the physician's prognosis, although less so now than in previous times. Those born between 1922 and 1927 came of age during World War II. The highest status many of these individuals ever achieved was during this war. They are generally great patients because they trust and accept authority. A final major cohort includes those born between 1928 and 1945, who came of age during the Eisenhower era. It was a time of conformity, and people in this cohort have a great trust in institutions and authority. Each of these cohorts has differing needs and expectations that marketing-oriented organizations can meet.

TIPS FOR MARKETING TO SENIORS

The following tips apply to most, if not all, marketing endeavors to the senior population.

DO NOT CALL THEM "OLD"

First and most important, never call an older buyer "old." Nobody likes to think that he is getting older, and reminding someone of this fact will hurt marketers' chances of success in promoting their products and services. Marketers themselves break this rule by referring to the older segment as the "gray market." In some areas, marketers cling to the outdated concept of the elderly as sick, feeble, and opposed to new ideas and ways of thinking. This conception is no longer accurate—and might never have been.

Members of the current older population view themselves as younger in age and outlook (irrespective of chronological age) than traditional seniors and more in control of their health, their lives, and their environment. They may be coping with hair loss, menopause, or osteoporosis, but they want to be seen as active, involved, vital, sophisticated, and interested. One study found that seniors prefer ads that portray older people as sharp and vibrant, with a sense of humor (Ball State University 2005).

KNOW YOUR BUYERS' INFLUENCERS

Many seniors rely on their grown children for advice. Often a daughter is the caregiver for one or both parents and will influence or actually make decisions such as which nursing home or assisted living facility to choose. The decision-influencing adult child is typically a 45- to 65-year-old married female who lives and works near her parents (Pearce 2007). Research has shown that women in their thirties and forties are the key healthcare decision makers for four generations: themselves, their children, their parents, and their grandparents (Ghent 1994). Ministers, siblings, friends, and grandchildren also help in the decision-making process and should be included where appropriate.

(?) DID YOU KNOW?
More About Cohorts

If you'd like to know more about cohorts, consult any of the following sources:

- Rick Hicks and Kathy Hicks, *Boomers, Xers, and Other Strangers: Understanding the Generational Differences That Divide Us* (Wheaton, IL: Tyndale, 1999)
- Claire Raines and Jim Hunt, *The Xers and the Boomers: From Adversaries to Allies—A Diplomat's Guide* (Berkeley, CA: Crisp Publications, 2000)
- Geoffrey E. Meredith, Charles D. Shewe, and Janice Karlovich, *Defining Markets, Defining Moments* (New York: Hungry Minds, 2002)
- J. Walker Smith and Ann Clurman, *Rocking the Ages: The Yankelovich Report on Generational Marketing* (New York: Harper Business, 1997)
- Richard D. Thau and Jay S. Heflin, *Generations Apart: Xers, Boomers, and the Elderly* (Amherst, NY: Prometheus Books, 1997)

Using mystery shoppers is one way to assess staff competency. A marketer needs information about how potential customers view the organization if he is to approach each market strategically. Information about competitors enables a provider to identify threats and opportunities in the marketplace. A mystery shopper visit can provide this information. This technique is particularly relevant for the assisted living industry. Mystery shopping, which can be conducted by phone or on-site, is a procedure in which an individual with an eye for detail poses as a potential customer and makes an assessment of a facility and its sales presentation. Some market researchers view mystery shopping in services industries as questionable because it may mislead employees into thinking that they are interacting with a real customer (Wilson 2001). However, if the shoppers simply make inquiries instead of positioning themselves as real sales leads, they can obtain enough information to evaluate the level of service the LTC organization provides.

DO NOT USE SCARE TACTICS

Stay away from advertising that uses fear. Advertising has increased in the LTC sector following the example of acute care systems. For years, healthcare organizations have barraged seniors with facts intended to cause fear. An advertising message that says, "If you are 75 years old or older you have a 50 percent chance of having cataracts," may be true, but older consumers tend to filter out promotional messages that use fear as a motivator. "Get your eyes checked so you can read to your grandchildren" may be a better approach. Using fear in an advertising message to seniors could also be interpreted as a form of intimidation and possible elder abuse, so it should be avoided at all costs. General guidelines for successful advertising include keeping the message simple, clear, relevant, well paced, and repetitive. Ads aimed directly at potential clients should use language they can understand. Words like *multiphasic* and *intraocular* should be avoided in favor of everyday vocabulary. The ads that are remembered most frequently are those that provide information about specific services, not image ads, which contain graphics along with text and are matched to a web page's content. Most important, ads should be based on a solid market plan with measurable goals and evaluated results.

EMBRACE COMPLAINTS

Complaints are good. As Microsoft founder Bill Gates says, "Your most unhappy customers are your greatest source of learning" (Hurley 2008). Complainers offer free market research to the savvy marketer. An analysis of complaints or errors can allow marketers to eliminate future problems. The average service never hears about the vast majority of its unhappy consumers. If an organization can recover from a customer complaint by listening carefully to the customer and handling the complaint expeditiously and fairly, that customer's loyalty will likely increase, and she will tell others about the positive treatment she received. Unhappy customers who do not complain are likely to go elsewhere. According to Christopher Lovelock and Jochen Wirtz (2007), the impact of this defection goes beyond the loss of that customer's revenue stream. Not only does it cost much more to attract new customers than to retain current ones, but angry customers often end up giving the organization bad publicity. It makes perfect sense for an organization to prefer customers to complain directly to it rather than to millions of other customers all over the world on the Internet.

HIRE EAGLES, NOT OSTRICHES

Hire solution-oriented people. Most of LTC is a service industry. Because services are produced and consumed simultaneously, the quality of the provider and the quality of the service provided must be measured together. In a facility that provides LTC, residents usually spend more time with facility employees than they do with most family members. Residents are rarely equipped to judge the clinical quality of healthcare services. They can, however, judge their interactions with staff members. Positive interactions strongly influence client perceptions of service quality. How can organizations ensure that service employees are motivated to deliver excellence? One way is hiring the right people. An organization can do this by ensuring that it is the preferred employer and utilizing the selection process to make prudent decisions.

Dr. John Branch (2008) categorizes employees as either eagles or ostriches. He says that eagles circle around in the sky, and when they see a problem they swoop down and fix it. Ostriches, on the other hand, bury their head in the sand when they see a problem. It is easier to hire eagles to begin with than to change an ostrich into an eagle. Hiring a good employee and then providing sound, ongoing training and rewards for good performance are critical. Phyllis Thornton (1994) suggests that employee job descriptions and performance reviews emphasize the employee's role as a customer service representative. Jack Cooper and John Cronin (2000) have found that internal marketing, an effort to train and motivate employees, is essential in LTC. They concluded that training and motivation to provide high-quality service creates a positive perception among the staff and residents of nursing homes. This positive perception spreads throughout the community, reaching potential employees and potential residents.

MANAGE THE ENVIRONMENT

Manage physical cues carefully, as they can have a profound impact on customer impressions. Sights, sounds, smells, and general ambience are important and often indicate the level of quality.

INCORPORATE THE INTERNET AND SOCIAL MEDIA

Over the last decade, access to vast amounts of market knowledge available on the web has given consumers greater control of the marketplace. Technological advances offer an extensive menu of new options to both marketers and consumers, and seniors are no exception. Today consumers have substantially more buying power and a greater amount of information about LTC services. A growing number of seniors are active users of the web. They are not resistant to or fearful of new technology. In fact, many enjoy surfing the web for information on medications, doctors, and service providers as well as taking advantage of the buying power and convenience it affords. It is not uncommon for seniors to turn on the computer first thing in the morning to review the news, access their stock portfolio, and check the weather forecast for their area. Members of the older generation use the Internet to chat with other seniors and e-mail their grandchildren. Furthermore, use of the Internet by the elderly is expected to accelerate as many late technology adopters from the workplace move into retirement. Smart marketers use this technology and such social media sites as Facebook and Twitter to promote healthcare products and services, to stay connected with their senior customers, and to gather marketing data. Seniors have time to surf the web, so when they log on, they tend to stay awhile.

Social media marketing
A form of Internet marketing that seeks to achieve branding and marketing communication goals through participation in various social media networks (MySpace, Facebook, LinkedIn), social bookmarking (Digg, StumbleUpon), social media sharing (Flickr, YouTube), review/ratings sites (ePinions, BizRate), blogs, forums, news aggregators, and virtual 3D networks (SecondLife, ActiveWorlds). Each social media site can be optimized to generate awareness or traffic.

Social media marketing is an ideal way to let older consumers know about products, services, and ideas. The Pew Research Center reports that 61 percent of US adults find health information online, and 60 percent of these e-patients (37 percent of US adults) use the interactive features of websites as a supplement to traditional information sources and to deepen their understanding of a condition and sharpen their questions for health professionals (Fox and Jones 2009). Social media advertising is growing at a faster rate than direct mail, newspaper, broadcast television, cable television, radio, or magazines (Elliot 2005). People who have access to a computer will often look online for information about eldercare options in their area before they search any other source. Whether an LTC provider chooses to create its own website or join others on a resource site, a social media presence for LTC providers is rapidly becoming commonplace.

A Look Ahead

The LTC market is constantly changing and creating new business opportunities. To be successful, marketers must have a strong marketing plan based on meeting the needs, wants, and tastes of seniors. Recognition that the senior market is diverse and heterogeneous supports the concept of segmentation. In healthcare, as in other industries, market segmentation can be based on any number of variables. Important segmentation variables in the senior healthcare arena include age, health status, payer status, income, ethnicity, and some measure of activity level. Segmentation allows an organization to research, advertise, and design services more effectively and efficiently. Use of new marketing strategies such as outreach via the web and social media campaigns will become commonplace in the future for LTC facilities and in the promotion of services for seniors.

The senior market of the future will be different, and strategies that work today may not work tomorrow. The market is large and is growing in number and in political and social power. Marketing strategies based on consumer needs will always allow LTC leaders to survive and to transform challenges into marketing opportunities.

FOR DISCUSSION

1. Define *market segmentation*.

2. Describe the difference between a marketing orientation and a selling orientation.

3. Why do organizations segment markets?

4. List some of the major segmentation variables for the senior market.

5. What are the chief characteristics of an ideal market position?

6. What is the alternative to market segmentation?

7. Is fear a useful technique when advertising to the elderly?

8. List three ways an organization can use the Internet to market to the elderly.

9. How should an LTC organization choose the most attractive market?

10. Where does the communications strategy fall in the marketing mix?

11. Why should consumer needs be the driving force in segmenting a market?

12. Is age alone a good predictor of behavior in the elder market?

CASE STUDY: FOX MEADOW ASSISTED LIVING

Mary Jane Martin, CEO of Fox Meadow Assisted Living Facility, is concerned about the facility's occupancy rate. At one time, the facility enjoyed a dominant position in the area, but its occupancy rate has declined from 90 percent to 70 percent in three years. This erosion is at the hands of other local competitors. Their key market is the baby boomers. The baby boomers are those individuals born during the post–World War II euphoria of 1946 to 1964. The aging of this group has created numerous opportunities for assisted living marketers. The segment numbers almost 80 million Americans and accounts for close to 30 percent of the US population. Mary Jane has directed Tomas Rodriguez, her marketing director, to institute a promotional campaign directed specifically toward this segment. Tomas's advertising objective was to increase requests for information about the facility by 30 percent in three months by using meaningful, believable, and distinctive print advertisements. The execution style for the message was to take a "slice of life" approach. With a promotional print budget of $8,000, Tomas ran a half-page ad in the local weekly free newspaper in four communities surrounding the facility. The ad provided contact information about the facility and pictured a 75-year-old grandmother type sitting in a comfortable rocking chair, doing needlepoint in front of a wood-burning fireplace. The caption read, "Rest and Relax, your time has come!" Following multiple iterations of this ad, the marketing director received a negligible increase in telephone inquiries. He said, "What happened? We did the research."

CASE STUDY QUESTIONS

1. Did this ad clearly target the baby boomer generation? Why or why not?
2. What alternative method of marketing would you suggest? Please include a short draft of your marketing proposal and cost estimate.
3. Who should long-term care providers market to, and why?

CHAPTER 11

Long-Term Care Human Resources

Reid Oetjen, PhD

LEARNING OBJECTIVES

After studying this chapter, you should be able to

➤ provide an overview of human resources, including its essential functions;

➤ provide an overview of legislation that governs human resources;

➤ offer some fundamental advice for managers to consider when conducting the human resources function; and

➤ examine the future trends affecting the long-term care workforce.

INTRODUCTION

Human resources
The practices and poli-
cies that are necessary
to keep the people
side of a business
operating.

Human resources is the lifeblood of all organizations. Human resources refers to practices and policies that are necessary to keep the people side of a business operating. Nowhere is this more critical than in long-term care (LTC), where residents rely on direct care workers to provide some of the most intimate care in healthcare. To be successful, LTC organizations must be noted for the quality of the product they provide, and that quality is directly related to the quality of the organization's workforce. Human resources provides the human capital to meet the needs of clients in LTC.

An organization's human resources team is responsible for developing a human resource plan, recruiting and screening workers, managing training and staff development programs, developing fair compensation guidelines, conducting performance appraisals, terminating employees, developing workplace policies that govern how employees interact within the organization, and ensuring that the organization complies with employment and antidiscrimination laws. Before examining these functions, it is necessary to look at the LTC workforce and the nature of human resources departments in LTC.

Human resources is especially critical to LTC because projections indicate that the elderly population will grow substantially over the next 40 years, which will significantly affect the demand for health and LTC services (Wunderlich, Sloan, and Davis 1996). Additionally, personnel costs are the largest expenditure for any LTC organization, and facilities are facing decreased reimbursement. Thus, LTC organizations must manage this crucial resource effectively to maintain profitability and properly care for residents and consumers. Hiring the right people, training them, keeping them productive, and retaining them as satisfied employees are critical activities.

This chapter explores human resources in the LTC sector. Topics discussed include the five basic functions of human resources, the human resource legal environment, challenges facing human resource professionals, and future trends affecting the LTC workforce. We start the discussion of human resources with a description of the LTC workforce.

THE LONG-TERM CARE WORKFORCE

LTC is a highly labor-intensive service industry, thus human resources plays a large role in its operations. Providing care to frail older adults is physically, mentally, and emotionally challenging. The personal nature of the work underscores the need for a special type of person. The LTC workforce is made up mostly of dedicated individuals who are called to the profession and are committed to working with this vulnerable segment of the population. Fulfilling the human resource role in this environment is one of the greatest challenges in LTC. Thus the human resource functions must be carried out effectively.

The LTC workforce is also a diverse group with a wide range of skills, from highly trained clinicians who may work as consultants to full-time **direct care workers** with little education. The LTC workforce can be divided into four broad categories: direct care workers, other healthcare workers, administrative staff, and other service personnel. The direct care worker category can further be subdivided into professional and paraprofessional. Professional direct care workers include registered nurses (RNs) and licensed practical nurses (LPNs). Paraprofessional direct care workers include certified nursing assistants (CNAs), nursing assistants, home care workers, and other paraprofessionals who work one-on-one with clients in institutional and noninstitutional settings. The majority of these direct care workers (90 percent) are women over the age of 45, more than half are nonwhite, and 20 percent are foreign born (Montgomery et al. 2005). Direct care workers provide an estimated eight of every ten hours of paid care (Paraprofessional Healthcare Institute 2009). Providing patient care in the LTC setting is physically demanding—so much so that the direct care workers in LTC face some of the highest injury rates among all US workers and experience the second highest number of occupational injuries (US Bureau of Labor Statistics and US Department of Labor 2003; Scherzer, Chapman, and Newcomer 2004). Organizations must treat these workers with respect and consider them valued assets.

The second category, other healthcare workers, includes personnel other than direct care workers who are involved in the patient care processes, such as physicians and therapists. The third category, administrative workers, is responsible for managing the direct care and other patient care workers and the service personnel. These individuals include nursing home administrators, directors of nursing, other department heads, and other administrative support personnel who are responsible for the daily operational decisions of LTC organizations. The fourth category, service personnel, includes individuals who work behind the scenes to ensure the smooth operation of facilities and other types of LTC organizations. This group includes dietary personnel, cleaning staff, maintenance personnel, transportation specialists, social workers, and nutritionists.

According to the US Bureau of Labor Statistics (BLS), the LTC industry employs more than 4.7 million workers. In 2009, 2.2 percent of the US workforce was employed as direct care workers, most of whom were employed in LTC settings; these workers make up the largest occupational category in LTC, accounting for almost 62 percent of that workforce. The largest single group of workers in this category is composed of nursing aides, orderlies, and attendants, who make up 42 percent of all direct care workers. Exhibit 11.1 breaks down the LTC workforce by service setting and occupational category.

Direct care workers
Professional and paraprofessional personnel who work one-on-one with clients in institutional or non-institutional settings. Examples include registered nurses, licensed practical nurses, certified nursing assistants, nursing assistants, and home care workers.

DESCRIPTION OF LTC HUMAN RESOURCE DEPARTMENTS

Providers of LTC services include residential institutions, LTC facilities (such as nursing homes and assisted living facilities), and nonresidential service providers or agencies

Exhibit 11.1
Estimates of
Employment in the
Long-Term Care
Delivery System,
2009

Total LTC Employment	4.7 million
Percentage of LTC Employment in the US Healthcare Sector	29.3%
Percentage of LTC Employment in Total US Jobs	3.6%
Total Number of LTC Direct Care Workers	2.9 million
Registered Nurse (RN) & Licensed Practical Nurse (LPN)	644,850
Nursing Aide, Orderly, Attendant, and Home Health Aide	2.2 million

SOURCE: Data from US Bureau of Labor Statistics and US Department of Labor (2009).

that provide home health and hospice care. These organizations either are part of a chain (multifacility organization) or are independent operators. Larger organizations such as chains tend to have dedicated human resource professionals at their corporate office and designated personnel at large facilities such as skilled-nursing facilities and assisted-living facilities.

These centralized human resource departments are responsible for ensuring compliance with human resource law and regulations, determining staffing levels and compensation, developing policies and procedures, conducting or coordinating new hire orientation and training, and maintaining proper employment records.

The human resource function at most other LTC organizations is decentralized and managed at each individual location. These organizations depend on a small core group of managerial staff to oversee the human resource function, including the day-to-day decision making involved in recruitment, hiring, promotions, and accountability for such activities. Typically these duties are the responsibility of the administrator of the facility or agency.

Goals and Functions of Human Resources

The main function of human resources in LTC is to ensure that the organization is properly staffed with qualified personnel who can provide care efficiently and effectively. Additional functions include improving productivity, improving the quality of work life, and ensuring the organization's compliance with laws and regulations. Human resource experts generally refer to the following five basic functions of human resources:

Planning
Forecasting and planning for the short-term and long-term human resources needs of the organization, and establishing standards (skills, knowledge, and ability) necessary for each position.

1. **Planning** refers to two major activities: (a) forecasting and planning for the short-term and long-term human resources needs of the organization and (b) establishing standards (skills, knowledge, ability) for each position. Without this critical function, the other functions would not be necessary.

2. Staffing refers to the recruitment and selection of qualified individuals. This function includes performing job analyses, writing job descriptions, setting compensation levels, and recruiting, screening, and interviewing potential employees.

3. Training and development refers to orienting new employees to the organization's policies and procedures, providing ongoing training and mentoring, and developing employees for promotion.

4. Evaluation involves addressing the issues of job performance at the employee level. This function includes conducting performance appraisals and motivating and counseling employees.

5. Human relations refers to helping to establish and maintain effective working relationships among personnel throughout the organization. This function includes recognizing and respecting employee rights (e.g., nondiscrimination, worker safety), monitoring unionization activities, retaining productive employees, and helping to build a culture of mutual respect whereby employees are committed to the organization.

PLANNING: THE STRATEGIC ROLE OF HUMAN RESOURCES

Most successful LTC organizations understand that human resources is perhaps the most important component in the creation and maintenance of a competitive advantage. However, these same organizations often fail to take human resources into account when making strategic decisions. Human resources needs to be a key player in the strategy formulation process rather than just the group who is responsible for implementing the plan (Tracey and Nathan 2002).

To be successful, human resources must align itself with the key issues and challenges facing the organization. Human resources is responsible for interpreting and managing the key initiatives and organizational strategy defined by the **strategic planning** process. As such, human resources must link staffing, training and development, evaluation, and human relations decisions to the strategic plan.

People are invaluable strategic assets in LTC because they create the culture of caring that is perhaps the most important competitive advantage in this service-intensive industry. Human resources can best fulfill its role as a strategic partner by hiring the best employees and training and developing the workforce in support of this competitive advantage.

Strategic planning
The process of analyzing and identifying the need and availability of human resources to accomplish an organization's objectives.

STAFFING

The most important human resource function is arguably making the correct hiring decisions. All subsequent decisions are subject to failure if the wrong person is selected for the

Staffing
The recruitment and selection of qualified individuals, including performing job analyses, writing job descriptions, setting compensation levels, screening, and interviewing.

Job analysis
The process of collecting information about a job by determining its particular tasks and duties, including the general importance of each.

job. The discussion of **staffing** that follows includes performing job analysis, writing job descriptions, establishing compensation, recruitment, screening applicants, and interviewing applicants.

Job Analysis

Job analysis is the process of collecting information about jobs by determining the tasks and duties of a particular job and the general importance of each task. Specifically, job analysis involves collecting information on the work environment, which may have a significant impact on the physical requirements to perform the job, and noting the tools and equipment employees use to complete the tasks of each job. It also outlines supervisory and reporting relationships and details the knowledge, skills, and abilities the job requires.

The purpose of conducting a job analysis is to improve the organization's performance and productivity. Job analysis focuses on positions within the organization and not individual employees. This process is time consuming and entails a systematic investigation of each position using a framework to guide the process.

The product of a job analysis is a document that details the employment requirements for the position and thus dictates recruitment, compensation, training, and performance appraisals. For instance, a job analysis can identify training needs, such as the content to be included and the method of training. It also helps determine the required skill and educational levels, level of responsibility, and compensation scales.

One typical method organizations use to perform a job analysis includes interviewing current employees to ascertain their tasks and duties; the work environment; the tools and equipment they use; their reporting relationships; and the knowledge, skills, and abilities required to do their job. Once the interview process is complete, the interviewer drafts an analysis, and current employees and supervisory staff review it for accuracy. Like a strategic plan, the job analysis is a living document and should be updated regularly to reflect changes in the job. The information obtained through the job analysis is used to create the job description.

Job Descriptions

Job description
A detailed description of the minimum qualifications and skills necessary to perform the duties of a job.

To select the correct personnel, managers must know what job skills and talents correlate with success in a given position. For instance, compassion and a service orientation are appropriate skills for direct care workers. However, these skills may be less essential to a successful administrator, who would have greater need for vision and strategic thinking. Thus, the first task in the selection process is to establish the prerequisites for success in a particular position. Skill expectations are established by writing **job descriptions**.

Job descriptions are essential to the human resource function. They guide recruitment, selection, and compensation; help communicate job expectations to employees;

		EXHIBIT 11.2 Essential Elements of a Job Description
General Purpose	The job description should list the major responsibilities and the basic purpose of the position, along with goals and how they relate to company objectives.	
Tasks to Be Performed	The job description should list the specific tasks to be performed and the criteria by which they will be judged.	
Related Areas of Responsibility	The job description should list responsibilities related to other departments and divisions. This list helps clarify an employee's role within the organizational structure.	
Standard Duties	The job description should list the standard duties that all employees are expected to perform, such as providing excellent customer service to patients and their families.	

and serve as a foundation for performance appraisal. A job description details the minimum qualifications and skills needed to perform the duties of the job. These minimum qualifications help hiring managers to determine if applicants qualify and to determine compensation levels. The job description explains the duties of the job, including the tasks and responsibilities involved. It may also include job specifications that describe the skills required to perform the job and the job's physical demands. The job description has no set standard for content or format, thus each organization's set of job descriptions varies. Exhibit 11.2 lists the essential elements of a job description.

Like the job analysis, the job description is a living document used to guide performance appraisals, raises, and even dismissals. If the roles and responsibilities of a job change, these changes should be communicated during the performance appraisal process, which is covered later in the chapter.

Exhibit 11.3 shows a sample job description for the CNA position.

Compensation

Compensation includes salary or hourly pay and **benefits** such as health insurance, retirement options, and other fringe benefits such as education reimbursement. Compensation in LTC is low because most LTC positions are low skilled. Consequently, benefit packages are small or nonexistent, which contributes to the high turnover and transiency of these workers. For instance, the lowest-paid workers in the United States are direct care workers, who earned an hourly wage of only $9.56 in 2005, compared to the national average wage of $14.15 (US Bureau of Labor Statistics 2003; National Clearinghouse on the Direct Care

Compensation
The salary or hourly pay and benefits such as health insurance, retirement options, and other fringe benefits such as educational reimbursement that an employee receives.

Benefits
Indirect financial payments given to employees, including health insurance, vacation, and retirement benefits.

EXHIBIT 11.3

CNA Sample Job Description

The CNA is a key person responsible for delivering direct care to and providing a therapeutic environment for the residents under the supervision of the licensed nursing staff. Delivers direct care to residents of our nursing home in accordance with established facility routines, methods, and techniques.

Active certification as a CNA in Massachusetts required. Obtain 12 hours of Continuing Education annually, which includes attendance at mandatory yearly updates (Infection Control, Fire Safety, Resident's Rights, Sexual Harassment, and Hazard Communication) and CPR.

Three full-time positions are open. Position pays $11–$12 per hour requiring evening shift, 2:30 pm–11:00 pm. Excellent benefits package included. AA/EOE

SOURCE: Reprinted with permission of the Seven Hills Foundation.

Workforce 2011). This rate translates to an annual wage for full-time workers of $19,884 per year. However, considering that many direct care workers in LTC only average 30 hours per week, annual salaries are actually less than $15,000 per year (HRSA 2004).

CRITICAL CONCEPT
Avoiding Common Compensation Pitfalls

An organization's level of compensation compared to its competitors can directly affect its ability to recruit and retain employees. A wise approach is to continually scan the market for similar organizations and ensure that compensation packages remain competitive. Especially because many of the jobs in LTC are low skilled and low wage, organizations need to track the compensation of other industries that may also attract low-paid workers.

Avoid the common pitfall of developing rigid pay scales that prohibit raises for exemplary employees who are at the top of the scale. These policies may save money, but they drive employees to competitors with more flexible pay policies.

Recruitment

Recruitment

The process of searching for and attracting new employees to the workforce.

Once the job analysis and job descriptions are completed, human resources can recruit potential employees. **Recruitment** strategies include internal recruitment, word of mouth, advertising, use of internships, contracting with employment agencies, and looking overseas for international candidates. Other options include marketing at local job fairs and recruiting from local schools and educational organizations.

Internal Recruitment

When an organization has a job opening, human resources should conduct an internal search prior to seeking external candidates. LTC organizations typically post internal openings via a bulletin board, e-mail, or the organization's intranet. This method reduces hiring costs by minimizing advertising costs. The downside of recruiting internal candidates is that the organization must fill the job that was vacated by the promoted staff member and train two employees in their new positions, resulting in reduced productivity for a time.

However, a positive impact of seeking internal candidates is the message that the organization values its employees, giving them the opportunity to advance their careers or expand their skill set in a lateral move. Internal recruitment also allows the organization to fill positions with a known quantity, as it has access to the employment history of each internal candidate. Another advantage of selecting internal candidates is that it maintains the stability of the care environment, allowing employees already familiar with residents or consumers to continue these relationships.

Word of Mouth

Another low-cost way to advertise openings is through the informal network of friends, families, and even competitors. This method is especially beneficial because current employees will most likely recruit individuals with whom they get along—a definite boost to a caring and cooperative culture. In fact, research has shown that CNAs recruited by their peers are more likely to remain in their jobs and are more committed (LaPorte 2009). The downside to this method is that employees may develop cliques, which can be disruptive to the care environment.

Advertising

Advertising is another common method for recruiting employees. Forms of advertising include newspaper ads, advertising in trade publications, and Internet job site postings. Advertising can yield a deep field of candidates, but one downside to this recruitment method is that it can be costly, especially advertising in trade publications. Another downside is that newspaper and Internet advertising can flood organizations with résumés from unqualified candidates, especially if the publication and sites enjoy a large readership.

Educational Institutions

Contacting local schools to enquire about recent graduates is an additional method of finding and recruiting talent. These institutions often host job fairs at which employers can recruit students. Many also offer internships or preprofessional practice, whereby students gain real-world experience in the field by working with knowledgeable professionals who act as mentors. Internships can be a source of recruitment if the intern turns out to be an excellent fit with the organization.

Employment Agencies

The majority of staff members work directly for LTC organizations, but staff may also be recruited to fill openings through outside contractors or **employment agencies**. This approach enables an organization to find a qualified workforce while maintaining flexibility. For instance, a majority of LTC providers use agency nurses to augment schedules so that required nursing minimums are met. The downside is that costs for these outside workers can be almost twice as high as for those employed by the organization. However, the flexibility this arrangement offers is invaluable, and it allows organizations to avoid the long-term costs of employment, including retirement and health benefits, and some of the turnover inherent in direct care.

Employment agency
Outside contractors that provide temporary or permanent employees.

International Recruitment

Many LTC providers have been seeking direct care workers from overseas to fill openings, especially for professional roles. For instance, some skilled nursing facilities recruit registered nurses from the Philippines and Puerto Rico. This method can be time consuming and cost prohibitive. Another associated problem is that the candidate's first language is not typically English, thus language barriers may impede the caregiving process.

Screening

Because LTC providers work with a vulnerable population, the workforce undergoes extensive preemployment screening to ensure that candidates have the appropriate background to work with the population. **Screenings** include conducting extensive criminal background checks, reviewing registration boards for clinical personnel, performing drug testing, and extending on-the-job training. Federal regulations require nursing homes to check their state nursing registries to ensure that workers are certified to perform the work, meet all state requirements, and do not have a history of abusing or neglecting clients or misappropriating resources associated with their license (Lewin Group 2006).

Screening
Preemployment procedures to ensure that workers are qualified to work; includes conducting extensive criminal background checks, viewing registration boards for clinical personnel, and drug testing.

Interviewing

Once candidates have been screened and the number of applicants has been reduced to three to five potential hires for a particular position, human resources conducts the interviews. **Interviews** are extremely effective for evaluating potential hires. Interviewers should prepare well for the interview and should thoroughly understand the nature of the job. Each interviewer should study the job description so that he fully understands the requirements of the job and can make an educated hiring decision.

It is best to use open-ended questions so that the candidate has an opportunity to speak and relate personal experiences to the position in question. This format allows interviewers to pick up clues regarding the applicant's recurring patterns of behavior. A practiced interviewer can use open-ended questions to elicit information about how applicants handle stress, how they behave in various situations, their values, and the extent of their commitment to the field.

Each interviewer should have a copy of the questions to be asked, and all candidates should be asked the same questions. The list of questions should include space for interviewers to take notes and a rating scale so that they can rank the candidate. These notes are extremely valuable later in the selection process. Ensuring that each candidate is given the opportunity to answer the same questions minimizes the chance that discrimination occurs and protects the organization from charges of unfairness.

Interview
The process by which an interviewee (prospective employee) is asked questions so that the interviewer (prospective employer) can obtain information from the interviewee.

TRAINING AND DEVELOPMENT

One of the main human resource functions is training. The first step in the training process is to examine the development needs of the organization. For instance, what skills and knowledge are critical to achieving success on the job? What are the new trends in the industry? What changes in the law have occurred?

Training topics in LTC typically cover a wide range of information and skill sets. Many providers do not have the staffing or expertise to conduct all the trainings necessary to keep their workforce up to date with knowledge and skills. If in-house expertise is not available, one option is to outsource training needs. Contracting with a vendor to provide training is often beneficial to organizations because reputable vendors know how other LTC organizations have successfully addressed training issues (Enyeart 2008). This added expertise can be invaluable in tailoring a training program to meet the specific needs of the organization. Training often takes the form of DVD or web-based videos or occurs face-to-face via a seminar or workshop.

A common training situation is orientation. Orientation guides new employees through the basic procedures necessary to function on the job. It may include a tour of the facility, a review of drug use policies and other general employment policies, and information on how to enroll in health and retirement benefits. Additionally, human resources is responsible for ensuring that all employees receive appropriate on-the-job training.

EVALUATION

Evaluation
The determination of employees' job performance; includes performance appraisal, motivation, and counseling.

Another key function of human resources is to provide employees with feedback about their job performance through an **evaluation** that includes a performance appraisal, motivational incentives, and counseling. The **performance appraisal** is typically tied to compensation; thus, it is a serious undertaking and a useful tool in motivating the workforce. Employees want to be given objective feedback about their behavior, and delivering it takes skill and tact. A basic feedback tool is the job description, which provides a foundation by which the employee and employer can measure employee performance. If the roles and responsibilities of a job change, employees should be notified of these changes during their performance appraisals.

Performance appraisal
A systematic employee review that occurs on a regular basis in which the employee receives feedback about her job performance.

An effective performance appraisal clarifies the standards of performance for both the employer and the employee. Each party should understand how job performance is measured and how the appraisal process affects compensation. When employers follow these guidelines, employees tend to view the process as fair because no guesswork is involved in performing the job properly. When employers do not follow them, the impact on employees' morale and perception of management's fairness can be negative.

Behaviorally anchored rating scales (BARS)
A method of employee appraisal that uses numeric scales to measure various levels of effectiveness. This method of appraisal focuses on behaviors that are determined to be important for completing a job task rather than focusing on employee characteristics.

One employee appraisal method that helps simplify the process for supervisors and employees is **behaviorally anchored rating scales (BARS)**. The BARS method uses numeric scales to create various levels of effectiveness, and it focuses on behaviors considered to be important in completing a job task rather than on employee characteristics such as personality (Smith and Kendall 1963). In other words, this method measures performance and not the effectiveness of the person, which is influenced by many variables beyond the control of the individual.

BARS identifies each duty that is necessary for successful completion of the job. A committee should compile the list of duties for a specific job and write a descriptive statement for each duty. Next, it should develop a rating scale for each dimension of the job.

Conducting performance appraisals is time consuming; however, if done properly, they can improve employee behavior and work performance. Appraisals can improve communication between supervisor and staff and even strengthen organizational commitment. Exhibit 11.4 provides a list of tips to guide the performance appraisal process.

Probationary Period

Most states have laws that allow employers to set a 90-day probationary period for new employees. Many organizations make the mistake of ignoring this opportunity to help the new hire start her job in a position to succeed. This is the best time to help new hires understand the expectations of the job and determine if they are a good fit with the organization. In other words, when an employee is not performing adequately during the first 90 days and coaching sessions and on-the-job training do not seem to help, it is wise

EXHIBIT 11.4
Performance Appraisal Tips

1. Keep it simple.	Don't make the process complicated; make it simple and transparent so that all parties understand it.
2. Do not introduce surprises.	Management needs to provide continuous feedback about job performance so that issues raised in annual performance appraisals are not a surprise to the employee.
3. Point out strengths.	Do not focus only on areas in which the employee is deficient.
4. When deficiencies are present, clearly identify any problems.	Be prepared to share specific examples. Look for reasons behind the deficiencies. For instance, is this a training issue? Does the person have access to the necessary tools and resources to perform the job adequately?
5. Focus on the behavior.	Do not attack the person; rather, focus on the behavior in question.
6. Listen.	When conducting performance appraisals, listen to employees and allow them to provide feedback.
7. Do not assume.	Do not make assumptions regarding why employees behave in a certain way. Ask questions to understand their behavior. Too often, performance appraisals are completed prior to meeting with the employee. Be flexible and allow employees to contribute to the final document.

to cut ties with her. If employers allow the 90-day period to pass without taking action, termination becomes incrementally harder and more time consuming.

Counseling

Some employees need **coaching** to improve performance; some need it to correct violations of rules or standards of behavior. Typical issues addressed in coaching include problems with punctuality, lapses in professional behavior, inappropriate attire, inadequate job performance, and insubordination.

When these problems occur, they need to be addressed immediately. This action sends the message to all staff that management is aware of deficiencies and that they will not be tolerated. When employees are coached, the conversation and a plan of action need

Coaching
Feedback and advice given to employees by an immediate supervisor or human resource professionals.

EXHIBIT 11.5

Addressing
Employee
Behavioral Issues

1. Confront the employee. Do not procrastinate.
2. Identify the problem. Be prepared to share specific examples.
3. Listen to the employee, and solicit her feedback.
4. Address the behavior, not the person.
5. Reaffirm the duties and responsibilities of the job.
6. Develop an action plan that establishes goals with specific time frames.
7. Document, document, document. Keep a record of all conversations with employees so that they understand you mean business. As part of the documentation, have employees sign the action plan to confirm receipt.
8. Follow up with the employee at regular intervals to ensure that she understands the action plan and the desired behavior.

to be thoroughly documented in the employee file for two reasons. First, it puts the employee on notice that this problem is serious, and second, it serves as evidence in possible legal proceedings.

When an employee has violated a rule or standard of behavior, discipline must be used. A common approach is progressive discipline. Typically, progressive discipline involves three levels:

1. Verbal warning for the first occurrence
2. Written warning for a second offense
3. Final warning for repeated abuse

> ### ⓘ CRITICAL CONCEPT
> #### When Coaching Fails
>
> Some employees inevitably violate rules and standards of behavior in the workplace. They may repeatedly do so despite repeated coaching attempts. This continued violation is a clear signal that these employees do not value their employment enough to learn their job or change their behavior.
>
> These situations dictate that you terminate the employee as part of your duty as a manager. You may do so by inviting the employee to seek alternative employment or by terminating him outright. Failure to do so will negatively affect the morale of the organization and your ability to effectively manage. Assuming you have tried your best to correct an employee's behavior, you should not feel bad for terminating his employment, as the employee has chosen not to comply.

	2007 (%)	2008 (%)	2009 (%)	2010 (%)
Director of Nursing	37.8	18.1	25.3	26.0
Administrative RNs	28.7	34.2	36.3	28.9
Staff RNs	41.0	42.8	46.7	41.0
LPNs	49.9	43.0	41.8	34.7
CNAs	65.6	53.5	46.6	42.6

EXHIBIT 11.6
Nursing Staff
Turnover Rates in
Nursing Facilities

SOURCE: Data from AHCA (2012).

As employees progress through the discipline steps, they are placed on the levels for increasingly long periods. For instance, an employee may be placed on the first discipline level for 30 days, and if he continues to violate rules during that time, he is placed on the next level for up to 90 days. If the employee continues to violate the conditions of the written and final warnings, termination is warranted. Exhibit 11.5 provides general tips for coaching and disciplining employees.

HUMAN RELATIONS

Human relations encompasses many activities, including establishing and maintaining effective working relationships between managerial and nonmanagerial personnel throughout the organization. This function includes recognizing and respecting employee rights, retaining productive employees, and helping to build a culture of mutual respect and commitment to the organization. Challenges that human resource professionals face in the area of human relations include mitigating employee turnover, ensuring cultural competence, and monitoring unionization. Additionally, human resource staff must be familiar with the host of laws and regulations regarding nondiscrimination and worker safety. Although these challenges are not unique to LTC, they may be more difficult to address than in other sectors of healthcare because of the nature of the LTC workforce and working conditions.

Human relations
Establishing and maintaining effective working relationships among personnel throughout the organization.

Turnover

Turnover refers to the voluntary or involuntary termination of employment. It can also mean movement from one position to another by means of promotion or transfer. The high rate of turnover in LTC is a serious issue that exists throughout the care continuum (Seavey 2004). This problem disproportionately affects the direct care worker in LTC. Exhibit 11.6 presents turnover figures compiled by the American Health Care Association

Turnover
The termination of employment, which can be either voluntary or involuntary.

Exhibit 11.7

Nursing Staff
Vacancy Rates in
Nursing Facilities

	2007		2008		2010	
	Vacant Positions	*Vacancy Rate*	*Vacant Positions*	*Vacancy Rate*	*Vacant Positions*	*Vacancy Rate*
Director of Nursing	686	4.4%	300	1.8%	620	3.9%
Administrative RNs	5,343	10.4%	3,700	8.2%	1,800	4.5%
Staff RNs	19,431	16.3%	8,000	7.9%	8,300	7.0%
LPNs	24,152	11.1%	15,600	5.6%	11,700	4.3%
CNAs	60,266	9.5%	43,700	5.7%	40,000	5.1%
Total	109,877	10.5%	71,300	5.9%	62,420	5.1%

SOURCE: Data from AHCA (2012).

(AHCA) for nurse staffing in skilled nursing facilities. Due to the high turnover, vacancy rates for nursing positions have skyrocketed. Exhibit 11.7 provides AHCA estimates of nurse staffing vacancy rates for skilled nursing facilities.

High turnover significantly drains a provider's bottom line and has other indirect costs that tend to be overlooked. These costs include the likelihood that residents and consumers will receive a lower quality of care from inexperienced workers and decreased employee morale caused by the team's inability to remain intact. Another indirect cost may be incurred when workers are given more work to make up for the vacancy, resulting in greater stress and decreased job satisfaction. The direct costs of turnover in LTC are estimated to be between $4,200 and $5,200 per position (Seavey 2004). The cost of turnover for more highly skilled positions is progressively higher.

Nursing aide turnover is especially disruptive to the care process because aides provide the majority of the essential care to residents and patients. In fact, LTC staff and clients alike report that turnover negatively affects the quality of care (Bowers, Esmond, and Jacobson 2003). Exhibit 11.8 outlines costs associated with turnover.

Retention

Efforts to retain LTC workers pay for themselves. Little research has been conducted on LTC worker retention; however, certain factors can be linked to job loss in LTC, including (1) inadequate compensation, (2) poor working conditions, (3) lack of educational opportunities,

Direct Costs	Indirect Costs
Separation (exit interviews, legal fees, administrative processing)	Decreased productivity (inefficiencies incurred while new staff assume roles vacated)
Vacancy (overtime costs, use of temporary employees)	Decreased quality of care (gaps in service created by having to employ new staff may result in lower quality ratings from regulatory and monitoring agencies)
Replacement (advertising, interviewing, background verification, employment testing and certification, hiring-bonus costs)	Lost clients (consumers may choose to transfer or avoid the facility in response to deterioration in reputation)
Training (formal and on-the-job training)	
Injuries (lost time, workers' compensation costs)	Culture (employee morale may be negative because of increased strain and/or decreased service quality, which may further affect turnover)
$4,200 to $5,200 per job loss	

EXHIBIT 11.8
Indirect and Direct Costs of Turnover

SOURCE: Adapted from Seavey (2004).

1. Fair, knowledgeable, and caring supervisors
2. Nursing supervisors who listen
3. Opportunities for educational advancement
4. Strong sense of belonging to a team
5. Adequate resources

EXHIBIT 11.9
Key Issues in Retention for CNAs

SOURCE: Data from Dawson (2007).

(4) lack of teamwork, and (5) caregiver stress related to the provision of care (Wunderlich, Sloan, and Davis 1996).

CNAs represent one of the largest groups of direct care workers in LTC. A growing body of literature addresses retention of this group and may lend insight into retention of other direct care workers in LTC. Exhibit 11.9 outlines several key strategies for the retention of CNAs.

It is the job of human resources to keep employees motivated to avoid turnover. The following sections share several interventions that have been proven to increase retention in the LTC industry.

Compensation

Although compensation is a motivator, it is not the strongest predictor of retention. R. Tamara Konetzka and colleagues (2005) found that economic factors such as compensation had little or no impact on turnover. Wage and benefit consideration is a necessary component of retention, but it should not be the key strategy. A culture of mutual respect, including employees' relationship with their supervisors, is an important driver of retention.

For clinical staff, the relationship with nursing management is critical. Nurse managers in LTC often do not possess advanced degrees and are promoted based on their clinical expertise. The job of a nurse manager or nursing supervisor requires interpersonal skills. Overall, career development of supervisory staff has a positive impact on nurse retention in LTC facilities. Thus, nurse managers and other administrators must have the proper managerial training to ensure retention of clinical staff.

CRITICAL CONCEPT
The Importance of Creating a Culture of Respect and Caring

> Because compensation is not a lasting motivator, other incentives are necessary to retain staff. The literature indicates that clinical staff members, such as nurses and nursing assistants, stay at an organization when they perceive that they have access to support, resources, and information to succeed in their roles. Thus, employees typically remain with organizations in which they feel valued, listened to, and part of a team.

Culture
The collective values, beliefs, and norms of an organization that shape how it behaves.

Organizational **culture** is the collective values, beliefs, and norms that shape the way an organization behaves. Creating a culture of respect is necessary to retain workers. After all, the direct care workers in LTC should be afforded respect if they are expected to respect the residents and consumers during the provision of care.

Retention Specialist

Another approach to the retention problem is hiring or designating a retention specialist. The person in this role focuses his efforts on evaluating the needs and resources of employees and customizing a retention strategy for the LTC organization, working in conjunction with human resource personnel. Pillemer and colleagues (2008) found that using a retention specialist decreases turnover.

Recognition

One method to retain quality personnel is to provide employees with greater recognition. This can be done at the individual level or at the industry level. At the individual level, outstanding employees who exemplify and understand the importance of caring for frail elders should be celebrated and rewarded for their commitment. Supervisors need to engage frontline employees and recognize their outstanding efforts. When employees are recognized and rewarded for positive behavior, they are likely to repeat such behavior. At the industry level, the LTC industry needs to launch campaigns to share success stories with the community and other audiences.

Educational Opportunities

Opportunities for educational advancement affect retention. Unfortunately, LTC providers have neglected implementing a culture of learning so that their workers are left to pursue educational and career opportunities on their own, which frequently means leaving the field altogether.

Another method to boost retention and perhaps even recruitment, then, is to provide direct care workers with a career ladder program. LTC employers might offer entry-level workers educational opportunities to help them acquire the skills necessary to advance to better-paying jobs.

Cultural Competence in LTC

Cultural diversity is a major issue in LTC and one that must be addressed; otherwise, employee unrest may lead to turnover. **Cultural competence** can be defined as the ability of individuals or organizations to understand the global view of clients from diverse cultures and adapt their practices to ensure effective provision of care (Stanley et al. 2009). Ninety percent of the administrators in nursing homes are Caucasian, and the vast majority of direct care workers are of other ethnicities. Additionally, almost 90 percent of the residents in LTC facilities are Caucasian—the atmosphere is ripe for cultural clashes. As previously mentioned, the industry can ill afford to have direct care workers leave their job for any reason, let alone because of cultural conflict.

Human resource management in LTC must proactively educate workers about cultural competence as a matter of smart business. If an organization is perceived to be culturally competent, employees and clients will be attracted to it.

Cultural competence
The ability of individuals or organizations to understand the global view of clients from diverse cultures, and adapt their practices to ensure their effectiveness.

Cultural competence requires that employees learn to respect and value other cultures and includes how residents are viewed, attitudes toward self-care, perceptions of family visits, familiarity with food choices, level of reluctance to ask for help, and attitudes toward supervision. In other words, the recipient of care should feel as much at home as possible in the care setting. The LTC workforce must be culturally sensitive to the needs of residents, consumers, and coworkers.

Mandatory diversity training sends the message to all employees that cultural diversity is valued and respected. The organization's leadership must also embrace this message; otherwise, employees will not value or be committed to this effort. The goals of a cultural sensitivity training program should be to (1) foster good communication and (2) prevent discrimination and harassment. One example of such training is language training to foster communication.

Unionization

Employers in all industries, including LTC, have long expressed their displeasure with labor unions and have acted to prevent unionization. Administrators and other management personnel abhor the idea of unionization because it limits their ability to change work rules without consulting the union and the collective bargaining contract. In other words, unionization implies a loss of control for managers.

Labor union
A group of workers that organizes for the purpose of furthering the social and economic well-being of its membership.

A **labor union** is group of workers who organize to further the social and economic well-being of its membership. Unionization was made legal by the Wagner Act of 1935, which allowed workers to organize and to bargain collectively.

National Labor Relations Act (NLRA)
Originally called the Wagner Act, this 1935 act provides specific guidelines to govern the relationship between unions, organizations, and workers.

Despite the feelings of employers, workers have the right to organize or to refrain from joining a union. The **National Labor Relations Act (NLRA)** (later amended by the **Taft-Hartley Act**) governs the unionization process. Taft-Hartley was amended in 1974 to include coverage of employees working in nursing homes and private hospitals. According to the Bureau of Labor Statistics (2011), only 11.9 percent of workers, or one in eight, were union members in 2010. This number is projected to increase over the next several years because many manufacturing jobs—the traditional source of unionized workers—continue to be outsourced overseas.

Taft-Hartley Act
A 1947 act that defines and prohibits unfair labor practices by unions. Formally called the Labor–Management Relations Act.

Another factor that may spur unionization is that Medicare and Medicaid continue to reduce reimbursement to LTC providers. As a result, less money is available for workers' salaries and benefit packages. Coinciding with this trend is many states' establishment of minimum staffing levels, which has placed further financial pressures on employers. Also, many direct care workers feel the added stress of employer demands for higher productivity and cost containment. These pressures may drive workers toward unions to help increase salaries and establish reasonable workloads.

Working in a unionized organization adds a layer of complexity, so most organizations try to prevent workers—to the extent allowed by law (see the next section)—from unionizing. Perhaps the most effective method to do so is through open and honest communication with staff. When employees feel that their opinions are heard and valued, they identify closely with the organization. Another approach to minimizing unionization activity is to remain competitive with other employers in terms of compensation and work conditions. When an employer deals with workers in a fair and consistent manner and fosters a culture of openness and community, employees are less likely to unionize than if the employer maintains an undesirable environment in which to work.

Laws Governing Unionization

Numerous laws govern the unionization process and outline the rights of workers and employers. The following sections discuss key regulations of which human resource professionals should be aware to maintain compliance with the law, should a group of LTC workers decide to unionize (Gellatly 2007).

Ninety-Day Notice Requirement

Collective bargaining contracts that include healthcare organizations must provide a 90-day notice to the other party prior to contract expiration. Additionally, they must provide the Federal Mediation and Conciliation Service (FMCS) a 60-day notice. Other industries need only provide a 60-day and 30-day notice, respectively. The additional 30 days allows healthcare organizations to prepare so that patient care does not suffer.

Mandatory Mediation

Parties involved in a dispute are required to participate in mandatory **mediation** if the FMCS believes that the threat of a **strike** or an actual strike will "substantially interrupt the delivery of healthcare" (LMRA; 29 USCS Sec. 141–197, 1947). In such cases, the director of the FMCS has the authority to appoint a board of inquiry to investigate and issue nonbinding recommendations.

Mediation
An intervention in which a neutral third party attempts to assist two parties in reaching a mutually agreed upon solution.

Ten-Day Strike Notice

This amendment requires labor unions to provide a ten-day (including exact time and day) notice to the healthcare facility prior to striking or picketing. If this notice is not given, the facility may immediately terminate any employees involved in the strike. The purpose of this amendment is to give the healthcare provider ample notice to plan for the care of its patients. Unions can be exempted from this requirement if it is determined that the employer has abused this ten-day notice period by engaging in "preparatory steps"; however, the legislation does not provide examples of these steps.

Strike
An organized work stoppage orchestrated by a union.

Conditions Retaining Neutral Status

This rule applies to secondary strikes that could affect facilities that agree to accept transfer patients from a facility whose employees are on strike. This rule bars the union from picketing and requesting that workers at this facility strike to show solidarity.

Nonsolicitation Rules

Section 7 of the NLRA states that "employees shall have the right to self-organization, to form, join or assist labor organizations." It is unfair for employers "to interfere with, restrain, or coerce employees in the exercise of rights guaranteed" by Section 7. The National Labor Relations Board (NLRB) allows employees to solicit for unions during free time at work, as long as such solicitation is not conducted in patient care areas. Examples of areas where solicitation is prohibited include residents' rooms and sitting rooms on patient floors (Gellatly 2007).

Right to Work

Right to work
A statute that declares it to be unlawful to require union membership as a condition of employment; however, the union in question is responsible for representing all workers in the bargaining unit.

A **"right to work"** state is one in which it is unlawful to require union membership as a condition of employment but the union in question is responsible for representing all workers in the bargaining unit. Currently, 21 states have right-to-work laws. In effect, these laws make it harder for unions to become established in these states.

LEGAL AND REGULATORY COMPLIANCE

One of the most important duties of human resources is to ensure that the organization complies with federal labor laws. These laws protect the rights and safety of individuals. They can be grouped into two broad categories that cover hiring, compensation, promotion, and dismissal: Antidiscrimination laws prohibit discrimination in the workplace, and worker safety laws protect workers from performing their job in an unsafe environment.

These laws continually change, thus human resources must ensure that the organization remains in compliance with them. Each state and local municipality may have laws that further define antidiscrimination and worker safety.

TITLE VII OF THE 1964 CIVIL RIGHTS ACT

Civil Rights Act of 1964
A law that makes it illegal to discriminate in employment based on race, color, religion, sex, or national origin.

The intent of the **Civil Rights Act of 1964** was to prohibit and prevent discrimination against any individual in the employment process. Specifically, it prohibits employment discrimination based on race, color, religion, sex, and national origin (EEOC 1964). In 1967, the Civil Rights Act was amended to in order to prohibit age discrimination against those aged between 40 and 65. This was accomplished through the Age Discrimination in Employment Act of 1967. It has been amended since to include new protections and will continue to evolve.

EQUAL EMPLOYMENT OPPORTUNITY ACT OF 1972

The 1972 legislation expanded coverage established under Title VII of the Civil Rights Act to include public and private employers with 15 or more employees, labor organizations with 15 or more members, and public and private employment agencies. It created the Equal Employment Opportunity Commission, whose purpose is to enforce various antidiscrimination laws and to conduct investigations into allegations of discrimination (EEOC 2012).

Equal employment opportunity
A concept that assumes that all individuals are entitled to equal treatment.

PREGNANCY DISCRIMINATION ACT OF 1978

This act amends the sex discrimination section of the Civil Rights Act of 1964. It broadens the definition of gender discrimination to include pregnancy, childbirth, and related medical conditions. Employees cannot be terminated because they are pregnant or intend to become pregnant (EEOC 2008).

FAIR LABOR STANDARDS ACT (1936)

The **Fair Labor Standards Act (FLSA)** applies to "employees who are engaged in interstate commerce or in the production of goods for commerce, or who are employed by an enterprise engaged in commerce or in the production of goods for commerce." The FLSA established a minimum wage and guaranteed that workers would receive time-and-a-half pay for overtime in certain nonexempt jobs. Several exemptions free employers from the minimum wage, overtime, and record-keeping requirements, such as so-called white-collar jobs, which include salaried staff such as administrators.

Fair Labor Standards Act of 1936
A law that established standards for minimum wage, maximum hours, and overtime pay.

In 2004, legislation was passed that further defined which workers were exempt from overtime pay. These exemptions address exclusion of healthcare personnel from overtime standards. To be excluded, or exempted, employees must meet certain tests and be salaried, earning more than $455 per week. LPNs, nursing aides, and similar personnel do not typically qualify because they are not learned professionals (i.e., holding a specialized advanced academic degree is not a prerequisite for entry into these occupations). An argument for exempting RNs can be made because their work requires advanced knowledge in a field of science or learning and requires an extended course of specialized intellectual instruction (US Department of Labor Employment Standards Administration and Wage and Hour Division 2008).

Equal Pay Act of 1963

Equal Pay Act of 1963
An amendment to the Fair Labor Standards Act that requires equal pay for equal work, regardless of sex.

An amendment to the FLSA, the **Equal Pay Act** sought to eliminate wage differentials based on gender (sex). In other words, all employees are entitled to receive equal pay for equal work (Equal Employment Opportunity Commission 1963).

Age Discrimination in Employment Act of 1967

Age Discrimination in Employment Act of 1967
An act that prohibits age-based discrimination for applicants or employees over the age of 40.

This law prohibits discrimination based on age for applicants and employees older than 40 in hiring, promotions, wages, terminations, and layoffs. The **Age Discrimination in Employment Act** also requires that certain pensions and benefits be provided to employees and that the general public receive information about older workers' needs. Prospective employers are prohibited from posting statements regarding age preference and limitations. Employers are also prohibited from denying benefits to employees on the basis of their age, unless they can provide reduced benefits to older workers for the same cost as providing full benefits to younger workers. Lastly, this law prohibits mandatory retirement, except for executives meeting certain qualifications.

Family and Medical Leave Act of 1993

Family and Medical Leave Act of 1993 (FMLA)
An act that allows eligible employees to take off up to 12 workweeks in any 12-month period for the birth or adoption of a child, to care for a family member, or if the employee has a serious health condition.

This law provides eligible employees unpaid leave of up to 12 workweeks during any 12-month period for any of the following reasons: (1) birth and care of the employee's newborn child, (2) adoption or foster care of the employee's child, (3) care of an immediate family member of the employee (spouse, child, or parent) with a serious health condition, or (4) medical leave for a serious health condition of the employee. The **Family and Medical Leave Act** applies to all public employers and to private-sector employers with 50 or more employees within 75 miles. To be eligible, employees must meet the following conditions:

1. The employer must be covered by the act.
2. The employee must have worked for the employer for at least 12 months.
3. The employee must have worked at least 1,250 hours over the previous 12 months.
4. The work location must be in the United States or in any territory or possession of the United States, and the employer must employ at least 50 employees within 75 miles.

Employment at Will

This doctrine applies to any employment relationship in which either party can terminate the relationship without liability, provided no contract is in place that specifies a definite term and the employer is not part of a union. Thus, the employer may discharge individuals without cause, and the employee is free to quit, strike, or cease working. This doctrine is subject to other employment and antidiscrimination laws; if terminating an employee without cause violates an antidiscrimination law, the **employment at will** doctrine does not apply.

AMERICANS WITH DISABILITIES ACT OF 1990

The **Americans with Disabilities Act (ADA)** prohibits discrimination on the basis of disability. The act defines disability as a physical or mental impairment that substantially limits a major life activity. The ADA prohibits qualifying employers (those with 15 or more employees) from discrimination in job application procedures, hiring, advancement, termination, workers' compensation, training, and other terms or conditions of employment. Other forms of discrimination include

- adversely limiting or classifying an applicant or employee,

- denying employment opportunities to qualified persons,

- failing to make reasonable accommodations to the known physical or mental limitations of disabled employees in the course of employment or training, and

- not promoting employees with disabilities.

Employers must make reasonable accommodations for disabled persons who can otherwise perform the essential duties of the job. Reasonable accommodation is defined as actions that permit an applicant or employee with a disability to perform the activities involved in the job in a reasonable manner. This applies to, but is not limited to

- an accessible worksite,

- acquisition or modification of equipment,

- support services for hearing or vision impairments, and

- job restructuring and modified work schedules.

WORKER SAFETY LAW

Worker safety law is the second broad area of human resource law and was created to provide a safe environment for employees. The main law that governs workplace safety is the Occupational Safety and Health Act.

Employment at will
A doctrine of employment in which the employer is free to discharge individuals without cause and the employee is free to quit, strike, or cease working at any time.

Americans with Disabilities Act of 1990 (ADA)
An act that prohibits discrimination due to disability and applies to job application procedures, hiring, advancement, termination, workers' compensation, training, and other terms or conditions of employment.

OCCUPATIONAL SAFETY AND HEALTH ACT OF 1970

Occupational Safety and Health Act
This law was passed to ensure safe and healthful working conditions.

This legislation created the Occupational Safety and Health Administration (OSHA), whose primary responsibility is to enforce regulations that protect workers from safety and health hazards involved in completing the tasks their jobs require. OSHA oversees the work environment, taking into account its physiological, physical, and psychological effect on an organization's workforce (Schuler 1987). Organizations are less likely to experience lost productivity that results from worker injuries when they fully comply with environmental safety and worker health mandates.

LTC is one of the most injury-prone industries in the United States. In 2003, 10.1 injuries or illnesses occurred in the workplace per 100 full-time nursing and residential care facility workers. By comparison, only 6.8 such injuries or illnesses occurred per 100 workers in the construction industry and 5.0 occurred per 100 workers in all private workplaces (US Bureau of Labor Statistics 2008). If an organization can provide and maintain a safe work environment, costs associated with employee injury can be avoided, as can the cost of turnover.

WORKERS' COMPENSATION

Workers' compensation
Insurance that provides compensation for medical care and rehabilitation for, and provides settlements to, employees who are injured during the course of employment.

Workers' compensation insures workers against injury during the course of employment. Most states govern this process and require that employers purchase private insurance or provide self-coverage. Workers' compensation provides employees with medical care, rehabilitation services, and financial settlements for workplace injuries. In exchange for this coverage, workers forfeit the right to seek legal action and damages (US Department of Labor 2011).

CURRENT AND FUTURE DIRECTION IN LTC HUMAN RESOURCES

Workforce issues are perhaps the biggest challenge facing the LTC system and will continue to be for the foreseeable future. LTC in the long term depends on the ability of human resources to confront such issues as caring for an aging population and its increasing disease acuity, staff shortages and employee retention, cultural competence, and the globalization of healthcare.

AGING POPULATION AND DISEASE ACUITY

Individuals older than 85 constitute the fastest growing segment of the US population. These individuals are at an increased likelihood of needing LTC services and institutionalization. The projected growth of the elderly population will exacerbate current nursing shortages.

A by-product of the aging population is the increase in acuity of LTC clients' diseases. These residents and consumers of LTC services are predicted to require a higher level of skilled care (Hollinger-Smith, Ortigara, and Lindeman 2001). As a result, the industry will have to become more diverse than it is currently and attract more skilled workers and different clinical professionals than it does now. The skill and education required by direct care workers, both professional and paraprofessional, will need to increase substantially.

For example, more than 47 percent of all persons older than 85 are estimated to have a form of dementia (Evans et al. 2003). Thus, LTC organizations will rely more heavily on advanced practitioners to conduct the bulk of patient care processes. This reliance will increase human resource professionals' burden of providing training and educational opportunities to maintain employees' certifications.

LTC STAFFING SHORTAGES

A chronic shortage of direct care workers has plagued nursing facilities and other LTC providers in the United States for more than a decade.

The results of a 2008 survey conducted by the AHCA indicates that nearly 110,000 direct care positions were vacant in 2007, including 1 in 6 staff RN positions, 1 in 9 LPN positions, and 1 in 10 CNA positions. Despite LTC providers' desire to fill these positions, qualified candidates were scarce (AHCA 2008).

Currently, many states mandate minimum staffing levels for nursing personnel, and these nurse-to-patient ratios have been shown to positively affect the quality of care (Castle and Engberg 2007). As a result of these findings, states will most likely legislate increased staffing levels in institutionalized settings to improve quality, which will require more personnel than currently are in place. And the aging of the baby boomer population will require yet more personnel. The number of elders will increase from 35.9 million people older than 65 living in 2005 to more than 72 million by 2030 as the baby boomer population benefits from medical advances and the resulting increase in life expectancy (He et al. 2005).

Paraprofessionals such as nursing assistants, home health aides, and personal assistants are also in short supply, and shortages in the physician ranks will rise, as only 3 of the nation's 1,145 medical schools have geriatric departments and courses in geriatrics are required at less than 10 percent of medical schools (Kovner, Mezey, and Harrington 2002). Currently, only 1 percent, or 6,600, of the nation's physicians are certified in this field. Population growth projections of the elder population indicate that an estimated 36,000 geriatricians will be needed to meet the demand of our growing elderly popularization (Kovner, Mezey, and Harrington 2002).

Another factor affecting staff shortages in LTC is the aging of the workforce. Older workers will not likely be able to continue in their roles because of the physical and taxing nature of the job. The average RN is currently 45 years of age (US Bureau of Health Professions Division of Nursing 2001). The rate of new professionals entering the field is projected to decrease significantly over the next 20 years, compared with the retirement rate.

The collective effect of these trends is that the need for skilled personnel will skyrocket. Those responsible for human resources in the LTC industry will have to come together to address this critical need. Without decisive action by both private and public sectors to develop a qualified workforce, this problem will worsen, culminating in a crisis (Stone and Harahan 2010).

EMPLOYEE RETENTION

Retention will continue to be a major theme in LTC human resources, as a study by Miller, Booth, and Mor (2008) suggests. The 39 experts interviewed for the study indicated that the poor image of caring for the elderly that prevails among the US workforce will likely continue, further affecting the ability of LTC organizations to attract workers. Human resource professionals in the LTC industry face an almost insurmountable challenge in turning this image around. If they fail to create and adopt professionally rewarding work environments, LTC will be unable to attract and retain high-quality workers who have a passion for providing care.

CULTURAL COMPETENCE

The aging of the baby boom generation will drive demand for LTC service over the next 40 years. One sector of this population is minority elders, who constitute the fastest growing segment of the elderly. As a result, the US Census Bureau (Vincent and Velkoff 2010) has projected that by 2050, the nation's racial and ethnic diversity will have increased and the population will be much older. At a minimum, the increased diversity of our LTC population will require the workforce to be culturally sensitive. Exhibit 11.10 provides current population estimates and projections for elderly minorities.

Globalization
The increased interdependence of nations to produce and consume goods and services.

GLOBALIZATION

LTC is not immune to the globalization phenomenon affecting all other industries, including the acute care system. **Globalization** can be defined as the increased interdependence of nations to produce and consume goods and services. In the future, the United States will increasingly rely on other countries to provide LTC workers. Organizations

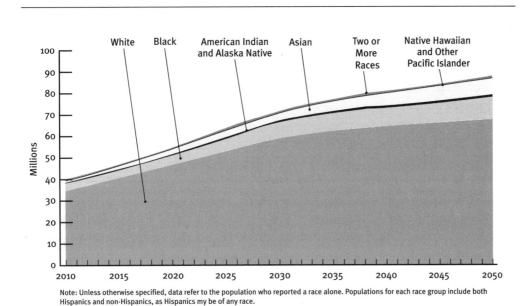

EXHIBIT 11.10
Projected US
Population Older
than Age 65, by
Race: 2010 to 2050

Note: Unless otherwise specified, data refer to the population who reported a race alone. Populations for each race group include both Hispanics and non-Hispanics, as Hispanics my be of any race.

SOURCE: US Census Bureau (2008c).

will have to adopt policies to address cultural competence and other issues related to staffing decisions. Additionally, LTC providers may face intense competition from providers overseas.

LTC WORKFORCE IMPLICATIONS

To meet these challenges and overcome unforeseen obstacles, the LTC industry must proactively expand the supply of qualified workers, invest in workforce education and development, and increase the level of competition for LTC positions (Stone and Harahan 2010).

EXPANDING THE LTC WORKFORCE

Expanding the LTC workforce will require the collaboration of private and public sectors to structure financial incentives, such as education loan forgiveness, to attract administrators and clinicians. Government entities should consider developing grants, scholarships, and federal traineeships in support of this effort.

One current example is the US Department of Labor's Long-Term Care Regional Apprentice Program. This program combines classroom instruction and on-the-job training with opportunities for career advancement for CNAs (US Department of Labor, Employment and Training Administration 2010). Other initiatives include training older workers and retirees to fill the gap between demand and supply of LTC workers. For instance, the Senior Community Service Employment Program, another Department of Labor grant initiative, has been successful in this effort (Hwalek, Straub, and Kosniewski 2008).

INVESTING IN THE LTC WORKFORCE

To develop and maintain a high-quality workforce, the private- and public-sector entities will have to make a joint commitment. Failure to do so will send a clear signal that society does not value the aging population.

The starting point in this effort will be to review the formal system of training and licensing that currently guides the process. Educators and policymakers will need to objectively assess current curricula, training programs, and licensing standards to discern whether these efforts meet the developmental needs of the LTC workforce. From here, they should identify specific competencies and develop curricula to ensure that future workers have the proper skill set (Stone and Harahan 2010).

INCREASING THE LEVEL OF COMPETITION

Finally, policymakers and the long-term industry need to collaborate to ensure that LTC careers become competitive with the broader healthcare market. Their compensation and wages need to be commensurate with those in the acute care sector. One solution may be to create incentives via Medicare and Medicaid rate increases for employers who retain workers and, as a result, achieve better outcomes (Better Jobs Better Care 2005).

A LOOK AHEAD

The LTC industry relies on people, perhaps more than any other industry. The care that the LTC workforce provides is the competitive advantage that differentiates providers in the marketplace. As such, the role of human resources is critical.

The future of the LTC industry depends on the ability of human resource professionals to recruit and retain qualified personnel. To be successful, the industry as a whole will need to address the image problems that have plagued LTC since its inception. Human resources, in its strategic role, will need to be a major player in this initiative.

For Discussion

1. What characteristic of the LTC workforce makes managing this group unique in all of healthcare?

2. What are the four broad categories of the LTC workforce?

3. What group of employees makes up the majority of the LTC workforce?

4. What does the typical LTC human resources department look like?

5. What is the main function of human resources?

6. List and briefly describe the five basic functions of human resources.

7. What are several methods to recruit employees?

8. Why is it necessary to screen workers entering the LTC workforce? What does screening entail?

9. What are the direct and indirect costs associated with turnover?

10. What key issues are related to turnover of the LTC workforce?

11. What key issues are related to retention of the LTC workforce?

12. What are the requirements necessary for employees to take advantage of family and medical leave as provided by the Family and Medical Leave Act of 1986?

Case Study: Retaining Certified Nursing Assistants

Certified nursing assistants (CNAs) are the backbone of long-term care. CNAs are tasked with the basic tasks that nurses used to perform, including toileting, bathing, changing diapers, and other "dirty" jobs. The turnover rate for these direct care workers is more than 70 percent (Bishop et al. 2008). LTC administrators spend time and money and lose productivity because of this turnover. CNA turnover has been estimated to cost more than $2,500 per occurrence (Seavey 2004). In addition to these direct costs, CNA turnover negatively affects residents' quality of life (Bishop et al. 2008). As such, it is critical for LTC administrators to be proactive and develop programs to retain these valuable employees. However, to develop effective programs, administrators need to understand the underlying factors that help retain CNAs.

Christine E. Bishop and colleagues (2008) found that the quality of CNAs' relationships with their direct supervisors was a key factor in remaining in their positions. Additionally, CNAs were more likely to remain in their positions when the proportion of CNAs that were committed to their jobs was high—if morale among CNAs was good, CNAs remained in their positions. The Iowa CareGivers found that the main reasons CNAs leave the job are short staffing, poor wages and benefits, lack of respect, and inadequate training and education (Iowa CareGivers Association 2000).

Several states have launched initiatives to retain CNAs. One Iowa initiative to retain CNAs offered focused training on topics such as caring for Alzheimer's patients. This program was effective in increasing CNA retention because it showed CNAs that they were valued enough for their organizations to invest in training. Another effective method for increasing job satisfaction and retention was instituting a lead CNA program in which experienced and top-performing CNAs were recognized and rewarded for their knowledge and dedication to their profession. Such programs typically involve a small pay increase, but more important, they give CNAs the recognition that is typically lacking (Iowa CareGivers Association 2000).

Other initiatives, such as including CNAs in decision making, may also be promising. For instance, administrators might consider including CNA supervisors in daily staff meetings and strategic decision making. After all, CNAs spend more time working directly with residents and much can be gained from their unique insight. Such efforts would help address the lack of respect that causes CNAs to leave the profession.

Better Jobs Better Care, a national initiative aimed at solving issues facing the direct care workforce, sponsored demonstration projects, including one that provided CNAs with subsidized housing. In addition, CNAs in the program had access to free transportation to and from the home, healthcare benefits, as well as a childcare stipend (BJBC 2008). Programs such as these go a long way to showing that CNAs are a valuable part of the long-term care workforce.

CASE STUDY QUESTIONS

1. What are the four main reasons CNAs leave their jobs?

2. Using the answer from the previous question, design a program to retain CNAs in your long-term care facility. Remember to provide citations for any sources used.

3. State how your initiative resolves two or more of the four main reasons that CNAs leave the profession.

CHAPTER 12

Legal Issues in
Long-Term Care

Edward L. King, RN, JD, EdD

LEARNING OBJECTIVES

After studying this chapter, you should be able to

➤ differentiate between statutes, common law, and natural law;

➤ explain the concept of federalism as it applies to the US legal system;

➤ differentiate between criminal and civil law cases and identify common legal cases healthcare administrators encounter in an LTC setting;

➤ explain the use of advance directives, such as the healthcare proxy, living will, and physician orders for life-sustaining treatment forms in the LTC setting; and

➤ use principles of healthcare ethics when confronted with an ethical dilemma.

INTRODUCTION

Healthcare administrators in long-term facilities are confronted with myriad federal, state, and local regulations. Even lawyers recognize that the vast body of healthcare law and regulation cannot be memorized. The policies and procedures set by the LTC facility must follow these regulations to avoid legal sanctions. With experience, administrators can gain understanding of the specific regulations that pertain to their industry.

This chapter provides an overview of healthcare law as it applies to LTC.

! CRITICAL CONCEPT
Code of Ethics

When confronted with a legal issue that is difficult to address immediately, the healthcare administrator's best response is to remain calm, take a deep breath, and indicate he will report back on this issue in a timely way. Before leaving the immediate situation, the administrator should make sure he has a thorough understanding of all the facts related to the issue at hand. He should not alter or move any item to make the situation appear more favorable to the institution. Any cover-up is more egregious than the original violation, and falsifying paperwork is a crime.

As the administrator's career advances, mistakes are inevitable, and he should view them as learning opportunities, not as a reflection of his character. His level of integrity, however, must be constant and above any degree of suspicion.

The American College of Health Care Administrators (ACHCA), a membership association for LTC leaders, created an ethics code for its members. If an administrator is asked to perform any activity that is illegal or in violation of the ACHCA's code of ethics (see www.achca.org/index.php/about-achca), he must refuse. Instead, he should refer to the institution's written policy and procedure manual to determine how to report this request to management. Superiors or other administrators seldom, if ever, overtly ask another professional to do something illegal or unethical. Beware, however, of the seemingly innocuous favors requested or the expressed desire to cut corners, as these incidents are the ones that usually lead to trouble.

Introduction to Legal Issues

The Concept of Federalism Within the United States

The United States' statutes, or laws, are based on the concept of **federalism**. Each state is free to pass its own laws as long as those laws are not prohibited by and do not contradict the US Constitution. The Tenth Amendment to the Constitution, the last amendment in the Bill of Rights, states: "The powers not delegated to the United States by the Constitution, nor prohibited by it to the States, are reserved to the States respectively, or to the people" (US Constitution 1791).

The federal government's ability to compel a state to enforce **federal law** is limited. In *New York v. United States*, for example, the US Supreme Court invalidated a portion of the Low Level Radioactive Waste Policy Amendments Act of 1985 because it mandated the state to enforce federal regulations. The federal government may encourage the states to adopt regulations by providing federal funds (spending power) or by preempting state law through federal law (commerce power) (*New York v. United States* 1992), but it cannot require a state to administer a federal program. In 1997, the Supreme Court struck down the Brady Handgun Violence Prevention Act because it forced the states to administer a federal program. Justice Antonin Scalia cited *New York v. United States* in the majority's opinion (*Printz v. United States* 1997).

Civil Law

Civil cases are brought by individuals, corporations, or governmental authorities to enforce a right or collect damages when injuries have occurred. The party bringing the lawsuit to court is the **plaintiff**. The party being brought to court is the **defendant**.

Many civil cases in healthcare arise from care, or lack of care, provided to residents that deviates from the written care plan and results in injury to the resident. The plan of care should conform to standard-of-practice guidelines, and the staff should follow the plan precisely. The institution can also face fines and legal sanctions affecting licensure if it violates the civil rights of residents or breaches their privacy rights under the **Health Insurance Portability and Accountability Act of 1996 (HIPAA)**.

In the event that an individual loses his job, Title I of HIPAA protects that worker's health insurance coverage. Title II of HIPAA, the Administrative Simplification provisions, requires national standards to be established for electronic healthcare transactions. It also mandates the establishment of national identifiers for healthcare providers, insurance plans, and employers. Those who violate HIPAA face monetary sanctions.

Another federal law with which healthcare providers must comply is the **Americans with Disabilities Act of 1990 (ADA)**. Residential facilities may not discriminate against the disabled in their admission policies. Their buildings must allow access for wheelchairs and other assistive devices; facilities must provide reasonable accommodations to any individual needing care within or entry to the institution. In addition to federal guidelines, the organization must meet local fire safety codes concerning the space and provide for parking availability. Federal and local requirements are complex, but compliance is mandatory. The federal government disseminates information regarding the ADA online at www.ada.gov.

An LTC institution can be sued for breach of contract by any individual or entity with which it has contracted, for negligence or malpractice by its patients, or under labor laws for its dealings with its employees. In some institutions, unions represent the workers. In a union setting, the contract between the employer and the workers is a binding document; breaching its regulations can lead to costly litigation. The freedom to form a union within an institution is set forth in the proposed Employee Free Choice Act. The proposal mandates counting worker union cards and provides guidelines regarding the union officials' election process. As such, unionized workers have the right to sue in order to enforce contracts with their suppliers, patients' families, or unions.

Civil cases are initiated when the plaintiff serves the defendant with a summons and complaint. The summons indicates which court is hearing the case, and the complaint contains the sworn allegations of fact that form the basis for the case. The defendant has to prepare an answer, and the summons must be served within a certain period of time. An administrator who is served with a summons and complaint should immediately turn it over to the organization's legal department or insurance company to avoid a **default judgment**. A default judgment occurs when the defendant fails to answer the summons and the complaint. In the event of a default judgment, the court may find in the plaintiff's favor, but **due process** safeguards built into the system protect defendants.

The choice of court at which the case is heard depends on the subject matter of the case. Civil cases involving the LTC industry are usually heard in the state's civil trial court. If a federal issue is involved, it may be heard in the federal district court for that location. The jurisdiction of the federal courts is set forth in the Seventh Amendment to the US Constitution, but access to these courts is limited by local rules. Each court has its own set of civil procedure laws, and these differ among the states.

Civil Cases

A case in which a patient, or his family as **guardian** of the individual, sues the institution for money damages is a civil case. Civil cases are also known as **torts**, defined as civil cases for money damages. The plaintiff must establish four elements to win a civil lawsuit for money damages:

HIPAA
Protects health insurance coverage for workers and their families when they change or lose their jobs. Title II of HIPAA requires the establishment of national standards for electronic healthcare transactions and national identifiers for providers, health insurance plans, and employers.

Default judgment
A ruling that occurs when the defendant fails to answer the summons and complaint. At that time, it is possible for a court to find in the plaintiff's favor, but there are due process safeguards built into the system to protect defendants.

Due process
The proper, official way to do things in a legal case such that the rights of all people involved are protected.

Guardianship
The office, duty, or authority of a guardian; the relation between guardian and ward.

Tort
A civil case for money damages.

1. A duty was owed by the institution to the patient.
2. An employee of the institution violated that duty toward the patient.
3. The violation of that duty caused injury to the patient.
4. The patient suffered actual injuries.

Medical Malpractice

Medical malpractice is a form of civil case. Malpractice occurs when a doctor or another medical professional causes damage or harm to a patient through negligence (e.g., an error in diagnosing or treating a patient, mismanagement of a patient's illness) or omission. This error must be a breach—a deviation from the generally accepted standard of practice—of the care that a medical professional is expected to deliver under the circumstances. If such an error injures a patient, the patient may be able to win a judgment against the care provider. The civil case may also name the healthcare institution as a defendant in the malpractice action. Negligence can include problems with the administration of medications, sanitation, or nursing care. Patients may bring cases against local, state, or federal agencies that operate healthcare facilities, but special requirements must be met before filing such a suit in any court.

Administrators have a duty to ensure that the proper level of care is being delivered to each resident in the facility. The resident's right to privacy, including the ability to engage in an intimate relationship, must be maintained. Patient behavior is monitored to the extent that safety requires, but patients' residency does not constitute a waiver of their humanity and all that it entails. The individual maintains her right to respectful treatment. As a resident's physical or mental capacity diminishes, her chart must document the interventions and evaluations the facility performed to ascertain the cause of the decline. There is no excuse for ignoring the decline, even when competent residents refuse medical intervention; caregivers must record this refusal in the chart. In certain cases, HIPAA permits caregivers to notify the designated healthcare agent of a resident's refusal.

When a resident declines, the level of care the institution delivers must meet the resident's physical, mental, and emotional needs. If the institution cannot meet her needs, the resident must be transferred to an appropriate facility. During this evaluation process and at the time of transfer, the administrator must follow the written transfer policy and cooperate with the resident's family.

Most legal problems can be avoided with open, honest communication between the parties. When family members are not realistic in their expectations, administrators should use the healthcare team in continuous efforts to engage the family. At all times, documentation of the interventions and evaluations must continue, because the facility may have to go to court, and documentation is the key to avoiding liability.

Wrongful Termination

Sometimes an administrator must terminate an employee. The decision to do so must be made with a great deal of forethought, and proper documentation is necessary to justify the termination. Documentation is required, whether the termination is a result of the employee's wrongful conduct or of the economic needs of the institution. It is critical in justifying the termination action and must include a paper trail of prior conferences, warning notices, and other communications with the employee.

Wrongful termination
Firing or laying off an employee for illegal reasons in violation of existing civil law.

> (!) **CRITICAL CONCEPT**
> Terminating Employees and Administrator Safety
>
> Terminating employees is a necessary part of an administrator's job. Terminations are life-altering events for the affected employees under any circumstances. The administrators should anticipate a negative reaction from the employee and institute measures to ensure the administrator's safety. One recommendation is to always have trained security personnel present in the room at the time of the termination.

Every effort must be made to avoid wrongful termination cases, not only because of their cost to the institution but also because of their negative impact on the other workers' morale. A **wrongful termination** occurs when an employer terminates an employee for reasons that violate existing civil law. Reasons for termination considered wrongful include the following:

- The termination violates federal or state antidiscrimination laws. Employers may not discriminate on the basis of race, national origin, sex, age, or, in some localities, sexual orientation.

- The termination has occurred as a form of sexual harassment. These types of cases may arise when employees or administrators date and then one of the parties believes he is being discharged because of the relationship, not his job performance. They may also occur when an employee rejects an administrator's advances or when a coworker's use of sexual innuendo or overt sexual references makes the workplace uncomfortable for another employee. Sexual harassment can be either hetero- or homosexual. The healthcare institution should have written policies in place that are consulted in any potential sexual harassment situation.

♦ The termination violates oral or written employment agreements between the institution and the employee. These agreements confer contractual rights and terms on both parties. When the terms are breached by one party, the other party can sue in court for breach of contract.

♦ The termination violates labor laws, including collective bargaining laws if union representation of the employee is present. The collective bargaining agreement is a contract. It must be followed, or the breaching party can be liable for damages.

♦ The employee has filed a complaint or claim, usually with a government agency, against the employer, and the employer has terminated the employee in retaliation. These types of cases, more than any other, require a comprehensive paper trail to prove the termination was caused by independent factors and not as retribution for the complaint.

Some violations can result in statutory penalties to the employer. For others, the employer may be required to pay damages to cover lost wages and other expenses the employee incurred. In certain wrongful termination cases, more than one wrongdoer may be held responsible for damages. Damages are dependent on the type of case and jurisdictional rules.

CRIMINAL LAW

Criminal law is enforced by the appropriate governmental agency at the local, county, state, or federal level. Criminal laws are designed to protect individuals from harm and to prevent fraud. They differ among the states, and the information presented here is based on general principles that may vary. A violation of criminal law usually will not result in a criminal record for the individual or the corporation. For instance, if a long-term care provider submits a claim to Medicaid or Medicare that they know is false, they are subject to a penalty of $10,000 per item or service, in lieu of criminal penalties.

Misdemeanor
A crime that is punishable by a term of imprisonment of no more than one year.

A **misdemeanor** is a crime punishable by a term of imprisonment of no longer than one year. A **felony** is a crime punishable by a term of imprisonment of longer than one year. The term of probation for a felony is longer and can impose more restrictions than that for a misdemeanor.

Felony
A crime that is punishable by a term of imprisonment of more than one year.

Both individuals and corporations can be charged with a crime. In the case that the corporation is charged, the officers of the corporation may face legal sanctions for their individual actions or for the actions of others for whom they were responsible.

A person charged with a crime is known as the defendant and is presumed to be innocent until she either pleads guilty or is found guilty after a trial. The defendant has certain protections derived from the US Constitution. For example, the Fourth Amendment protects against unreasonable searches and seizures. The government must obtain a search warrant to search an institution if the administrator does not consent to the search, except in the case of an emergency. The Fifth Amendment provides for a grand jury in the case of a felony charge, protects defendants from being charged with the same crime twice, and protects the defendant from being forced to testify against himself. This last protection is called the privilege against self-incrimination. It does not stop the government from obtaining physical evidence or evidence from business records to be used against the defendant. The Sixth Amendment provides for a speedy and public trial with a jury in the jurisdiction where the crime occurred. It contains procedural guidelines to ensure that the charges are public, not secret; that the defendant has the right to cross-examine the witnesses against him; that the defendant can subpoena witnesses on his behalf; and that he has the right to an attorney at all stages of the criminal proceeding. The Eighth Amendment protects against excessive bail and fines and protects defendants from cruel and unusual punishments.

> ### (!) CRITICAL CONCEPT
> Case for Careful Supervision
>
> An administrator may find herself in a situation in which the criminal and civil laws overlap. Say an employee of the organization assaults a resident and is found guilty of criminal assault. The conviction establishes that the employee is guilty beyond a reasonable doubt and that the patient sustained actual physical injuries beyond a reasonable doubt. As a result of the conviction, the healthcare institution can expect to be sued in a separate civil case, as it is responsible for its employees' actions at work. This is one reason to monitor and supervise employees on a continuous basis.

ETHICAL ISSUES

PRINCIPLES OF HEALTHCARE ETHICS

Natural law is a set of expectations for human behavior that is derived from God or is considered to come from nature. Ethical decision making is often derived from natural law. Healthcare ethics can be viewed as a means of interpreting God's will to determine how we care for our fellow human beings.

Reasonable people will disagree on how to proceed when faced with actual clinical scenarios. Rather than base decisions on feelings or even common sense, the learned individual will base them on ethical principles. Ethical principles can be traced to Ancient Greece; Aristotle's writings on ethics form the foundation of this field of study.

Natural law
A philosophical system of legal and moral principles purportedly deriving from a universalized conception of human nature or divine justice rather than from legislative or judicial action; also known as law of nature, natural justice, or divine law.

Autonomy
The right of a competent patient to make her own healthcare decisions.

Beneficence
The responsibility of those caring for any patient to "do good" for the patient, but above all, to do no harm to the patient.

Fidelity
The faithful discharge of one's duty toward the patient's care.

Justice
A legal and ethical responsibility to care for all people without discrimination as to race, creed, color, or sexual orientation.

A code of ethics is a profession's written values that set forth the standards of conduct for individuals in that profession. Each profession has its own code of ethics. Physicians trace their code of ethics to the Hippocratic Oath (American Medical Association 2009). Registered nurses trace theirs to Florence Nightingale (American Nurses Association 2001). The ACHCA's code of ethics, mentioned earlier, is shown in Exhibit 12.1.

The ethical principles discussed most often in the healthcare field include autonomy, beneficence, fidelity, and justice. **Autonomy** is the right of a competent patient to make healthcare decisions for herself. Separate rules apply to incompetent patients and children whose decisions are made by legal guardians (including parents) and courts. **Beneficence** is literally the responsibility of those caring for any patient to "do good" for the patient and, above all, to do no harm to the patient. This principle gives rise to ethical dilemmas in healthcare because people's understanding of cultural values differs. **Fidelity**, derived from the Latin word *fidelis*, stands for the faithful discharge of one's duty toward the patient's care. **Justice** is a legal and ethical responsibility to care for all people without discrimination on the basis of race, creed, color, or sexual orientation. These principles are found within the ACHCA's code of ethics.

The patient or her healthcare agent can request or demand certain medical procedures, but it is up to the healthcare practitioner, as the expert, to determine what care is appropriate to be delivered to the patient. A medical doctor cannot be forced to deliver medical care that he does not consider warranted under the circumstances. On the other hand, a competent adult patient cannot be forced to undergo a medical procedure unless her condition presents a danger to others. Examples of patients who can be forced to receive medical treatment against their wishes include a patient with a contagious disease, who may be treated against his wishes to prevent the spread of that disease, or a person who is forced to receive a vaccination to prevent the outbreak of a disease. In these instances, negotiation between the parties can become heated, and court intervention may be necessary to resolve the issue.

ETHICAL DILEMMAS

This section discusses the particular ethical dilemmas concerning ordinary care versus extraordinary care. With the introduction of new technology, such as respirators for artificial breathing, ethical dilemmas arose. Two early court cases involved Roman Catholic patients, Karen Quinlan and Brother Joseph Fox, SM. In both cases, the courts acknowledged that the Catholic Church did not require extraordinary care to avoid an inevitable death. In the 1980 Brother Fox case, Justice Milton Mollen of the Appellate Division of the New York State Supreme Court wrote:

> In the Quinlan case, a position statement by Lawrence B. Casey, Bishop of Paterson, contained in the amicus curiae of the New Jersey Catholic Conference, made clear the official position of the Catholic bishops of New Jersey (see Matter of Quinlan, 70

NJ 10, 30-33, supra). As in the Quinlan proceeding, the position of the Diocese of Rockville Centre on the moral implications of withdrawal of Brother Fox's respirator has been expressed by Bishop John R. McGann in a statement reproduced in the brief amicus curiae of the Catholic Lawyers Guild of the Diocese of Rockville Centre (*Matter of the Application of Phillip K. Eichner* 1980).

EXHIBIT 12.1
ACHCA Code
of Ethics

American College of Health Care Administrators

PREAMBLE

The preservation of the highest standards of integrity and ethical principles is vital to the successful discharge of the professional responsibilities of all long-term health care administrators. This Code of Ethics has been promulgated by the American College of Health Care Administrators (ACHCA) in an effort to stress the fundamental rules considered essential to this basic purpose. It shall be the obligation of members to seek to avoid not only conduct specifically proscribed by the code, but also conduct that is inconsistent with its spirit and purpose. Failure to specify any particular responsibility or practice in this Code of Ethics should not be construed as denial of the existence of other responsibilities or practices. Recognizing that the ultimate responsibility for applying standards and ethics falls upon the individual, the ACHCA establishes the following Code of Ethics to make clear its expectation of the membership.

EXPECTATION I

Individuals shall hold paramount the welfare of persons for whom care is provided.

Prescriptions: The Health Care Administrator shall:
- Strive to provide to all those entrusted to his or her care the highest quality of appropriate services possible in light of resources or other constraints.
- Operate the facility consistent with laws, regulations, and standards of practice recognized in the field of health care administration.
- Consistent with law and professional standards, protect the confidentiality of information regarding individual recipients of care.
- Perform administrative duties with the personal integrity that will earn the confidence, trust, and respect of the general public.
- Take appropriate steps to avoid discrimination on basis of race, color, sex, religion, age, national origin, handicap, marital status, ancestry, or any other factor that is illegally discriminatory or not related to bona fide requirements of quality care.

Proscription: The Health Care Administrator shall not:
- Disclose professional or personal information regarding recipients of service to unauthorized personnel unless required by law or to protect the public welfare.

EXPECTATION II

Individuals shall maintain high standards of professional competence.

Prescriptions: The Health Care Administrator shall:
- Possess and maintain the competencies necessary to effectively perform his or her responsibilities.

(continued)

Exhibit 12.1
ACHCA Code
of Ethics

- Practice administration in accordance with capabilities and proficiencies and, when appropriate, seek counsel from qualified others.
- Actively strive to enhance knowledge of and expertise in long-term care administration through continuing education and professional development.

Proscriptions: The Health Care Administrator shall not:

- Misrepresent qualifications, education, experience, or affiliations.
- Provide services other than those for which he or she is prepared and qualified to perform.

EXPECTATION III

Individuals shall strive, in all matters relating to their professional functions, to maintain a professional posture that places paramount the interests of the facility and its residents.

Prescriptions: The Health Care Administrator shall:

- Avoid partisanship and provide a forum for the fair resolution of any disputes which may arise in service delivery or facility management.
- Disclose to the governing body or other authority as may be appropriate, any actual or potential circumstance concerning him or her that might reasonably be thought to create a conflict of interest or have a substantial adverse impact on the facility or its residents.

Proscription: The Health Care Administrator shall not:

- Participate in activities that reasonably may be thought to create a conflict of interest or have the potential to have a substantial adverse impact on the facility or its residents.

EXPECTATION IV

Individuals shall honor their responsibilities to the public, their profession, and their relationships with colleagues and members of related professions.

Prescriptions: The Health Care Administrator shall:

- Foster increased knowledge within the profession of health care administration and support research efforts toward this end.
- Participate with others in the community to plan for and provide a full range of health care services.
- Share areas of expertise with colleagues, students, and the general public to increase awareness and promote understanding of health care in general and the profession in particular.
- Inform the ACHCA Standards and Ethics Committee of actual or potential violations of this Code of Ethics, and fully cooperate with ACHCA's sanctioned inquiries into matters of professional conduct related to this Code of Ethics.

Proscription: The Health Care Administrator shall not:

- Defend, support, or ignore unethical conduct perpetrated by colleagues, peers, or students.

SOURCE: American College of Health Care Administrators (2007).

On November 24, 1957, Pope Pius XII delivered an address to a group of anesthesiologists concerning the moral consequences of withdrawing "modern artificial respiration apparatus in cases of deep unconsciousness, even in those that are considered completely hopeless in the opinion of the competent doctor." The Pope stated, essentially, that it was not morally sinful to use such extraordinary treatment for a terminal patient. However, neither was it required since such a patient need be given only ordinary treatment. Specifically, the Pope stated that as the use of a respirator went "beyond the ordinary means to which one is bound, it cannot be held that there is an obligation to use them or to give the doctor permission to use them. There is not involved here a case of direct disposal of the life of the patient; nor of euthanasia in any way; this would never be licit. Even when it causes the arrest of circulation, the interruption of attempts at resuscitation is never more than an indirect cause of the cessation of life."

Catholic doctrine holds no religious obligation for the Catholic patient to accept extraordinary care, nor does it place the physician under a religious obligation to deliver such care.

Other religions also have doctrines on and expectations of the healthcare system concerning extraordinary care for the terminally ill. For example, two nurses published an article discussing the Jewish view of death and what they termed "terminal dehydration, i.e., withholding or withdrawing food and fluid as a means to allow a terminally ill patient to die" (Bodell and Weng 2000):

The [Jewish] tradition views death as a part of life and teaches there is a time to die. However, when is a person considered to be dying and what does Jewish law teach about this? Gordon states: The law concerning a goses [dying person], defined by the rabbis as "one who is within three days of death," is that one may not do anything to shorten the person's life, even to relieve his or her suffering.

The dilemma of withdrawing food and fluid becomes tied into the limited time frame of three days before death to say that one is a "dying person."…Thus, even for the terminally ill patient who is not yet considered a goses by Jewish law, that commandment is to live every moment to the fullest, which includes taking in food and fluid naturally or, in many cases, artificially.

While individual Catholic and Jewish patients may disagree with their religion's doctrines and expressed viewpoints, the preceding examples are presented to demonstrate to the new healthcare administrator that individual religions have their own sets of ethics.

The same end-of-life ethics issues can be seen playing out across racial lines. African Americans are less likely than Caucasians to have advance directives, but this cultural difference goes further. Similar to patients who practice their faith in the Catholic and Jewish traditions, African-American patients may feel that pain and suffering are simply part of life. White patients choose to undergo treatments that improve their quality of life but that may reduce their longevity twice as often as African-American patients do. However, whites refuse life-sustaining treatments more often than Hispanics or African Americans do in the case of dementia. Some African Americans see illness as a test of faith. The belief in carrying on through adversity contradicts the common idea in the healthcare system that suffering should be alleviated whenever possible (*Cruzan v. Director* 1990).

In the case of Nancy Cruzan, the US Supreme Court refused to differentiate between artificial nutrition and hydration and any other medical treatment. The Court wrote, "[f]or purposes of this case, we assume that the US Constitution would grant a competent person a constitutionally protected right to refuse lifesaving hydration and nutrition"(*Cruzan v. Director* 1990).

Ethical dilemmas also extend to situations in which patients participate in research and clinical trials. The healthcare administrator must ensure that the ethical guidelines her institution follows are in compliance with the National Institutes of Health (NIH). The dilemmas presented in any clinical trial are exacerbated when the population being tested is at risk for manipulation or coercion. Vulnerable populations include the terminally ill, patients desperate for a cure, children, the elderly, and the developmentally disabled. NIH has set forth several safeguards to protect them. Any institution performing research must be aware of the current regulations and follow them scrupulously. This requirement is also set forth in the four expectations in the ACHCA's code of ethics.

END-OF-LIFE ISSUES

THE OREGON DEATH WITH DIGNITY ACT

Oregon Death with Dignity Act (ODWDA) A statute that provides physicians with protection from liability if they choose to prescribe medications for physician-assisted suicide, provided that: (1) the patient has an incurable and irreversible disease that will cause death within six months, (2) the patient has given written informed consent, and (3) the attending physician's conclusions are confirmed by a second physician.

In 1994, Oregon enacted the **Oregon Death with Dignity Act (ODWDA)**. The statute's format protects physicians who prescribe medications in physician-assisted suicide from liability, provided they comply with the following safeguards and meet certain other eligibility determinations (Sclar 2006):

- The patient has an incurable and irreversible disease that will cause death within six months.

- The patient has given written informed consent.

- The attending physician's conclusions are confirmed by a second physician.

It must be noted that "ODWDA legally prohibits **euthanasia** in which a physician or another person actually administers the medication to end another person's life" (Chin et al. 1999). The law faced several legal challenges, including an immediate injunction against it enacted by the US District Court for the District of Oregon. This injunction was later lifted by the Ninth Circuit Court of Appeals (*Lee v. State of Oregon* 1995). The US Supreme Court refused to hear that case (*Lee v. Harclerod* 1997).

The next time the Supreme Court addressed the ODWDA was in *Gonzales v. Oregon*. This decision was six to three to uphold the law. Justice Scalia, who struck down the Brady Bill on federalism grounds, sought to strike down this state statute, not because it was not a question of federalism but in deference to Attorney General John Ashcroft's interpretation of the 1971 Controlled Substance Act (CSA). The majority decision, written by Justice Anthony Kennedy, discussed the aspect of federalism, but the ruling was limited to the statutory interpretation of the 1971 CSA. The constitutionality of the ODWDA under the doctrine of federalism has yet to be reached. Washington State enacted an identical statute to ODWDA in 2008.

The American Medical Association and the American Nurses Association have published official positions against their members helping patients take their own life.

Euthanasia is still considered murder in the United States.

ADVANCE DIRECTIVES AT THE END OF LIFE

The living will and the healthcare proxy form allow patients to make their wishes clear to healthcare providers in the event the patient is not able to directly communicate them. The patient's use of these forms is within the ethical principle of autonomy and the legal right of a competent patient to refuse medical care when such refusal does not present a danger to others. **Do not resuscitate (DNR) orders** issued by physicians and the **physician orders for life-sustaining treatment form (POLST)** in no way advocate euthanasia. These orders recognize that patients have the right to decide which medical treatments they wish to receive and which they wish to refuse.

Patient Self-Determination Act

In 1990, the federal government passed the Patient Self-Determination Act (USC 1990). It mandated that patients be given access to information about the healthcare proxy and living will when admitted to a hospital or facility receiving Medicare funds. Patients need not complete the form, but they must be made aware of its existence. These advance directives are intended for competent adults.

Euthanasia
The act or practice of killing or bringing about the death of a person who suffers from an incurable disease or condition, especially a painful one, for reasons of mercy. Euthanasia is sometimes regarded by the law as second-degree murder, manslaughter, or criminally negligent homicide. Also termed mercy killing or assisted suicide.

Do not resuscitate order (DNR)
A legally binding document that states resuscitation should not be attempted in the event of a cardiac or respiratory arrest.

Physician orders for life-sustaining treatment (POLST)
A document that expresses a person's end-of-life wishes for medical treatment.

Advance Directives: The Healthcare Proxy and the Living Will

The **healthcare proxy** form permits a competent adult to designate a healthcare agent. This designated agent can make healthcare decisions for the patient when he can no longer communicate his wishes to the healthcare provider. The healthcare proxy form includes a section in which the individual can specify his wishes to accept or refuse artificial nutrition and hydration. It is designed to provide clear and convincing evidence about the individual's wishes. The healthcare proxy also contains a section wherein the individual can express his preference to donate or not donate his organs after death, and it allows room for the individual to write specific instructions regarding end-of-life care. The states of New York and Ohio have developed a conservative approach to end-of-life care for competent adults, which requires written advance directives, especially in the case of artificial hydration. This statutory scheme is in compliance with federal law but differs from the more liberal approach adopted by the **Uniform Health Care Decisions Act**. This act is intended to help individuals and medical professionals ensure a person's right to determine the course of treatment; however, only several states have adopted these provisions. The provisions of this act state that the healthcare agent may not be one of the two subscribing witnesses. Other states do not require written advance directives and permit family members or spouses to make decisions on the basis of the patient's earlier oral directions.

At the time of the resident's admission it is important to ensure that her healthcare proxy form is entered into her chart. It is unwise to wait until an emergency has occurred because the resident may no longer be able to communicate. Planning ensures that her wishes are being followed and will permit the institution to communicate with the designated healthcare agent without any violation of privacy. Furthermore, if the resident becomes legally incompetent because of illness or trauma, the healthcare proxy remains in effect.

The **living will** is a legal form that details the patient's wishes regarding the type of medical care he desires or, more specifically, the medical procedures he does not want performed when he can no longer communicate and medical care is artificially prolonging his life. It usually states that the person wishes to be kept comfortable with medications to avoid pain at the end of life. This form must be signed by the patient and two subscribing witnesses. Subscribing witnesses are individuals who witness the execution of an instrument and sign their names as proof of such an execution.

Many states now use POLST forms when transferring a resident to a hospital for treatment or to an LTC facility.

POLST forms are distinctive, sometimes printed on pink paper, and completed by the treating physician. Some states, such as New York, permit a nurse practitioner or physician's assistant to complete this form when the physician is not available. It can be considered the corollary form to the living will completed by the patient to detail her wishes for end-of-life care.

The POLST form is completed once the physician understands the patient's wishes concerning the scope of treatment he wishes to have. This understanding can come from conversations with the patient, an examination of the living will, or talking with the healthcare agent. This communication by the physician should be documented in the patient's medical chart. In some jurisdictions, the POLST form may be completed after conversations with family members. This order communicates the end-of-life care ordered by the attending physician to any facility in which the patient is being cared for or in a subsequent facility to which the patient is transferred. The more specific the order is, the easier it is for subsequent healthcare providers to comprehend and follow. Depending on the local statute, this order may be considered a DNR order within a hospital or nursing home. The use of these orders is governed by individual state statutes. In New York State, it is referred to as a medical order for life-sustaining treatment form.

USE OF ETHICS COMMITTEES WITHIN HEALTHCARE INSTITUTIONS

In 1983, the President's Commission for the Study of Ethical Problems in Medicine and Biomedical and Behavioral Research called for ethics committees within healthcare institutions to help families with end-of-life decisions. The commission wrote (President's Commission for the Study of Ethical Problems in Medicine and Biomedical and Behavioral Research 1983):

When patients are incompetent to make their own decisions, others must act on their behalf. The Commission found that existing legal procedures can be adapted for the purpose of allowing people while competent to designate someone to act in their stead and to express their wishes about treatment. When it is not possible to know what a particular patient would have chosen—as, for example, with seriously ill infants—those who make the choices should attempt to serve the patient's best interests, judged from the patient's vantage point. To ensure that the interests of incompetent patients are protected, the Commission urges that healthcare institutions develop and utilize methods of internal review that will permit all relevant issues to be explored and all opinions to be heard and that will improve communication among the full treatment team and patients' family members.

The ethics committee is interdisciplinary, and the membership varies among institutions. Members usually include a healthcare administrator, a physician, a registered nurse, a specialist in healthcare ethics, a lawyer, and a representative of the local community. This committee is independent in its conclusions; thus, conclusions are not binding on any party, but they are generally followed. In any subsequent court case, the committee's findings become part of the judicial record.

The ethics committee's purpose is to clarify the issues and improve communication between healthcare providers and patients or their family members while helping to resolve issues regarding healthcare decisions at the end of life. Research in multiple hospitals has found that these committees cut costs and improve communications and are effective in helping families through this difficult process (Gilmer et al. 2005).

A LOOK AHEAD

Legal and ethical issues in long-term care are especially complex because they involve a vulnerable population. In addition, long-term care is the most regulated sector of healthcare as the majority of its customers have little or no recourse, thus adding to the complexity. This chapter provided a primer on the difference between statutes, common law, and natural law and also explained the concept of federalism as it applies to the US legal system. The reader should also be able to differentiate between criminal and civil law cases and identify common legal cases faced by long-term care administrators in a variety of long-term care settings. Finally, this chapter provided future long-term care administrators with the principles of healthcare ethics to assist them as they confront ethical issues throughout their careers.

FOR DISCUSSION

1. Discuss how the US Constitution's Supremacy Clause interacts with the Ninth and Tenth Amendments in the Bill of Rights.

2. The Tenth Amendment protects the states from intrusion by the federal government on the powers reserved to the states. Discuss how this concept of federalism affects the state's ability to regulate healthcare today.

3. The LTC institution you work for just received a summons and complaint suing it for alleged negligence in the care of a patient that resulted in a bedsore. Discuss the legal and ethical tasks the healthcare administrator must undertake upon receipt of the summons and complaint.

4. Discuss the difference between natural law, statutory law, and common law.

5. Discuss how the different advance directives serve to inform the healthcare team as to the patient's wishes concerning the delivery of healthcare.

6. What is a POLST form?

7. Discuss how the four expectations of an LTC healthcare administrator presented in the American College of Health Care Administrators code of ethics affects professional behavior on a daily basis.

8. Discuss the role of an ethics committee in an LTC institution in helping families and physicians reach an ethical decision.

9. Discuss end-of-life care as it relates to do not resuscitate (DNR) orders by physicians versus the use of passive euthanasia in Oregon and Washington.

10. Discuss the various types of euthanasia and suicide.

11. Discuss the difference between palliative care, rehabilitation care, and acute care at the end of life.

CASE STUDY: END-OF-LIFE CARE AND THE FAMILY

An 80-year-old man in a coma, with no hope of recovery, is admitted to an LTC facility where you are employed as a healthcare administrator. The man has not prepared an advance directive such as a living will or a healthcare proxy. The patient's religion does not require artificial nutrition or hydration, and all members of the patient's family agree that the patient does not want to die with tubes attached to him. The attending physician has met with the family prior to completing the POLST form to determine what orders he will write. The physician informs the family that the patient will die in a few days without having a feeding tube inserted for water and liquid food. The feeding tube may keep him alive for a number of years. If there is no feeding tube for hydration, his death might be painful or uncomfortable. The physician and the facility's religious affiliation would prefer to treat the patient with artificial hydration via a feeding tube rather than do nothing. The family has refused the feeding tube, and the physician has referred the matter to the institution's ethics committee.

CASE STUDY QUESTIONS

1. As a member of the healthcare ethics committee, explore the following options:

   a. Transfer the patient to an inpatient hospice, where he can die a natural death and any pain will be treated with medications.

   b. Keep the patient at your facility and go to court for an order to insert a feeding tube under the contention that, without the feeding tube, he will die.

2. Discuss how keeping the patient at your healthcare institution or having this physician treat the patient would violate the religious stance of both the organization and the physician.

3. How is this discussion changed if the patient has both a living will and a healthcare proxy that specifically state he does not want a feeding tube and he wishes his death to be peaceful, even if that means using medications to keep him comfortable at the expense of shortening his life?

CASE STUDY: REFUSING TREATMENT

A 35-year-old woman with chronic disease is admitted to your LTC facility. She has developed a problem requiring a transfusion, and if she does not receive one, she will die. Her religious beliefs preclude her from receiving blood products. After a thorough explanation by the physician, she understands that she is likely to suffer permanent physical injury and possibly die if she refuses to accept the transfusion. Her family, which shares the same religious affiliation, supports her decision. The physician refers the matter to the healthcare ethics committee on which you sit as the healthcare administrator. The committee members all agree that the law permits a competent adult to refuse medical care.

CASE STUDY QUESTIONS

1. Is it ethical to speak to this patient in private, away from her family, and offer her the option of a secret transfusion so that nobody knows of it, or is this coercion into sinful behavior?

2. Is it ethical to meet with the family and patient to attempt to convince them to change their minds regarding the transfusion? What can and should be said to them? What should not be said?

3. How does this discussion change if the patient is a child or a ward of the state?

4. What are the legal facts of which the healthcare administrator must be aware in such a case?

CHAPTER 13

Regulation of Long-Term Care

JoAnn Nolin, JD, RN

LEARNING OBJECTIVES

After studying this chapter, you should be able to

➤ track the historical development of regulation as it applies to LTC services;

➤ examine political and social influences affecting the development and implementation of LTC services;

➤ compare the role of public and private regulation of LTC providers and organizations;

➤ identify social and demographic changes that have influenced the development of assisted living options; and

➤ explore the actions and political impact of public interest groups that are focused on LTC quality.

INTRODUCTION

The US long-term care industry has evolved from its origins as an unorganized and un-regulated effort to provide homes for elders who were unable to care for themselves and lacked family systems able or willing to provide those services. Prior to the passage of the Social Security Act (SSA) in 1935, seniors without family or financial resources were relegated to state-run almshouses that provided little actual care. The SSA included Old Age Assistance (OAA) grants that, for the first time, provided the elderly with income that could be used to pay for care (Ogden and Adams 2009). These grants were not available to individuals receiving public assistance, such as shelter in state-funded homes. Thus, a new cottage industry arose with individual homes opening their doors to retired elderly who now had funds to pay for services.

Employment opportunities for women, expanded by World War II and the robust economy that followed, changed the face of the American workforce and contributed to the decline in private homes providing shelter for the aged. Following the war, many young families moved in search of employment opportunities, leaving older Americans to age without the social supports available to prior generations. The decline in home care options fueled by changing demographics and growing numbers of women joining the workforce in the second half of the twentieth century led to the emergence of privately and publicly owned facilities that provided institutional care. Regulation and financing of this care, where it existed, varied greatly.

Today, a rapidly growing senior population poses new challenges for the delivery of high-quality LTC services that cannot be ignored. In response, the LTC arena may see the development of new models of community-based care.

ORIGINS OF REGULATION

Federal, state, and private regulation of LTC service providers and agencies came about as an expression of societal and political expectations for care. During the twentieth century these expectations coincided with and reflected the scientific advancements that changed medical care and the role of the physician in people's lives. **Licensure** of physicians, other healthcare professionals, and the institutions that provide acute and LTC services established a minimum standard for delivery of health services. Financial support for LTC evolved from self-pay and charity care to include private and public insurance programs. Many current regulations that affect LTC services are directly linked to the financing of care by the federal and state governments.

The regulation of physicians in the United States began prior to the twentieth century; discussion of physician licensure began as early as the establishment of the 13 colonies. Regulations mandating criteria for practice were first instituted at the city level. State regulations, which were drafted to limit uneducated or poorly educated individuals

Licensure
Permission granted by an agency of the government that provides an exclusive right to practice certain legally defined functions; states license healthcare facilities to provide long-term care services.

Flexner report
A study of medical education in the United States and Canada.

Accreditation
The act of giving credit or recognition to organizations that maintain suitable standards.

American College of Surgeons Hospital Standardization Program
A list of standards developed by the ACS for accreditation of hospitals; this evolved into the Joint Commission for Accreditation of Healthcare Organizations.

The Joint Commission
A private, not-for-profit organization that operates accreditation programs for a fee to subscriber healthcare organizations in the United States. Formerly the Joint Commission for the Accreditation of Healthcare Organizations (JCAHO).

from practicing medicine, followed. Efforts by physicians to self-regulate grew with the development of the state medical societies, which had the authority to license physicians in some states. However, these early efforts were unsuccessful in limiting practice by unqualified individuals, as regulation of medical education was virtually nonexistent. The situation did not change until the American Medical Association (AMA) gained control of medical education standards following publication of the **Flexner report** in 1910, which issued a scathing indictment of the state of medical education in the United States (Cooke et al. 2006; Starr 1982).

Hospital regulation also began at the local level, with little state or federal intervention before the early twentieth century. Until that time, most hospitals were private institutions, owned and managed by religious or philanthropic organizations, and they primarily served the indigent population. While the owners of these institutions operated them with good intent, well into the twentieth century hospitals were dangerous places because their staffs lacked knowledge about infectious processes and effective treatments were scarce. The death rate from infections alone was high, and a majority of hospital patients did not survive. Individuals with the funds to be treated at home did not generally seek hospital services.

Early discussions proposing municipal regulation of hospitals were primarily led by physicians (Dorr 1912). As states began to license hospitals, they adopted many of the standards established by the AMA for physician education. They also drew on the American College of Surgeons' (ACS) Minimum Standards for Hospitals, which were initially published in 1917. ACS's original one-page list of standards evolved into the **ACS Hospital Standardization Program**, which served as the model for **accreditation** review programs until 1952. At that time, the program was transferred to a new organization formed for that purpose. This organization, the Joint Commission on Accreditation of Hospitals, continues today as **The Joint Commission** and offers accreditation programs for a wide variety of healthcare organizations, including nursing homes.

The regulation climate for nursing homes changed as government mandates were developed in response to a series of scandals in the 1950s, ranging from deadly fires in poorly built facilities to widespread allegations of fraud, abuse, and poor care. These allegations were addressed in 1967 with the passage of the **Mossman Amendments**, which provided a legislative basis for the standardization of nursing home regulations and denial of Medicare and Medicaid funding for facilities that failed to comply (Smith and Moore 2008). Standards for nursing services were also established for custodial and medical care and staffing. In addition, nursing homes were now required to meet National Fire Protection Association safety standards. By the time of implementation, the Mossman Amendments had undergone significant changes and were less effective than originally intended in bringing significant changes to nursing home practices.

The passage of the **Omnibus Budget Reconciliation Act of 1987 (OBRA 87)** was the first legislation to effectively impose reforms on the nursing home industry. This act mandated the provision of certain services to ensure that residents achieve and maintain the highest practicable level of well-being. It also established a patient bill of rights and an outcome-focused, resident-oriented survey process. This process replaced an earlier effort that focused on facilities rather than resident care or condition.

BASICS OF LICENSURE, CERTIFICATION, AND ACCREDITATION OF LTC SERVICES

State governments now license LTC facilities and providers under their right to dictate and police activity necessary to ensure the health and safety of their residents. However, prior to 1950, states were not required to license nursing homes. That year, amendments to the SSA mandated licensure for states wishing to receive matching federal funds for construction of new nursing homes. The amendments required increased levels of safety and standard of care in these facilities, which were considered understaffed, underfinanced, and poorly constructed for their intended use. The states were eventually mandated to establish an agency or authority to develop and maintain standards for these institutions. The initial federal requirement for licensure standards did not identify the standards to be met and did not provide a mechanism for ensuring that states enforced the standards once they were established, but it led to state regulations that, in some cases, resulted in the closure of facilities and the replacement of substandard buildings with new construction.

While the states regulate nursing home activity by virtue of their police power, the federal government regulates though its financing authority. Significant federal financing of nursing home care and related home-based services for the elderly came about with the establishment of the Medicare and Medicaid programs in the 1960s. Facilities and providers wishing to participate in these programs are required to meet the Conditions of Participation set by federal law.

Enrollment in Medicare has gone from 19 million at its enactment in 1966 to almost 36 million in 2008 (CMS 2011). Medicaid enrollment has increased from 10 million in 1967 to more than 58 million in 2007. In 2007, Medicare and Medicaid program funds paid for almost 60 percent of all nursing home care. With hundreds of millions of federal dollars allocated to nursing homes on an annual basis, it is not surprising that the federal government has promulgated rules and regulations that affect every aspect of care and activity in the nursing home setting.

Private regulation is also in place, having arisen from the efforts of individuals and groups to establish standards and measure efforts to provide high-quality services. The most widely recognized of the private regulators is The Joint Commission, which has accreditation processes in place for not only hospitals but also nursing homes, assisted living facilities, and home health services. Most US hospitals are accredited by The Joint Commission, which accords hospitals deemed status by the US government, meaning that they have met the Conditions of Participation for Medicare and Medicaid without undergoing

Mossman amendments
A legislative basis for standardization of nursing home regulations and denial of Medicare and Medicaid funding for organizations that fail to conform to them.

Omnibus Budget Reconciliation Act of 1987
This act mandated the provision of certain services meant to ensure that residents achieve and maintain "highest practicable" physical, mental, and psychosocial status; also established a patient bill of rights and an outcome-focused, resident-oriented survey process.

a state and federal survey. Joint Commission–accredited nursing homes are not accorded the same status and must still submit to a state and federal survey to be eligible for federal funds.

NURSING HOME LICENSURE AND CERTIFICATION PROCESS

Nursing homes are among the most highly regulated healthcare facilities in the United States. While state licensure standards for nursing homes vary, they generally cover the same areas. New facilities must be licensed, and the licensure inspection process begins before construction. Nursing homes must demonstrate that they meet or have the ability to meet all the standards required for an operational facility prior to admitting patients. Once the facility opens, it must continue to demonstrate compliance with state standards. A state survey team (made up of individuals with backgrounds in healthcare) surveys licensed facilities annually. Survey team members include nurses, social workers, pharmacists, dieticians, healthcare administrators, fire and safety professionals, and other allied health practitioners.

Nursing homes are licensed as either skilled nursing facilities (SNFs) or intermediate care facilities (ICFs). SNFs provide 24-hour nursing care for residents requiring medical, nursing, rehabilitative, and nutrition services; activity programs; and medication management. To participate in Medicare, a nursing home must be licensed as an SNF.

ICFs provide 24-hour residential care but are only required to provide 8 hours of nursing supervision per day. ICF residents are generally ambulatory and require less assistance with daily activities and little nursing care. SNFs and ICFs are eligible for **certification** as Medicaid providers.

While state standards can vary, federal legislation under the SSA mandates minimum standards that all facilities must meet to participate in Medicare and Medicaid, regardless of location. These standards are found in the **Code of Federal Regulations**. The federal government contracts with the survey agency of each state to perform initial surveys and periodic resurveys to ensure compliance with the federal standards. The surveys take place concurrently, in most cases, with the state licensure survey during a 9- to 15-month window. The surveys are unannounced. During a nursing home's survey window, the staff knows the survey team can walk in any day of the week, including weekends, and at any time of the day or night to start the survey. The scope and specificity of the state and federal regulations and the fact that the nursing home staff must be prepared for survey any day and at any time make this process stressful for staff and administrators.

Congress passed the first federal nursing home standards in 1967 and updated them in 1980, 1987, and 1990. Early regulations established a process-focused survey that asked nursing homes to demonstrate that the necessary processes and procedures were in place to care for facility residents. Key elements of the legislation include (1) an emphasis on a resident's quality of life, (2) new expectations for activities of daily

Certification
A process of external review or assessment upon which a designation is awarded to ensure qualification to perform a job or task; long-term care facilities are certified to provide care by the federal Medicare and Medicaid programs.

Code of Federal Regulations
Title 42 sets minimum standards for participation in the Medicare and Medicaid programs that must be met by all facilities regardless of location.

living (ADLs) that residents can perform (absent medical reasons that would prevent this), (3) individualized care planning and a time frame for completion, (4) the right to return to the nursing home after a hospital stay, (5) the initiation of a family council, (6) the right to have a safely managed resident bank fund, (7) the right to be free of physical and chemical restraint, and (8) uniform standards for homes accepting Medicare and Medicaid funds.

With passage of OBRA 87 the focus shifted to quality of life. The resident became the focus of the survey, and states were charged with establishing effective monitoring and enforcement mechanisms to ensure that state licensure requirements and federal standards were met. OBRA 87 also mandated staffing levels and education programs for caregivers. These regulatory changes held nursing homes accountable for the outcomes of the care they delivered. The resident's right to safe and competent care became the core issue of the survey process (Walshe and Harrington 2002).

The survey team begins preparation for the survey by reviewing the facility's prior survey report, complaint investigations, quality indicators, and other documents related to operation of the facility. The intent behind the unannounced surveys is to be able to view the normal daily operation of the nursing home. Upon entering the facility, the survey team alerts the administrator to the purpose of the visit. In most cases, the team meets briefly with administrative leadership before beginning the observations, record reviews, and interviews that make up the majority of the process. The observations portion of the survey attempts to construct an understanding of the quality of care delivered and includes observing delivery of clinical care, such as medication administration, dressing changes, and therapy sessions, and interactions between staff and residents.

The state survey team evaluates all facets of the nursing home's operation. It inspects the physical plant, conducts fire and safety checks, reviews disaster and evacuation plans, addresses infection control issues, and reviews the organization's personnel and financial records. The facility must produce evidence of adherence to local ordinances and regulations and the currency of all required operational and staff licenses. Some states require mandatory, ongoing training for staff that must be documented. While much of the surveyor's activity is focused on those federal standards that overlap with state requirements, each state has specific regulations that the surveyor must also address.

All state surveyors attend mandatory training conducted by state and federal agencies in preparation for their roles in the survey process. Despite this training, concerns about the reliability of survey results persist, voiced by providers, policymakers, facility residents and their families, and surveyors themselves. Studies have examined the performance of these survey teams, but they have not been able to answer questions about the validity of differences in regional and state outcomes (Harrington et al. 2008; Lee, Gajewski, and Thompson 2006; Walshe and Harrington 2002).

> ⓘ **CRITICAL CONCEPT**
> Nursing Home Accreditation
>
> While all nursing homes must undergo state licensing surveys and those seeking participation in the Medicare and Medicaid programs must submit to federal certification surveys, accreditation is a voluntary process. The Joint Commission (TJC) accredits LTC organizations that are certified by Medicare and Medicaid and licensed by the state as nursing homes in addition to units in hospitals with beds licensed as LTC beds. It also accredits nursing home units operated by the VA and other government agencies.
>
> Unlike the licensure and certification process, the focus of accreditation by TJC and other private, nonprofit accrediting organizations is performance improvement. The cost of accreditation is borne by the organization and is seen as an investment that can help improve organization performance, demonstrate facility achievement in the areas of quality and safety, and help market facility services. The accreditation survey is based on an on-site evaluation of the systems and processes in place for the delivery of care and maintenance of the facility and environment. The surveyors evaluate the facility using standards developed in consultation with industry providers, residents, families, LTC experts, and other relevant stakeholders. The standards cover residents' rights, ethical treatment, medical and nursing care, infection control, information management, human resources, environmental services, and overall organizational performance. TJC approaches the survey as an educational endeavor, with surveyors serving in a consultant role.
>
> The difference in TJC's accreditation process and the licensure and certification process is in their respective focus. Licensure and certification are enforcement processes that measure performance against minimum state and federal standards. Inadequate performance can result in deficiency citations at the state and federal level. Subsequent to the enactment of OBRA 87, federal deficiency citations can include **civil money penalties**. The same legislation enabled other intermediate sanctions, such as the denial of payment for current residents or new admissions and the appointment of temporary managers where needed to ensure resident safety and continued facility operation (Harrington et al. 2008).
>
> The public can access safety and quality information about Joint Commission–accredited LTC organizations, including detailed performance data and comparisons with other institutions, at www.qualitycheck.org.

Civil money penalties
A punitive fine imposed by a civil court on an entity that has profited from illegal or unethical activity.

Assisted Living Facilities

In the United States, assisted living developed as an alternative to more expensive nursing home care for individuals who needed supervision and assistance with ADLs but did not necessarily require skilled nursing services. The nursing home's medical model did not provide a positive environment for the senior who was healthy enough to live in a less restrictive setting. The loss of independence, privacy, and connections to friends and the community and the institutional surroundings did not foster positive perceptions by residents, their families, or senior advocates. With increasing demands for an alternative to institutionalization of frail seniors, a new model of care was envisioned that bridged the gap between senior housing, which was intended for elders capable of living independently, and nursing homes, which provided institutional care. Efforts to develop a more senior-friendly living alternative reflected the need to construct living arrangements that provided a homelike environment while making essential support services available. The result was a model that featured resident choice and decision making in an environment that allowed independence and connections with family and community.

In the early 1980s Oregon began applying for Medicaid waivers for community-based LTC services that emphasized client decision making, dignity, and independence (Wilson 2007). State officials began seeking waivers for home care and adult foster care programs and eventually opened apartment-style congregate housing that was designed to provide a level of services previously seen only in licensed settings. Oregon policymakers termed these settings *assisted living*. Within a few years the term was being applied to a wide range of facilities and services with no common definition. Early proponents of assisted living saw a clear need for an alternative to the sterile and restrictive environments of licensed nursing homes. However, Oregon's efforts to bridge the gap between home and nursing home with use of federal housing dollars and Medicaid waiver programs were not uniformly followed as the assisted living arrangement evolved in the United States. Other residential arrangements labeled as assisted living included private homes converted to congregate living facilities, commercial construction of retirement communities, and existing senior housing units adapted for that purpose. The stated intent of most of these early providers was to offer a variety of services on site that would allow autonomy and individual choice and prevent premature nursing home admission. Development of assisted living on the East Coast differed from the Oregon model in that it was driven more by a combination of private investment and adaptation of nonprofit senior housing. Despite coming from different philosophical viewpoints, both groups recognized client choice, autonomy, and supportive care as key elements of successful aging in residential settings.

While a single, specific definition of assisted living has not been adopted nationally, a commonly cited definition (Hawes et al. 2003; Phillips et al. 2003; Zimmerman et al. 2003) is the following:

A congregate residential setting that provides or coordinates personal services, 24-hour supervision and assistance (scheduled and unscheduled), activities and health related services; designed to minimize the need to move; designed to accommodate individual residents changing needs and preferences; designed to maximize residents dignity, autonomy, privacy, independence, and safety; and designed to encourage family and community involvement. (ALQC 1998)

Other definitions are offered by provider organizations and state licensure regulations. The Assisted Living Federation of America (2009) defines assisted living as "a long-term residence option that provides resident-centered care in a residential setting . . . designed for those who need extra help in their day-to-day lives but who do not require the 24-hour skilled nursing care."

What these definitions do not address is the oversight or regulation of the providers or the services offered. The following federal laws affect assisted living, as they affect all employers:

◆ Americans with Disabilities Act

◆ Civil Rights Act of 1991

◆ Rehabilitation Act of 1973

◆ Family and Medical Leave Act

◆ Fair Labor Standards Act

◆ Occupational Safety and Health Act

The impact of these regulations varies by type of business and number of employees.

In most cases, corresponding state laws address many of the same issues. As significant federal funding has not been allocated for assisted living, federal oversight specific to this area is minimal and state licensing requirements vary. State regulations can affect every aspect of assisted living situations, from services offered to participation in Medicaid waiver programs. For example, regulations in a few states do not allow individuals to reside in assisted living facilities if they meet the criteria for admission to a nursing home. Individuals in these states cannot qualify for Medicaid Home and Community-Based Services waivers, as waiver applicants must be nursing home eligible. Other differences in state licensure include regulations that address every aspect of care and services and in some cases provide for different levels of facility licensure based on the services offered.

Regulation of these facilities varies by state, but assisted living providers across the nation generally agree that any level of regulation needs to be limited to allow the flexibility to address the changing service needs of residents as they age. Proponents of increased regulation, on the other hand, cite examples of poor care and exploitation of the elderly. The fact that elders and their families pay for the majority of assisted living services has given them a voice that the assisted living industry has heeded in development of a wide variety of residential settings and services. Thus, assisted living providers would be wise to listen to this group of stakeholders in order to avoid increased regulation by state and federal legislators.

Continuing Care Retirement Communities

LeadingAge, formerly the American Association of Homes and Services for the Aging (AAHSA), defines a continuing care retirement community (CCRC) as an organization that offers a variety of services ranging from housing to residential and healthcare services in order to serve changing needs of residents as they age. This definition is similar to that of an assisted living facility. While CCRCs offer assisted living services, assisted living is only one of their three levels of service. The other levels are independent living and skilled nursing care. Residents contract with the CCRC for a continuum of services that allow the resident to age in place. This contractual agreement, which is unique to CCRCs, guarantees that the resident receives services on the basis of individual need as he ages. CCRC arrangements differ, but generally CCRCs provide the resident with assisted living or nursing home services once he is unable to live independently. Depending on the contractual arrangement, the resident may pay a portion or none of the cost of care beyond his monthly service agreement once he advances to a higher level of care.

The same licensing laws that cover nursing homes and assisted living facilities also apply to nursing home and assisted living beds located in CCRCs. In addition, 38 states regulate continuing care contracts. These regulations resemble insurance regulations in that they address the financial arrangements between the resident and the CCRC and require financial disclosure by the CCRC. In many cases the regulatory agency assigned oversight of CCRC contracts is the state department of insurance (GAO 2010).

CCRC contract regulation primarily protects the residents' rights related to prepaid entrance fees and refund policies and ensures that the facility uses standard accounting practices for required reporting of facility operating and investment capital. Regulations may require that some or all of the entrance fees be placed in escrow to ensure that a refund will be available if one is due under the provisions of the contract. Some states also require CCRCs to maintain a cash reserve to help protect against a loss of services during times of financial difficulty (Bogutz et al. 2005).

The inconsistency of states' approaches to CCRC regulation limits people's ability to assess the quality of services in an individual community and to compare quality between communities. The formation in 1985 of the Continuing Care Accreditation Commission (CCAC) was an effort to address the questions of financial stability and quality of

Pennsylvania	50	Virginia	15
California	28	Illinois	14
Florida	23	Maryland	13
North Carolina	21	New Jersey	10
Ohio	20	Connecticut	9

SOURCE: CARF International (2012).

care offered by CCRCs. Initially sponsored by the AAHSA, the CCAC was taken over by the Commission on Accreditation of Rehabilitation Facilities (CARF) in 1996.

Since that time, continuing care retirement communities and other aging services networks have been accredited under CARF-CCAC standards through submission of a comprehensive self-study and an on-site survey process. The process is similar to The Joint Commission process and includes observation, record reviews, and interviews with administrators, staff, residents, and other stakeholders. Of the approximately 2,100 CCRCs in the United States, only 311 (14.8 percent) are accredited by CARF-CCAC (CARF 2009), leaving potential residents and their families with little information about the vast majority of these communities.

Participating communities market their participation as evidence of quality in that they have gone beyond any applicable state and federal requirements for oversight and are committed to continuous improvement. It is not surprising that four of the five states with the largest numbers of accredited CCRCs (see Exhibit 13.1), Florida, Pennsylvania, North Carolina, and Ohio, are also among the top ten states in percentage of population older than 65 years of age (He et al. 2005). California, with the largest over-65 population, leads in number of accredited CCRCs. However, Florida, which is the fifth most populated state with 18.3 million residents, is second in the number of over-65 residents (3.0 million to California's 3.9 million) and has the highest-percentage population older than 65, at 16.9 percent (see Exhibit 13.2).

The aging baby boomer generation will add significantly to the need for quality housing and supportive care for the elderly population. As their numbers swell the Medicare rolls over the next decade, the need for acute and LTC services will grow proportionally. States with disproportionally large numbers of seniors face significant challenges related to provision of health and residential services.

HOME AND COMMUNITY-BASED SERVICES

Home and community-based services are federal- and state-sponsored programs that support community-dwelling seniors and their caregivers. These programs also receive private funding. The Administration on Aging (AoA) oversees the promotion and development of coordinated home and community-based LTC services at the federal level. Many of these

	Total Population (millions)	Over-65 Population (millions)	Over-65 Residents as % of Total Population
California	38.2	4.4	11.5
Texas	24.8	2.6	10.5
New York	19.9	2.7	13.6
Florida	19.1	3.4	17.8
Illinois	12.9	1.6	12.4
Pennsylvania	12.9	2.0	15.5
Ohio	11.7	1.6	13.7
Michigan	10.2	1.3	12.8
Georgia	9.8	1.0	10.2
North Carolina	9.7	1.2	12.4
New Jersey	8.8	1.2	13.7
Virginia	8.0	1.0	12.4

EXHIBIT 13.2

Twelve US States with the Highest Over-65 Population

SOURCE: ProximityOne (2011).

programs arise from the Older Americans Act (OAA), which authorizes and provides funding for the administration of programs that deliver social and nutrition services to seniors through the National Aging Network. This network is made up of 56 state agencies on aging, 629 local-area agencies on aging, 244 tribal organizations, 2 native Hawaiian organizations, and approximately 20,000 service providers. Programs funded under the OAA include multipurpose senior centers, nutrition centers (which provide congregate meals), adult day care, home-delivered meals, respite care and support programs for volunteer caregivers, health and wellness programs, legal services, abuse prevention services, and many offerings.

Additional legislation that authorized funding for programs and services for seniors includes Section 398 of the Public Health Service Act, which established Alzheimer's disease demonstration grants to states. The AoA administers two other acts, the Health Insurance Portability and Accountability Act, which funds fraud and abuse control efforts, and Title XXIX of the Public Health Service Act, which authorizes funding for respite care programs. These programs undergo regular, planned evaluations to assess their effectiveness, efficiency, and cost related to the services they provide. The evaluation efforts provide current, relevant data to policymaking bodies as they allocate limited resources to care for a rapidly growing senior population.

ACCOUNTABILITY AND QUALITY IN LTC

The demand for accountability across the LTC industry has led to greater availability of information about the scope and quality of services at the state, federal, and private levels. Reporting of nursing home data mandated by the Centers for Medicare & Medicaid Services (CMS) provides information on quality outcomes for the approximately 17,000 nursing homes participating in Medicare and Medicaid programs. CMS's web-based reporting program, Nursing Home Compare, provides user-friendly access to data on quality ratings and measures, health outcomes, and nursing home staff, and results of fire safety inspections. The intent is to provide the public with information that can aid in making decisions related to nursing home placement. Reporting began in 2002 in response to a broad quality initiative that also mandated reporting of quality indicators for hospitals, dialysis facilities, and home health agencies at similar websites.

At the same time, CMS began contracting with **quality improvement organizations (QIOs)** in each state to work with hospitals, nursing homes, home health agencies, and other health service providers to improve quality of care for Medicare beneficiaries and to protect the Medicare Trust Fund through accurate service reimbursements. In nursing homes, much of the QIO activity focuses on work with physicians and nursing staff and includes consultative and educational components. While some questions about the impact of mandatory reporting and QIO efforts have arisen, early studies show some improvement in measures such as use of restraints, pain management, and prevalence of pressure sores (Arling 2007; Shih, Dewar, and Hartman 2007; Rollow et al. 2006). Overall, the gains have been modest, and attention remains focused on efforts to improve care.

Individual states have taken different approaches to reporting care outcomes in nursing homes. In each case, however, the intent is to help people select high-quality health facilities. State scoreboards may include state ranking systems for high-performing nursing homes. Accrediting organizations post lists of accredited programs and, in some cases, detailed information on their facility reviews. One example is The Joint Commission's Quality Check site, which provides information on the safety and quality performance of accredited nursing homes and comparisons to similar facilities.

Another response to concerns about the quality of care offered in nursing homes was to amend the OAA in 1978 to establish the Long-Term Care Ombudsman Program (LTCOP). All 50 states now have **ombudsman programs** that are responsible for addressing complaints about care by nursing home residents and interested parties. The ombudsman role includes advocacy for policy and regulatory change to improve care and provision of information and education for clients and their families. The programs are funded by federal and state monies and are operated by a variety of state agencies and nonprofit organizations. The mandated investigatory and advocacy roles of ombudsman programs are carried out by individuals in paid and volunteer positions (Estes et al. 2004; Nelson et al. 2004).

Quality improvement organization (QIO)
A private, not-for-profit organization staffed by trained professionals who review medical care and help beneficiaries with complaints about the quality of care and implement improvements in the quality of care available throughout the spectrum of care.

Ombudsman program
A program that includes advocacy for policy and regulatory change to improve care and provision of information and education for consumers; funded by federal and state monies and operated by a variety of state agencies and nonprofit organizations.

Concerns about the effectiveness of ombudsman programs have been investigated by researchers at the state and national levels. Carroll Estes and colleagues (2004) looked at the perceptions of ombudsmen related to factors affecting their ability to effect positive change. The study found that two factors negatively affect LTCOP effectiveness: limitations on funding and the placement of ombudsmen in agencies that also regulate nursing homes or make Medicaid payment decisions.

Efforts are also in place to ensure that assisted living facilities and other community-based LTC programs provide high-quality services. As mentioned earlier, the federal government oversees all programs that are reimbursed through Medicare or Medicaid. Private foundations that support many community-based services also require accounting of funds and reporting of program outcomes. Public interest in safety and quality of life for the nation's seniors has risen as seniors themselves, who make up an increasingly large proportion of the population, have gained a voice in the national discourse about LTC. This generation of seniors is better educated and more affluent than preceding generations. They exert influence through their purchasing power and political activism as they seek to affect the quality, availability, and affordability of health and residential services.

(!) CRITICAL CONCEPT
Campaigns for Nursing Home Quality

The development of ombudsman programs occurred at the same time as a growing list of private and consumer-based health quality initiatives. Many of these programs addressed specific health issues or conditions; few focused on specific healthcare settings. An exception is the National Citizens' Coalition for Nursing Home Reform. This organization and its many constituent citizens' advocacy groups have played significant roles in informing the public of concerns related to nursing home care and influencing the passage of legislation related to improving care (Phillips et al. 2008). One such effort is a campaign called **Advancing Excellence in America's Nursing Homes.** It is backed by a public/private coalition that includes providers, government agencies, facility clients, health professionals, private foundations, and other quality care advocates. The coalition supports a program that attempts to increase the quality of nursing home care by challenging nursing homes to address major problem areas, including pressure ulcers, the inappropriate use of physical restraints, and pain management for long- and short-term residents. The coalition's goals include identifying specific targets for quality improvement, assessing satisfaction with care, improving consistency of staff assignment, and staff retention.

(continued)

Advancing Excellence in America's Nursing Homes
A public/private coalition of long-term care providers, government agencies, consumers, health professionals, private foundations, and other quality care advocates that attempts to improve the quality of nursing home care by challenging nursing homes to address major problems in care, identify specific targets for quality improvement, assess satisfaction with care, improve consistency of staff assignment, and enhance staff retention.

> ⓘ **CRITICAL CONCEPT**
> Campaigns for Nursing Home Quality (continued)
>
> The nursing home industry is accountable for the care provided to its residents. Pressure brought by regulation and private oversight has affected care and care delivery models. New initiatives are designed to improve the quality of life for institutionalized residents and the working conditions for care staff by changing the nursing home setting and culture. These efforts, which seek to move nursing home care from a medical model to a resident-centered model, show promise. Early studies have found improvement in quality-of-life measures and in the quality of care provided. Additionally, improvement in staff satisfaction has translated into lower turnover rates, a key factor in the delivery of high-quality care (Koren 2010; LeRoy, Treanor, and Art 2010; Wilson 2009).

A LOOK AHEAD

Early regulation of healthcare services came about as individuals and communities sought to address physician competence and safety and care issues in hospitals. Initial regulatory activity included development of standards by professional organizations, state licensure laws, and private accreditation efforts. When the Medicare and Medicaid programs were launched in 1965 and the US government began to finance LTC services, federal standards were developed for covered services, including home care and institutional care. Congress passed the first set of nursing home standards in 1967. Since that time the number and complexity of regulations that address LTC services have grown, along with oversight activity by state, federal, and private regulators.

While care has improved markedly in LTC residential facilitates, problems still exist. Well-reasoned efforts to change the culture in nursing homes and to move payment for LTC services to more community-based models shows promise in improving quality of life for many elderly people. However, oversight of home and community-based care paid for by public funds will be difficult, and some will see it as intrusive. As the government extends payment to new models of care, that effort will be accompanied by regulatory processes that attempt to address provider accountability and ensure services. A large and politically active senior population can be expected to weigh in on the development and delivery of these services individually and through local, regional, and national consumer interest groups.

FOR DISCUSSION

1. Each state has health facility surveyors who are trained in state and federal survey protocol, regulations, and procedures. What are the qualifications, position description, and job responsibilities for individuals serving in this role in your state?

2. State requirements for the education and certification or licensure of nursing home administrators and assisted living facility administrators vary greatly. Select three states and create a chart comparing requirements for licensure or certification and education or training for each.

3. Laws regulating skilled nursing facilities and assisted living facilities vary by state. However, most states' regulations address emergency/disaster preparedness, fire safety, staff training, medication management, resident privacy, and background checks. What do the regulations in your state say about these issues? Where do you see the greatest differences in regulations? Why?

4. What was the significance of the passage of the Omnibus Budget Reconciliation Act of 1987?

5. What are the differences in the primary mandates assigned to state and federal health facility surveyors and state ombudsmen?

6. What public interest groups, aging services, or professional organizations have the most influence on political decisions related to LTC? Why?

7. Conduct research on one public interest group and one professional organization to determine the three highest-ranking issues on their political agendas. Are their focus areas similar?

8. What are the differences in services provided by skilled nursing facilities and intermediate care facilities?

9. What role do quality improvement organizations play in ensuring quality in LTC organizations?

10. Identify the federal legislation you believe has had the most significant impact on care for the elderly, and explain why.

CASE STUDY: JOINT COMMISSION ACCREDITATION

As the new administrator of Golden Oaks Nursing Home, you have been approached by the facility owner and asked to prepare a report discussing your recommendation as to whether the facility should seek accreditation by The Joint Commission. Golden Oaks is a 120-bed skilled nursing facility located in a midsized city and has four competitors within a five-mile radius. Three of those competitors have been in business for less than five years and have new buildings with upgraded furnishings. Your building is 40 years old. It was last renovated ten years ago and is in good repair but a little dated in appearance. You are hoping to convince the owner to spend money on cosmetic fixes that would be helpful in marketing the facility's services.

CASE STUDY QUESTIONS

1. What is the perceived or real value of Joint Commission accreditation?
2. Identify the pros and cons of accreditation as you frame the argument that your facility should or should not commit the time and expense required to participate in the accreditation process.

Financing Long-Term Care Services

Robert Spinelli, DBA, and Mary Helen McSweeney-Feld, PhD

LEARNING OBJECTIVES

After completing this chapter, you should be able to

➤ distinguish the characteristics of public versus private sources of financing long-term care services;

➤ understand the role of long-term care insurance as a source of payment for long-term care;

➤ understand how public and private sources of long-term care service reimbursement complement each other;

➤ understand the process of assessing individuals to determine their need for long-term care services;

➤ discuss the links between quality and reimbursement for long-term care services; and

➤ distinguish differences in approaches to financing long-term care services in the United States and other countries.

INTRODUCTION

Payment for long-term care services determines an individual's access to and use of those services in the United States and other parts of the world. A government's decision to pay for certain services can also be a factor in that person's ability to age successfully and live a productive life in his community.

The phrase "form follows financing" means that the availability of money or financing determines the accessibility and level of care for individuals. To fully understand the structure of the LTC service delivery system in the United States, one must look at the public and private payment systems for these services that have evolved throughout much of the twentieth century and into the twenty-first. Unless significant payment system reforms are implemented, the prospect of an overburdened, patchwork LTC financing system will become reality as individuals throughout the world live increasingly longer lives and as many face the likelihood that they will outlive their financial resources.

DEMOGRAPHIC TRENDS AND FINANCING

LONG-TERM CARE

As the baby boom generation ages, the US elderly population is expected to experience rapid growth over the next few decades. Estimates by the US Census Bureau indicate that the elderly population will more than double between 2010 and 2050, and by 2050, 20.2 percent of the population will be aged 65 years or older, compared with 12.9 percent in 2010 and 8.1 percent in 1950 (US Census Bureau 2011b). This trend is a global phenomenon (see Exhibit 14.1). Those aged 65 or older worldwide (projected to be 545 million people) in 2011 will account for about 8 percent of the world population. That number is expected to rise to 1.55 billion, or 17 percent of the world population, by 2050 (US Census Bureau 2011a). Developing countries are also aging, frequently at a faster rate than in the developed world (Kinsella and He 2008). All of these changes will dramatically increase demand for long-term care services at a global level.

Substantial resources are already devoted to LTC services. Recent estimates by H. Stephen Kaye, Charlene Harrington, and Mitchell LaPlante (2010) indicate that approximately $33.7 billion (2009 dollars) were spent annually on LTC services delivered at home (over a broad period from 2004 to 2006), and $113.7 billion were spent annually on care for nursing home residents over the same period. Ari Houser and Mary Jo Gibson (2009) estimate that the value of family caregiving (including donated or unpaid care) totaled more than $375 billion in 2008. Although the value of donated care is difficult to measure, it is the largest financing source for LTC. Medicare and Medicaid payments and out-of-pocket expenditures follow. Private LTC insurance currently accounts for a small portion of financing.

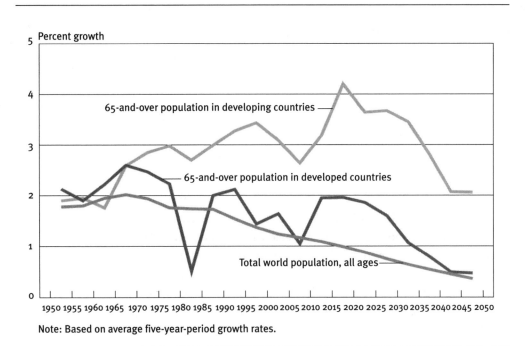

EXHIBIT 14.1
Average Annual
Percent Growth of
Older Population
in Developed
and Developing
Countries: 1950 to
2050

Note: Based on average five-year-period growth rates.

SOURCE: Kinsella and He (2009).

> ⚠ **CRITICAL CONCEPT**
> Long-Term Care Costs in the United States Continue to Rise
>
> The cost of LTC services continues to grow in the United States. According to the 2011 MetLife Market Survey of Nursing Home, Assisted Living, Adult Day Services and Home Care Costs, costs for nursing home care range from an average of $214 daily for a semiprivate room to $239 a day for a private room, a monthly average stay in an assisted living facility runs $3,477 dollars, hourly rates for home care attendants are $21 per hour, and adult day services are estimated at $70 per day for an individual (MetLife Mature Market Institute 2011). Given the growing potential retirements of the baby boomers and the probability of flat economic growth for the next several years, individuals will have to shoulder a greater portion of LTC costs in the future.

The rules that govern the provision of LTC programs influence financing patterns by creating incentives for people to rely on government programs to cover the costs of long-term care.

The US government has only recently created demonstration programs (e.g., Cash and Counseling, Money Follows the Person) that permit more flexibility in the use of funding dollars for services. If left unchanged, such incentives will increase the financial burden that government programs already face as a result of the aging of the population and the increase in healthcare costs.

FINANCING LONG-TERM CARE IN THE UNITED STATES

LTC in the United States is financed through private resources and public programs. Private resources include unpaid or donated care from family members or friends, out-of-pocket spending, commercial insurance payments (although these payments are typically limited), and private LTC insurance. **Medicaid** and **Medicare** are the public programs primarily responsible for financing LTC; the Department of Veterans Affairs and the Social Services Block Grant program also fund some of the costs. In contrast, most European countries finance LTC expenses through public benefit or insurance programs, unpaid care from family members and friends, and out-of-pocket resources.

Private Sources of Payment

Most impaired residents of a given community rely heavily on donated or unpaid care from friends and family. As Exhibit 14.2 shows, only one-fifth of LTC expenditures in 2004 were paid out-of-pocket. The federal government subsidizes some of this spending. Taxpayers with impairments and those whose dependents have impairments may deduct the portion of their LTC, medical, and dental expenses that exceeds 7.5 percent of their adjusted gross income from taxable income.

Long-term care insurance
A specialized private insurance policy that pays the cost of nursing home care and home and community-based care but typically specifies a maximum daily benefit level of reimbursement; can be purchased by individuals and on a group basis through an employer who chooses to offer this benefit.

Employer-sponsored health insurance plans and managed care plans offer some reimbursement for LTC services, although the level of reimbursement is typically limited. Plans can offer payment for home care services or a limited period of nursing home days or rehabilitation care within a nursing home, but these plans are not intended to provide comprehensive coverage of LTC services.

Private **long-term care insurance** entered the insurance markets relatively recently, and payment for care depends on the extent of coverage selected by the policyholder. Less than 10 percent of the population currently has private coverage because they cannot afford it, underestimate the risk of LTC events, or perceive that government programs will provide sufficient coverage. While private LTC coverage is growing, an accurate measurement of subscribers is difficult to obtain. Payments that insurers make directly to providers can be captured, but insurers' reimbursements to policyholders for out-of-pocket payments may be missed. Thus, estimates of LTC insurance payments should be interpreted with caution.

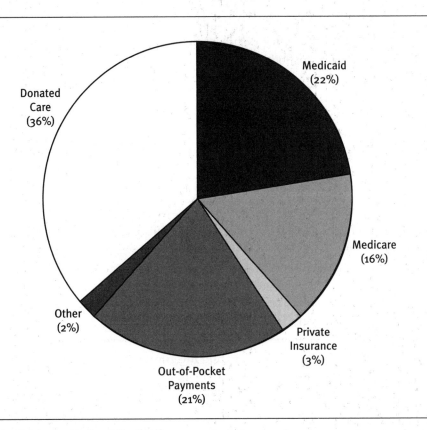

EXHIBIT 14.2
Estimated
Percentage Shares
of Spending on
Long-Term Care for
the Elderly, 2004

SOURCE: Congressional Budget Office (2005).

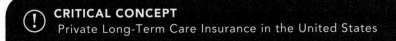

⚠ CRITICAL CONCEPT
Private Long-Term Care Insurance in the United States

Currently, approximately 7 million private LTC insurance policies are in force, covering about 10 percent of those age 65 or older (Stevenson et al. 2010). While growth in the LTC insurance market has slowed considerably, policies have changed substantially and now provide similar coverage for residential, home and community-based care and other services such as assistive technology.

A typical LTC insurance policy covers nursing home care and home and community-based care up to a daily expenditure limit (such as $150) and may include other restrictions. Policies may protect against inflation by increasing benefits by a specific percentage (such as 5 percent) each year or offering a nonforfeiture benefit, which continues protection based on the length of time the policy was in force and the premiums paid if a policyholder cancels her policy. While some policies offer coverage without a time limit, most cover a specific period, such as two to five years, or include a preestablished maximum lifetime benefit amount. Eligibility to collect benefits generally begins when the policyholder reaches a certain level of impairment, most often loss of ability to perform two or three activities of daily living (ADLs) or a cognitive impairment that causes him to need substantial supervision. The policy can be purchased on either an individual or a group basis. A growing number of employers are offering this coverage as an option in their benefits package.

Younger people pay lower premiums for LTC policies, which reflects the lower risk that they will require the services covered in the short term and the likelihood that they will pay more premiums before they need LTC. Individuals who select more comprehensive policies with longer periods for payment of benefits as well as inflation and nonforfeiture protection will have higher premiums. Premium guarantees, which are a feature of some LTC policies, prevent premiums from increasing over time, even though the risk of needing services rises. Insurers calculate these premiums so that total payments over the policy's life, combined with the interest earned through investment of the premiums, will cover the policyholder's claims and the costs to the insurer. However, if new information is released that indicates current premiums and investment returns for a specific group of policyholders (e.g., all policyholders in a state) will not cover the expected expenditures, insurers may raise the premiums of all members of that group.

Government Programs: Medicaid and Medicare

The Medicaid Program

Medicaid

A state-administered, means-tested federal insurance program that pays for medical care and other supportive services for low-income individuals, the disabled, and poor elderly persons. Within broad federal guidelines, the states establish eligibility standards; determine the type, amount, duration, and scope of services; set the rate of payment; and administer their own programs.

Government funding sources pay for most formal LTC services in the United States. Medicaid, which is funded jointly by the states and the federal government, is the largest of these sources. **Medicaid** provides medical benefits for certain groups, including low-income, impaired seniors. Working within guidelines set at the federal level, each state administers its Medicaid program and determines standards for eligibility, payment rates, and type, amount, duration, and scope of services. A statutory formula determines how much of a state's Medicaid expenditures the federal government will pay; for LTC, the number is about 56 percent.

While specific Medicaid benefits differ by state, the program generally covers services provided in nursing facilities, at home, and in the community.

In 2007, of the $190.4 billion in estimated spending for nursing home and home health care in the United States, Medicare paid for 25 percent, while Medicaid and other public funds paid for 42 percent and private insurance paid for 11 percent (Ng, Harrington, and Kitchener 2010). Medicaid's state and federal expenditures for seniors in institutional settings totaled about $58.3 billion. Spending for LTC accounted for about one-third of total Medicaid expenditures, which was about the same amount in 1999.

Medicaid spent less on home and community-based services (HCBS) than on nursing home care, but HCBS spending, which includes personal care services, home health care, and HCBS waiver programs, is growing rapidly. The waiver programs give states the option to provide enhanced community support services not included under federal statutes for people with impairments. HCBS expenditures under Medicaid in 2007 totaled $41.8 billion, representing a 95 percent increase from 1999 levels; however, need for these services remains unmet in communities, and access to Medicaid programs and spending vary tremendously across states.

The Medicare Program

Medicare covers care given at home and in skilled nursing facilities (SNFs) for individuals older than 65, those who have received Social Security disability benefits for more than two years, and those with amyotrophic lateral sclerosis (Lou Gehrig's disease) or end-stage renal disease.

Medicare is composed of four parts. Part A covers hospital and SNF stays of up to 100 days; it is noncontributory for plan participants until day 21, when a daily out-of-pocket coinsurance comes into effect, assuming plan participants still meet the need for nursing home care. Medicare Part B, commonly known as medical insurance through the Medicare program, covers physician and outpatient services; it is a voluntary program for which recipients pay a monthly premium. Medicare Part C is a managed care version of Medicare that replaces benefits in Parts A and B with a comprehensive managed care network, and Part D covers some prescription drug expenses depending on the level of coverage selected by the participant and level of expenditures that are currently subject to limitations (the gap in coverage is known as the doughnut hole).

The primary purpose of Medicare is to assist beneficiaries in recovering from acute episodes of illness, not to finance long-term care. However, the program offers a home health benefit, which essentially provides LTC coverage. Beneficiaries who are homebound and need a licensed professional, such as a registered nurse or physical therapist, to provide intermittent care are eligible for this benefit. Such beneficiaries are also reimbursed for care from a home health aide, who provides services typical of LTC.

Medicare home health spending was an estimated $15.6 billion in 2007, a 59 percent increase from 1999 (Ng, Harrington, and Kitchener 2010). A growing portion of Medicare spending is for short-term post-acute care (after hospitalization), hospice care, nursing home care, home care, or care received in other settings, such as assisted living facilities. In 2007, total Medicare spending on post-acute care totaled $37.8 billion, a 75

Medicare
The federal health insurance program for individuals over age 65, those on Social Security disability benefits for more than two years, and those with Lou Gehrig's disease or end-stage renal disease. It has four parts and covers care provided in skilled nursing facilities (SNFs) for up to 100 days as well as home care.

> ⓘ **CRITICAL CONCEPT**
> Spending Projections: Medicare and Medicaid
>
> The Congressional Budget Office (CBO) has projected that by 2040, total LTC expenditures for seniors will reach $540 billion (in 2000 dollars), including the value of unpaid family caregiving or donated care. This estimate assumes a 1.1 percent decline in impairment per year. If impairment levels remain the same, 2040 LTC expenditures will be closer to $760 billion and will account for about 3.3 percent of gross domestic product. If impairment levels increase, expenditures will be even higher. Furthermore, if the current economic downturn leaves individuals needing care with diminished ability to pay for that care, they may be even more likely to outlive their savings and assets.
>
> Researchers call for greater coordination of LTC needs between the Medicare and Medicaid programs (Programs of All-Inclusive Care for the Elderly, or PACE, and some managed care waiver demonstrations are exceptions). Greater interaction between public programs and private LTC insurance is also necessary, as they can serve complementary roles in the reimbursement of LTC services (Stevenson et al. 2010).

percent increase over that spent in 1999, and hospice spending totaled $10.3 billion, a 229 percent increase over 1999. Medicare spending for nursing home care also experienced a 32 percent increase, to $22.1 billion, by 2007 (Ng, Harrington, and Kitchener 2010).

Medicare Prospective Payment System for Long-Term Care Facilities

A key component of Medicare payment for services delivered in LTC facilities is its prospective payment system, which was implemented in 1998. The primary instrument for determining the level of care need, and consequently payment, for long-term care expenses in nursing homes as well as swing bed providers (hospitals that have beds that can be used to provide long-term care or acute care) is the **Minimum Data Set** 3.0 (MDS) survey questionnaire. This is a standardized screening, assessment, and data collection tool that forms the foundation for assessment and (ideally) should be completed by an interdisciplinary team on admission of all residents to long-term care facilities certified for participation in Medicare and Medicaid, with the results submitted to CMS. The MDS contains items that measure physical, psychological, and psychosocial functioning. The items in the MDS give a multidimensional view of the patient's functional capacities and identify specifically which of the resident's

Minimum Data Set
A standardized screening, assessment, and data collection tool for determining the level of care need for long-term care expenses in nursing homes and hospitals.

needs must be met by the nursing facility. A discharge plan for each resident is also required by the MDS 3.0.

The data collected as part of the MDS 3.0 assessment process are also used in the calculation of CMS Quality Indicators, or QIs (used to point out potential problem areas in care); **Resource Utilization Groups,** or **RUGs** (used to determine level of payment; and **Care Area Assessments,** or **CAAs** (used to further identify and evaluate the resident's strengths and potential problems). These reports contain information at the state and county level for every Medicare- and Medicaid-certified nursing home in the country. The quality indicators are published, along with information about nursing home surveys and staffing information, in Medicare's Nursing Home Compare database on the CMS website (www.cms.gov/nhcompare). Due to the significant number of changes in the MDS 3.0 and RUGS (now in Version IV), nursing homes and other facilities accepting Medicare residents will have ongoing challenges in the implementation of these new assessment and data collection tools.

Resource Utilization Groups (RUGs)

A prospective payment system used under Medicare to determine the level of payment for resident care, based on care and resource needs, under Medicare Part A. Skilled nursing facilities determine a RUG based on 108 items on the Minimum Data Set (MDS) resident assessment tool.

Care assessment areas (CAAs)

A standardized screen used in Medicare's minimum data set survey to further identify and evaluate a resident's strengths, problems, and needs and to help identify the need for further specialized services for the resident.

> ## (!) CRITICAL CONCEPT
> Quality Management in Long-Term Care: CMS Initiatives
>
> The issue of quality management in the delivery of LTC services has been a primary focus of CMS in recent years. On the basis of data collected from providers under the Medicare system, CMS has developed a comprehensive system whereby nursing homes, home care agencies, dialysis centers, and hospitals can compare their performance on key quality indicators with the performance of their primary competitors, state averages, or national statistics. Laypeople also have access to the system, as the indicators are published on the CMS website and updated periodically.
>
> CMS's focus on quality management has also spurred the development of private, industry-based initiatives to create tools for measuring LTC quality, such as the Alliance for Quality Nursing Home Care and the Advancing Excellence in Nursing Home Care Campaign. These projects have led to a multidimensional approach to measuring quality in LTC facilities, in which clinical indicators are combined with resident and family caregiver satisfaction, staffing indicators, and other financial and operational indicators.

Policy Issues: How to Pay for Long-Term Care in the Future

Government programs currently contribute a significant share of LTC financing, which increases the pressure the federal budget will experience as the baby boomers age. These programs offer incentives that make the use of private resources such as private insurance a less attractive means for seniors to finance care. If those incentives are changed or eliminated, more people might use private resources rather than government assistance to finance their care.

Federal Spending Limits

The pressures on federal finances could be relieved through a reduction of the role of Medicaid and Medicare. Tighter financial qualifications for Medicaid coverage would reduce Medicare's coverage of home health care and improve coordination of care and services between the two government programs.

Medicaid is intended to finance healthcare for the poor and poor elderly, but many applicants get around the income restrictions by spending down their resources and disposing of their assets in such a way that they protect their wealth but still qualify for government assistance, a practice called Medicaid estate planning. Strengthening the qualification rules to prohibit this strategy, and encouraging individuals with assets to purchase long-term care insurance early, would help prevent those who do not need Medicaid benefits from receiving them.

Currently the Medicaid program conducts a five-year "look back" to identify inappropriate transfers of assets intended to protect those assets from the state. Some individuals who encounter a roadblock in their application for Medicaid seek advice from their attorneys or attorneys in their communities who specialize in this area. The look back discourages some people from applying but has little impact on Medicaid spending.

Once a person qualifies for Medicare home health care coverage, he is not required to contribute copayments or coinsurance of any kind. If a cost-sharing requirement were included in the program, expenditures would decrease because beneficiaries would be less eager to use services for which they had to pay.

Encouragement to Privately Finance Long-Term Care

Another method of decreasing future federal spending on LTC is to encourage reliance on private resources and to promote the view that private insurance and government programs are complementary. As mentioned earlier, private insurance accounts for very little LTC spending. According to CBO estimates, private insurance will pay for about 17 percent of LTC spending in 2020—less than Medicaid or Medicare will pay. This limited increase is the result of several factors that affect availability and quality of insurance, such as administrative cost issues, unstable premiums, adverse selection, and inability to insure against certain risks unique to LTC. Group LTC insurance policies purchased through an employer can only be purchased on a posttax basis, unlike employer-sponsored health insurance, for which employees pay with pretax dollars. The interaction between private insurance and Medicaid also affects demand for private insurance.

ADMINISTRATIVE COSTS IN LONG-TERM CARE INSURANCE

Most LTC policies are individual rather than group policies, leading to high administrative costs. Marketing to and enrolling individuals cost about twice as much as doing so for groups, where administrative costs can be spread among more beneficiaries.

Administrative costs as a percentage of premiums will probably decrease as group policies begin to account for a larger share of the private LTC insurance market. If employers offer LTC benefits, employer-paid premiums are excluded from employee participants' taxable income. This factor may provide an incentive for employees to enhance their level of coverage under policies provided by their employer.

INSTABILITY OF LONG-TERM CARE INSURANCE PREMIUMS

Although LTC premiums typically do not increase as the policyholder ages or experiences a decline in health, insurers may increase premiums for all policyholders in a rating class if the insurer has miscalculated the expected cost of that class's claims. Multiple increases of this kind by some insurers have led policyholders to cancel their coverage and have most likely also deterred potential purchasers.

Nonforfeiture benefits offer policyholders some protection against large premium increases by enabling them to recoup some of their paid premiums from the insurer when they cancel coverage. However, even with these benefits, policyholders lose the associated returns on the investment of the money they get back.

ADVERSE SELECTION

Because the market for LTC insurance is still new and the number of policies being sold is small, adverse selection may affect the market. Expectations of using LTC services in the future drives purchasing decisions, but the information insurers collect during enrollment fails to capture those expectations. The belief that adverse selection is occurring might lead insurers to charge higher premiums. Those higher premiums might deter potential purchasers who would purchase coverage if premiums reflected their lower expectations of using LTC services. A continuing problem exists in the current marketplace as claims for individuals with Alzheimer's disease have increased substantially due to the potential length of this illness, and this trend may have led some insurers to increase premiums to balance these risks.

THE INABILITY TO INSURE AGAINST CERTAIN RISKS

In general, private LTC insurance does not protect against significant price increases, making it unattractive to some. Most policies specify the benefits that will be provided if the policyholder becomes impaired. Consumers may also purchase a policy rider that specifies a rate of growth in the policy's benefits each year (usually 5 percent). Over 20 years, a benefit of $100 per day would grow to $265 per day (in today's dollars) with an annual inflation protection rider of 5 percent. However, if costs continue to grow at an annual rate of 6.7 percent, the benefit would need to grow to $366 per day to cover the costs of care.

The policy could also become obsolete. As the market for LTC services and private insurance matures, the care and insurance evolve, which may cause individuals to think twice about purchasing an LTC policy. They might also hesitate to purchase insurance if they expect that future public policy changes could render their coverage obsolete.

THE AVAILABILITY OF MEDICAID

Why would someone purchase private LTC insurance when Medicaid is available? While Medicaid is intended to serve low-income individuals, people with impairments, even those with significant savings set aside, can qualify for Medicaid by exhausting all of their private sources of financing for their LTC. Thus, people who do not have private insurance essentially use Medicaid as an alternative form of insurance when they become impaired for a significant period. Indeed, people may choose not to acquire significant assets or to give away or hide their assets in response to Medicaid's impoverishment requirement.

But the use of Medicaid coverage for LTC has drawbacks. Applicants must pay out-of-pocket for medical expenses until their savings are depleted. Medicaid pays lower fees than private payers, so beneficiaries may receive a lower quality of care. In some states, Medicaid covers fewer services and offers a narrower choice of providers and types of care than private insurers. Few physicians accept Medicaid patients because of the program's low and slow reimbursement, and now LTC facilities are discouraged from accepting Medicaid patients with the advent of Medicaid bundling. With Medicaid bundling, providers are required to absorb the costs of oxygen, therapy services (though Medicare Part B can be used until exhausted per the therapy cap), durable medical equipment, over-the-counter medications, and resident transportation.

Medicaid coverage does offer advantages as well. The beneficiary pays nothing for care services. Unlike private insurance, which guarantees a specific monetary benefit but not coverage for specific services, Medicaid covers a specified set of services.

While Medicaid differs from private LTC insurance, it may still reduce demand for this type of private insurance. According to a study by Brown and Finkelstein (2008), the availability of Medicaid substantially influences the decision to purchase private insurance and how much to buy, regardless of income level. Medicaid's rules for financial eligibility offer a low-cost LTC alternative to preparing financially for possible future impairment. Private insurance policyholders and those who have accumulated substantial savings are less likely to qualify for Medicare; such preparation means forgoing the government-provided benefits. The perceived cost of financial preparation rises as a result of the availability of Medicaid. This increased cost may seem small for those too wealthy to ever be likely to qualify for Medicaid, but the effect can be greater on others.

DID YOU KNOW?
Public-Private Partnerships for Long-Term Care

In February 2006, Congress approved legislation that encourages the expansion of existing public-private partnerships for LTC. This law authorizes changes in state law that permit individuals to purchase LTC insurance that coordinates with state Medicaid programs. Under these policies, when individuals exhaust the benefits provided under their LTC insurance policy, the state Medicaid program will pay for the remainder of their care without requiring them to spend down their assets. A number of these programs were initially created under the **Partnership for Long-Term Care** sponsored by the Robert Wood Johnson Foundation in the 1980s, but the limits of this program left only a handful of states with active programs. This legislation allows for program expansion with significant potential benefits. The AHIP Center for Research and Policy (2007) projects that expanding these partnerships could lead to potential savings of $6 billion annually by 2050. They may also increase the attractiveness of LTC insurance policies for individuals who wish to maintain their assets for their families or other future beneficiaries.

PUBLIC LONG-TERM CARE INSURANCE: GERMANY, JAPAN, AND THE CLASS ACT

The Partnership for Long-Term Care Program
A program authorized under the Deficit Reduction Act of 2005 that permits states to promote the purchase of private long-term care insurance by offering consumers access to Medicaid under special eligibility rules should additional long-term care coverage (beyond what the policies provide) be needed.

Many of the major industrialized nations have restructured their long-term care systems over the past 20 years. Some countries, such as Germany and Japan, have public LTC insurance programs that supplement their public health insurance programs by providing paid assistance to family members or others providing care or enhanced reimbursement for community-based services. In these countries, the "social insurance programs are universal, support family caregivers, and allow individuals considerable flexibility in securing the services they require" (Campbell, Ikegami, and Gibson 2010).

As part of the federal healthcare reform initiatives under the Affordable Care Act, the US Congress has passed the Community Living Assistance Services and Supports (CLASS) Act, a type of voluntary, public long-term care insurance that could pay for long-term care as well as other supportive services for people with disabilities. The intent of the CLASS Act is to provide long-term care insurance for individuals with severe disabilities who may be turned down for private long-term care insurance coverage and who then turn to their state Medicaid program for coverage for services critical to their independence, such as assistive technology, housing modifications, transportation, and other items. At the time of the publication of this book, the decision to fund the CLASS Act has met resistance in the US Congress, although the concept of government-provided long-term care insurance may be revisited in the future.

Germany and Japan have well-established, public LTC insurance programs. They introduced these programs in the 1990s because their frail older populations were growing, traditional resources for care were declining, and existing LTC programs were seen as costly, inefficient, and unfair. However, the models differ, as Japan pays for a high level of community services whereas Germany offers cash to support family caregiving services. An examination of the goals, eligibility process, scope, size, and sustainability of each program for application in other countries found that current US spending on LTC services is higher than in Germany and is slightly lower than in Japan (Campbell, Ikegami, and Gibson 2010). Consequently, efforts to expand public LTC insurance options in the United States may prove to be a practical solution for financing the population's growing LTC needs.

A Look Ahead

LTC services are currently financed through various sources, including private resources and government programs. The financing structure includes incentives to rely on government programs and may discourage reliance on private resources to prepare for LTC needs. The aging of the baby boom generation will increase demand for LTC and exacerbate budgetary strains. Greater coordination of resources under government programs such as Medicare and Medicaid, combined with incentives for individuals to purchase private or public LTC insurance, are potential solutions for more effective financing of LTC.

For Discussion

1. What are the main sources of payment for LTC services in the United States? How does the financing structure compare with that in many European countries?

2. What impact will the baby boom generation have on the cost of long-term care over the next decade and beyond?

3. Discuss the reasons LTC insurance has not become more popular in the United States.

4. Why isn't Medicare considered a major source of LTC reimbursement?

5. Can the growth in Medicaid spending for LTC services be expected to decrease in the next ten years?

6. How does Medicare assess a person's need for LTC services in a nursing home setting?

7. Why is family caregiving an important part of payment for long-term care needs?

8. What is the CLASS Act?

9. What is Medicaid estate planning?

10. What are public-private partnerships for LTC?

CASE STUDY: CMS FIVE-STAR QUALITY RATING SYSTEM

Launched in November 2010 by CMS, the Five-Star Quality Rating System awards nursing facilities a rating from one star (well below average) to five stars (well above average) on the basis of their performance on state surveys of their facility, levels of staffing, and performance on ten quality measures tracked by the system. These indicators, many of which are clinical in nature, include reducing new pressure ulcers, decreasing pain, maintaining mobility, decreasing urinary tract infections and the use of indwelling catheters, reducing the use of physical restraints, and reducing the incidence of delirium.

The rating calculation looks at the past three years' surveys, giving greater weight to more recent years and adjusting for any deficiencies or complaints. CMS then compares each facility to its peers within the state and assigns a star rating. Only 10 percent of the facilities in any state may receive a five-star rating, and facilities rated as five stars in one period may be downgraded to a lower star ranking in a future period, especially if another facility receives a better survey. The five-star ratings are published as part of the data on each nursing facility on the CMS Nursing Home Compare website. While the intent of the rating system is to provide people with more information on the quality of nursing homes in their community, it does not include certain key information about a facility's specialized services, such as whether it has a ventilator unit or specializes in particular types of rehabilitation care. In addition, measures of survey satisfaction data for each facility are not included, and CMS is hesitant to include such data in the absence of nationally standardized data.

CASE STUDY QUESTIONS

1. Is the Five-Star Quality Rating System helpful to potential residents and their families in making decisions about nursing home care? Why or why not?

2. Does a facility that receives a five-star rating in one period and then is downgraded to a lower number of stars in a later period face any financial consequences?

3. How might facility administrators use the five-star rating system to address issues of quality within their organization?

Epilogue

Mary Helen McSweeney-Feld, PhD, and Reid Oetjen, PhD

A s the global population continues to age, pressures on countries' healthcare delivery and pension systems will mount. The traditional model of retirement at age 65 will be replaced by a model that features a higher age at which people will become eligible for collecting retirement benefits from public pension systems, part-time employment subsidized by government system payments, and more limited employer-sponsored pension funds. Socialized medical systems will experience increased pressure to accommodate the healthcare demands of a fast-growing segment of the aging population—the oldest among us (those older than 85)—and new models for delivery of care emphasizing the use of technology, a social model of care, consumer education and self-help, and new payment mechanisms will be implemented and refined.

To better understand the challenges ahead, the long-term care community must conduct a needs assessment. What do we know, and what information do we need in order to facilitate successful aging and the provision of LTC services on a global basis? The following sections present areas for continued exploration.

GLOBALIZATION OF HEALTHCARE

The healthcare field is changing and will follow all other industries toward globalization. To confront—and embrace—this trend, the LTC community needs access to internationally comparative knowledge on basic health indicators as well as data on the living arrangements of elderly individuals, the demand for care, and the organization and supply of LTC. This information is currently fragmented, and comprehensive international data sets and concepts are not yet fully developed (Huber et al. 2009). The US Census Bureau, the United Nations, the Statistical Office of the European Communities, and other organizations have begun to issue reports on global trends in LTC to facilitate evidence-based policymaking in these areas.

As part of the Shaping Long-Term Care in America project, Brown University has received funding from the National Institute on Aging to create a comprehensive long-term care database in the United States (Brown University, Alpert Medical School 2009). Continued efforts to share information and data across nations are needed to address the challenges of global aging.

INNOVATIVE PAYMENT SYSTEMS FOR LTC NEEDS

Global economic trends and countries' ability to fund public pension systems will remain a challenge to financing LTC. Public-private partnership solutions will continue to be pursued, and the use of private insurance and other healthcare and retirement savings account mechanisms will continue to grow in importance as the needs of aging populations worldwide outpace the labor force that supports the tax base. Future generations will be increasingly called on to plan and invest in a variety of plans that will help ensure the provision of LTC services.

TECHNOLOGICAL INNOVATION

The use of technology to obtain care and LTC services will continue to grow. Groups such as the baby boomers and health seekers will join the wired retired in the pursuit of healthcare services (Coile 2002). Studies to determine the cost-effectiveness of new technological initiatives and the impact of electronic medical records systems and health information technology networks will grow in importance as governments, policymakers, and individuals examine best practices in these areas. Self-care technologies that allow seniors to age in place in the community will continue to be developed and marketed to new, more tech-savvy cohorts of boomers and others who follow.

Technological innovations may change the playing field, allowing providers to reach clients in new ways while reducing the cost of care. At the same time, advancements in healthcare may increase the cost of care as new treatments extend lives. The cost-effectiveness of these new technologies will need to be continuously evaluated.

CHRONIC HEALTH CONDITIONS

The United States spends a disproportionate amount (almost 75 percent) of healthcare dollars treating chronic conditions compared with other conditions (Partnership to Fight Chronic Disease 2011). Research on effective treatment protocols will continue to be a priority worldwide. Diseases of aging, such as Alzheimer's and other forms of dementia, will rise to the level of heart disease, cancer, obesity, and diabetes in relevance, and greater funding for research and new treatment options from the global medical community will need to be pursued. Prevention efforts directed at decreasing the prevalence of chronic conditions in nonelderly populations will also require attention.

INCREASED DIVERSITY

The need for LTC spans the age range from children to older people, and growth in the older population, especially those age 85 or older, has contributed to increased need (Ng, Harrington, and Kitchener 2010). At the same time, future older people may have lower disability levels than those in previous generations and may use fewer institutional services (Vladeck 2005). Future LTC providers who wish to remain competitive will need to be fluid to provide culturally competent care and new alternatives. Awareness and training in these new trends will be essential for current and future LTC administrators, students who are studying to become providers of LTC services, and human resources managers in workplaces where employees are balancing jobs and caregiving responsibilities.

QUALITY-OF-CARE CONCERNS

The early history of LTC delivery in the United States was plagued with scandal and stories of neglect and abuse. Although the LTC industry is arguably the most regulated sector of healthcare, many new forms of LTC services developed in recent years have largely escaped regulation and scrutiny. The LTC community needs to be vigilant so that vulnerable populations of elders, especially those who are economically challenged, do not suffer harm at the hands of unscrupulous and poor-quality providers. LTC provider organizations need to continue to develop measures of service quality; otherwise, regulatory agencies and government will be forced to step in, impeding the innovation necessary to meet future challenges.

Another quality challenge facing the global LTC community is leveraging technology to provide the aging population with evidence-based and value-based care. To date, the acute care system has not sufficiently used technology to provide evidence-based medicine. Perhaps the LTC sector of healthcare can lead the way on this initiative.

SUSTAINABILITY

The medical model of LTC delivery is no longer sustainable because of the looming insurmountable cost of institutionalizing the aging population. The challenge of sustainability addresses the spread of the culture change philosophy that is currently under way in the provision of LTC services in the United States. Most LTC recipients prefer to stay at home and in their communities. To create a sustainable model of care, the LTC community must pursue the client-driven model of care, emphasize self-directed options and choices, and develop more cost-effective alternatives to institutionalized care. The industry needs to provide the care that people want without building new facilities.

Another catalyst for this movement is the fact that today's and tomorrow's elderly are highly educated, vocal, and unafraid to flex their political will. Society and the LTC industry will serve their best interests by investigating and quickly adopting innovative methods and strategies.

Tremendous opportunities exist for individuals to train and retrain for new employment opportunities in this field and to develop new businesses and models of care that can address the needs of this new aging population. At the same time, the information about LTC issues and specialized training programs for services must be introduced into educational curricula to encourage students to choose careers in the LTC industry. Without these initiatives, efforts to meet the needs of our growing aging population will continue to be fragmented at best and unmet at worst. This is an exciting time to be working in the field, as those who embark on a career today will help to shape the future of the industry.

Accountability: The importance of the employee or team meeting established objectives as well as follow-through on the part of management in carrying out the team's recommendations.

Accreditation: The act of giving credit or recognition to organizations that maintain suitable standards.

Activities of daily living (ADLs): Routine daily activities; the basic ADLs are eating, bathing, dressing, toileting, and walking. A person's ability to perform ADLs is a determining factor in the level of long-term care he needs.

Administration: Those employees who manage the day-to-day operations of the organization and who carry out the policies of the governing body; also known as the management team.

Administration on Aging: A division of the US Department of Health and Human Services responsible for advancing the concerns and interests of older people and their caregivers.

Adult day services: Community-based facilities for individuals who need supervised care during the daytime, but who otherwise remain in their homes.

Advance directive: Information provided to a healthcare provider that details an incapacitated individual's wishes for medical care.

Advancing Excellence in America's Nursing Homes: A public/private coalition of long-term care providers, government agencies, consumers, health professionals, private foundations, and other quality care advocates that attempts to improve the quality of nursing home care by challenging nursing homes to address major problems in care, identify specific targets for quality improvement, assess satisfaction with care, improve consistency of staff assignment, and enhance staff retention.

Age Discrimination in Employment Act of 1967: An act that prohibits age-based discrimination for applicants or employees over the age of 40.

Age-segregated communities: Also known as age-restricted communities, this is housing, frequently gated, that restricts ownership of units to individuals over a set age, such as age 50 or 55, in order to provide a living area without the perceived problems of having children around.

Aging Network: Housed under the Administration on Aging, the Aging Network is a comprehensive and coordinated system of home and community-based long-term care services.

Aging process: The changes in the functions and capabilities of people's bodies over time; influenced by genetic and environmental factors.

Aging tsunami: The aging Baby Boomers' huge impact on society.

Alzheimer's disease: A progressive and fatal brain disorder that destroys brain cells and causes memory loss as well as problems with thinking and behaviors that can affect an individual's work and social activities.

American College of Surgeons Hospital Standardization Program: A list of standards developed by the ACS for accreditation of hospitals; this evolved into the Joint Commission for Accreditation of Healthcare Organizations.

Americans with Disabilities Act of 1990 (ADA): An act that prohibits discrimination due to disability and applies to job application procedures, hiring, advancement, termination, workers' compensation, training, and other terms or conditions of employment.

Assisted living facilities (ALFs): Facilities in which staff help residents with the activities of daily living, coordinate services from outside providers, and monitor activities to help to ensure residents' health, well-being, and safety.

Assistive technology: Hardware and software applications that help people with physical impairments or those managing chronic health conditions.

Autonomy: The right of a competent patient to make her own healthcare decisions.

Behaviorally anchored rating scales (BARS): A method of employee appraisal that uses numeric scales to measure various levels of effectiveness. This method of appraisal focuses on behaviors that are determined to be important for completing a job task rather than focusing on employee characteristics.

Beneficence: The responsibility of those caring for any patient to "do good" for the patient, but above all, to do no harm to the patient.

Benefits: Indirect financial payments given to employees, including health insurance, vacation, and retirement benefits.

Care assessment areas (CAAs): A standardized screen used in Medicare's minimum data set survey to further identify and evaluate a resident's strengths, problems, and needs and to help identify the need for further specialized services for the resident.

Caregivers: Individuals who provide healthcare and/or supportive long-term care services. Caregivers are an important part of the system of support that allows consumers to continue to live in the community.

Cash and Counseling programs: Programs in which consumers direct and manage their personal assistance services, including long-term care, according to their specific needs and receive reimbursement for these services.

Centers for Medicare & Medicaid Services (CMS): An agency of the Department of Health and Human Services responsible for regulating long-term care facilities.

Certification: A process of external review or assessment upon which a designation is awarded to ensure qualification to perform a job or task; long-term care facilities are certified to provide care by the federal Medicare and Medicaid programs.

Chronic illness: A long-lasting or recurrent illness that needs to be managed on a long-term basis.

Civil cases: Cases brought by individuals, corporations, or governmental authorities to enforce a right or collect damages when injuries have occurred.

Civil money penalties: A punitive fine imposed by a civil court on an entity that has profited from illegal or unethical activity.

Civil Rights Act of 1964: A law that makes it illegal to discriminate in employment based on race, color, religion, sex, or national origin.

Coaching: Feedback and advice given to employees by an immediate supervisor or human resource professionals.

Code of Federal Regulations: Title 42 sets minimum standards for participation in the Medicare and Medicaid programs that must be met by all facilities regardless of location.

Cohort: A group of people bound together in history by a set of events.

Cohousing community: A type of collaborative community designed and operated by the residents. The community may be multigenerational or exclusively for people aged 55 and older.

Compensation: The salary or hourly pay and benefits such as health insurance, retirement options, and other fringe benefits such as educational reimbursement that an employee receives.

Conflict resolution: Negotiation by the manager where compromise is the desired outcome in an LTC setting in which opposing goals between any combination of residents, families, and/or employees become counterproductive.

Congregate care facilities: Facilities typically designed for those aged 75 to 82 that offer social activities and homemaker services such as meals, housekeeping services, and transportation. These homes also provide assistance with the instrumental activities of daily living.

Continuing care retirement communities (CCRCs): Residential complexes for seniors that offer comprehensive nursing care and housing options to residents as they age and their needs change. Assisted living, skilled nursing, and independent living facilities, along with their respective nursing and service components, are all located in one community.

Continuous quality improvement (CQI): The ongoing critical examination of resident care processes within long-term care facilities through which team members identify problems, isolate the causes, and develop practical solutions for more effective methods.

Continuum of long-term care: A holistic system comprising services and mechanisms that assist individuals over time through a wide range of physical health, mental health, and social services needs, across all levels of care intensity.

Cultural competence: The ability of individuals or organizations to understand the global view of clients from diverse cultures and adapt their practices to ensure their effectiveness.

Culture: The collective values, beliefs, and norms of an organization that shape how it behaves.

Culture change: An evolving philosophy of providing long-term care services that surpasses the traditional long-term care medical model by nurturing the human spirit while meeting medical needs. Also known as person-centered care or resident-directed care.

Data mining: The analysis of data that has been stored in a data repository, such as a data warehouse.

Data warehouse: A repository of an organization's electronically stored data from which inquiries and analysis can be made.

Database management system: A software system that facilitates the creation, maintenance, and use of an electronic database.

Default judgment: A ruling that occurs when the defendant fails to answer the summons and complaint. At that time, it is possible for a court to find in the plaintiff's favor, but there are due process safeguards built into the system to protect defendants.

Defendant: The party being brought to court.

Defined benefit plan: A retirement plan, typically funded by an employer, that pays a retiree a set amount of money on a predictable schedule.

Defined contribution plan: A retirement plan to which an employer contributes money, such as a 401(k), while the person is employed there. Once that employee leaves the company, the company's obligation is over.

Dementia: An acquired persistent impairment of intellectual function that compromises at least three of the following spheres of mental activity: language, memory, visual/spatial skills, emotion or personality, and cognition.

Diagnostic and Statistical Manual of Mental Disorders: A manual published by the American Psychiatric Association (APA) that provides the standard classification of mental disorders used by mental health professionals.

Dimensions of care model: A nonlinear approach to long-term care that acknowledges the services identified in the continuum of care model, allows the consumer to have a single point of entry into the LTC delivery system, and encourages consumers to use technology in administering self-care and to use services within the community.

Direct care workers: Professional and paraprofessional personnel who work one-on-one with clients in institutional or noninstitutional settings. Examples include registered nurses, licensed practical nurses, certified nursing assistants, nursing assistants, and home care workers.

Disaster plan: A detailed written plan that includes procedures to meet all potential emergencies and disasters, such as fire, severe weather, and missing residents.

Diversity: The variation in cultural, personal, and lifestyle attributes of individuals, including ethnicity, race, age, sexual orientation, and socioeconomic status.

DNR (do not resuscitate) order: Instructions, usually written by a physician after discussion with a patient, telling other healthcare providers not to try to restart a patient's heart through cardiopulmonary resuscitation or other treatments if the patient's heart were to stop beating.

Due process: The proper, official way to do things in a legal case such that the rights of all people involved are protected.

Early Indicators Project: A long-term study of Union Army members that put forth a theory of "technophysioevolution," which posits that humans have gained a degree of control over their environment that has permitted rapid improvements in morbidity and mortality.

Eden Alternative: A philosophy of providing long-term care services in an environment that promotes quality of life for all involved, as opposed to the traditional institutional model.

Electronic medical record: A digital healthcare file composed of various individual data elements that is typically a historical view of one individual's healthcare information.

Emotional intelligence: The personal attributes of great leaders that involve "qualities of the heart" (Goleman 2004), such as empathy and self-awareness.

Employment agency: Outside contractors that provide temporary or permanent employees.

Employment at will: A doctrine of employment in which the employer is free to discharge individuals without cause and the employee is free to quit, strike, or cease working at any time.

Empowerment: Permitting people working within teams to exercise their own independent judgment and to make decisions regarding their work activities.

Encore career: Employment in the second half of life, often in positions of greater meaning and social impact in not-for-profit or public-interest fields.

End-of-life care: Care provided to patients approaching the end of life that is focused on pain relief, comfort, respect for the patient's decisions, support for the family, and interventions to help psychological and spiritual needs.

Enterprise-wide technology management system: A system that allows any division of an organization to access information and generate reports and to link clinical and administrative components of their management process.

Equal employment opportunity: A concept that assumes that all individuals are entitled to equal treatment.

Equal Pay Act of 1963: An amendment to the Fair Labor Standards Act that requires equal pay for equal work, regardless of sex.

Euthanasia: The act or practice of killing or bringing about the death of a person who suffers from an incurable disease or condition, especially a painful one, for reasons of mercy. Euthanasia is sometimes regarded by the law as second-degree murder, manslaughter, or criminally negligent homicide. Also termed mercy killing or assisted suicide.

Evaluation: The determination of employees' job performance; includes performance appraisal, motivation, and counseling.

Excess disability: Disability caused not by a disease but by disuse of a skill, which may lead to atrophy of that skill and ultimately increase the workload of staff.

Fair Labor Standards Act of 1936: A law that established standards for minimum wage, maximum hours, and overtime pay.

Family and Medical Leave Act of 1993 (FMLA): An act that allows eligible employees to take off up to 12 work weeks in any 12-month period for the birth or adoption of a child, to care for a family member, or if the employee has a serious health condition.

Federal law: The body of law consisting of the US Constitution, federal statutes and regulations, US treaties, and federal common law.

Federalism: The right of each state to pass its own laws as long as they are not prohibited by or contrary to the United States Constitution.

Felony: A crime that is punishable by a term of imprisonment of more than one year.

Fidelity: The faithful discharge of one's duty toward the patient's care.

Five stages of grief: A five-stage psychological model, first proposed by Dr. Elisabeth Kübler-Ross (1969) in *On Death and Dying*, that describes five emotional stages—denial and isolation, anger, bargaining, depression, and acceptance—that many people experience as they deal with the knowledge of their approaching death.

Flexner report: A study of medical education in the United States and Canada.

Four pillars of retirement income: The idea that postretirement employment provides additional income when the traditional three sources—Social Security, pensions, and savings—are insufficient.

Globalization: The increased interdependence of nations to produce and consume goods and services.

Governing body: The oversight and policymaking arm of the organization, with legal and fiduciary responsibility for how the organization functions; frequently referred to as the board of directors.

Green House Project: An innovative form of long-term care based on the social model of care that attempts to deinstitutionalize care and use small, ten-bed group homes for elders.

Green Houses: A deinstitutionalization movement for long-term care in which individuals who require care live in small homes and have access to clinical and personal care services on the level of those provided in high-quality nursing homes.

Guardianship: The office, duty, or authority of a guardian; the relation subsisting between guardian and ward.

Health Insurance Portability and Accountability Act (HIPAA): Protects health insurance coverage for workers and their families when they change or lose their jobs. Title II of HIPAA, known as the Administrative Simplification (AS) provisions, requires the establishment of national standards for electronic healthcare transactions and national identifiers for providers, health insurance plans, and employers.

Healthcare proxy: A form that permits a competent adult to designate another person as his healthcare agent. The agent will make healthcare decisions for him if he is unable to make them himself.

Healthcare surrogate: The person designated by a patient to make healthcare decisions for the patient in the event that he is no longer able to make decisions. If no one has been designated by the patient, by default the next of kin is the healthcare surrogate.

Home care: Healthcare or supportive services for individuals with a chronic disability or illness who live in the community.

Home infusion therapy: Drug therapy provided intravenously that is given to an individual at home.

Hospice: Treatment that provides support and comprehensive care for the dying and focuses on maintaining quality of life by relieving the patient's physical, emotional, or spiritual suffering.

Human relations: Establishing and maintaining effective working relationships among personnel throughout the organization.

Human resources: The practices and policies that are necessary to keep the people side of a business operating.

Inclusiveness: Making sure each member of the organization's team feels valued as an important contributing member.

Independent living: A category of housing options for individuals who are able to live without assistance, including adult communities and congregate housing arrangements. These residences often impose age restrictions and offer social activities, supportive services, and increased security.

Instrumental activities of daily living (IADLs): Activities such as shopping, house cleaning, cooking, and managing finances that are not necessary for fundamental functioning but allow people to function independently.

Interdisciplinary team: A group of individuals from different disciplines/areas of expertise within the long-term care setting who influence one another toward shared objectives to meet the needs of individual residents or groups of residents with related issues.

Interoperability: The ability to transmit and read data regardless of the technology platform (or operating system) or the software language.

Interview: The process by which an interviewee (prospective employee) is asked questions so that the interviewer (prospective employer) can obtain information from the interviewee.

Iterative process: A process in an information system that can be repeated as needed to ensure that the outcome meets the business requirements of the user.

Job analysis: The process of collecting information about a job by determining its particular tasks and duties, including the general importance of each.

Job description: A detailed description of the minimum qualifications and skills necessary to perform the duties of a job.

The Joint Commission: A private, not-for-profit organization that operates accreditation programs for a fee to subscriber healthcare organizations in the United States. Formerly the Joint Commission for the Accreditation of Healthcare Organizations (JCAHO).

Justice: A legal and ethical responsibility to care for all people without discrimination as to race, creed, color, or sexual orientation.

Labor union: A group of workers that organizes for the purpose of furthering the social and economic well-being of its membership.

Leadership: The process by which people are voluntarily and "imaginatively" guided (Dunn 2010) and influenced in choosing and attaining the goals of the organization.

Licensure: Permission granted by an agency of the government that provides an exclusive right to practice certain legally defined functions; states license healthcare facilities to provide long-term care services.

Life Safety Code: Established standards that address items that may cause fires or other issues that would affect resident safety.

Livable community: A community that include features such as reasonably priced housing, access to public transportation, easy navigation, and supportive services that help residents remain independent and engaged, civically and socially.

Living will: A legal document in which a person directs that his life not be artificially prolonged by extraordinary measures (such as life support) if there is no reasonable expectation of recovery. This is also called declaration of a desire for a natural death or directive to physicians.

Long-term care: A wide range of health services, supportive services, and other assistance, provided informally or formally to individuals who have a chronic illness or disability and are unable to function independently on a daily basis.

Long-term care insurance: A specialized private insurance policy that pays the cost of nursing home care and home and community-based care but typically specifies a maximum daily benefit level of reimbursement; can be purchased by individuals and on a group basis through an employer who chooses to offer this benefit.

Long-term care services: Services provided to consumers at any age and in a wide range of settings that correspond to problems in performing activities of daily living and instrumental activities of daily living.

Management: In long-term care entities, this is the process of reaching organizational goals by working with people and other resources to protect and address the special needs of the vulnerable individuals depending on the organization's care.

Market positioning: Choosing a market segmentation that provides the organization with the maximal opportunity to achieve a leadership position in the marketplace.

Market segmentation: Dividing a market into subsets in which each subset has characteristics in common.

Marketing mix: The product or service, price, promotion, and place or channels of distribution.

Mediation: An intervention in which a neutral third party attempts to assist two parties in reaching a mutually agreed upon solution.

Medicaid: A state-administrated, means-tested federal insurance program that pays for medical care and other supportive services for low-income individuals, the disabled, and poor elderly persons. Within broad federal guidelines, the states establish eligibility standards; determine the type, amount, duration, and scope of services; set the rate of payment; and administer their own programs.

Medical home: A care approach whereby a primary care physician, in conjunction with specialists and other healthcare providers, coordinates the access to healthcare services when and where they are needed.

Medical malpractice: A negligent act or omission by a doctor or other medical professional who has a duty to care for a specific patient that results in damage or harm to that patient.

Medicare: The federal health insurance program for individuals over age 65, those on Social Security disability benefits for more than two years, and those with Lou Gehrig's disease or end-stage renal disease. It has four parts and covers care provided in skilled nursing facilities (SNFs) for up to 100 days as well as home care.

Mhealth: The use of mobile technologies for healthcare purposes.

Minimum Data Set: A standardized screening, assessment, and data collection tool for determining the level of care need for long-term care expenses in nursing homes and hospitals.

Misdemeanor: A crime that is punishable by a term of imprisonment of no more than one year.

Money Follows the Person programs: A grant program that encourages a beneficiary discharged from an institutional care facility to remain in the community and receive services at home.

Mossman amendments: A legislative basis for standardization of nursing home regulations and denial of Medicare and Medicaid funding for organizations that fail to conform to them.

Motivation: The process by which organizational leaders arouse and energize the inner needs or drives of individuals working within the organization to promote organizational goals.

National Fire Protection Agency (NFPA): A nonprofit agency, established in 1896, whose mission is to reduce the burden of fire and other hazards on the quality of life by providing standards, codes, and training.

National Labor Relations Act (NLRA): Originally called the Wagner Act, this 1935 act provides specific guidelines to govern the relationship between unions, organizations, and workers.

Natural law: A philosophical system of legal and moral principles purportedly deriving from a universalized conception of human nature or divine justice rather than from legislative or judicial action; also known as law of nature, natural justice, or divine law.

Naturally occurring retirement communities (NORCs): Communities with a large proportion of older persons residing within a specific geographical area. These communities frequently offer supportive service programs administered under the US Administration on Aging.

Object-oriented database: A database that stores the data as well as the processing instructions, such as how to calculate certain quantities.

Occupational Safety and Health Act: This law was passed to ensure safe and healthful working conditions.

Occupational Safety and Health Administration (OSHA): The federal agency charged with the enforcement of safety and health legislation; part of the Department of Labor.

Older Americans Act (OAA): Legislation passed by the US Congress in 1965 that established the Administration on Aging and state agencies on aging to address the social services needs of older adults.

Ombudsman program: A program that includes advocacy for policy and regulatory change to improve care and provision of information and education for consumers; funded by federal and state monies and operated by a variety of state agencies and nonprofit organizations.

Omnibus Budget Reconciliation Act of 1987: This act mandated the provision of certain services meant to ensure that residents achieve and maintain "highest practicable" physical, mental, and psychosocial status; also established a patient bill of rights and an outcome-focused, resident-oriented survey process.

Oregon Death with Dignity Act (ODWDA): A statute that provides physicians with protection from liability if they choose to prescribe medications for physician-assisted suicide, provided that: (1) the patient has an incurable and irreversible disease that will cause death within six months, (2) the patient has given written informed consent, and (3) the attending physician's conclusions are confirmed by a second physician.

Organizational culture: A set of shared values, norms, and rituals that organization members have regarding the functioning and character of their organization.

Pain management: Comprehensive assessment of and plan for a patient's total pain, including physical, psychological, and spiritual pain.

Palliative medicine: The comprehensive, multidisciplinary care of patients with life-limiting illness. Palliative care extends the principles of hospice but begins at an earlier point in the disease process, and accepts that some curative therapies may be appropriate even though the patient has been diagnosed with a fatal disease.

The Partnership for Long-Term Care Program: A program authorized under the Deficit Reduction Act of 2005 that permits states to promote the purchase of private long-term care insurance by offering consumers access to Medicaid under special eligibility rules should additional long-term care coverage (beyond what the policies provide) be needed.

Performance appraisal: A systematic employee review that occurs on a regular basis in which the employee receives feedback about her job performance.

Physician orders for life-sustaining treatment (POLST): A document that expresses a person's end-of-life wishes for medical treatment.

Plaintiff: The party bringing the lawsuit to court.

Planned virtual retirement community (PVRC): A community in which the elderly live in their own homes, but receive information and services to help them remain independent.

Planning: Forecasting and planning for the short-term and long-term human resources needs of the organization, and establishing standards (skills, knowledge, and ability) necessary for each position.

Post-acute care unit: A unit in a skilled nursing facility or hospital that provides healthcare services to individuals who need additional support after a discharge from acute care services in a hospital setting. Also referred to as transitional care units.

Program of All-Inclusive Care for the Elderly (PACE): Nonresidential programs that provide healthcare, social services, and other services in a daycare setting to consumers who are eligible for nursing homes but choose to remain in the community instead. Reimbursement is a mixture, sometimes capitated, of funds from Medicare and state Medicaid programs.

Project manager: An individual who manages a systems development project. The project manager facilitates the process of the development and monitors the progress to determine the possibility for schedule delays, cost overruns, or other risks that would affect the delivery of the system.

Prototype: A sample information system or model built to test a concept or a process before final implementation.

Quality improvement organization (QIO): A private, not-for-profit organization staffed by trained professionals who review medical care and help beneficiaries with complaints about the quality of care and implement improvements in the quality of care available throughout the spectrum of care.

Recruitment: The process of searching for and attracting new employees to the workforce.

Relational database: A database that consists of related tables of data that are designed in a logical structure for storage and easy data retrieval.

Relationship marketing: A set of strategies that focus on the lifetime relationship with the customer rather than the individual transactions of the customer in order to increase profit. Relationship marketing captures customer share, or the share of the customer dollar, rather than the number of customers within the market share.

Resource Utilization Groups (RUGs): A prospective payment system used under Medicare to determine the level of payment for resident care, based on care and resource needs, under Medicare Part A. Skilled nursing facilities determine a RUG based on 108 items on the Minimum Data Set (MDS) resident assessment tool.

Retirement: Withdrawing from one's occupation, business, or office and pursuing new activities.

Right to work: A statute that declares it to be unlawful to require union membership as a condition of employment; however, the union in question is responsible for representing all workers in the bargaining unit.

Screening: Preemployment procedures to ensure that workers are qualified to work; includes conducting extensive criminal background checks, viewing registration boards for clinical personnel, and drug testing.

Section 202: A specialized housing subsidy program under the US Department of Housing and Urban Development that provides financing for construction of housing for low-income senior citizens and those with disabilities.

Section 8: An affordable housing assistance program under the US Department of Housing and Urban Development that provides funds to landlords who designate a portion of their property for Section 8 tenants and rental vouchers to individuals who then select their own housing.

Selling orientation: An organization's primary focus on the needs of the seller rather than the buyer.

Senior centers: Places where older adults come together for services and activities that reflect their experience and skills, respond to their diverse needs and interests, enhance their dignity, support their independence, and encourage their involvement in and with the center and the community.

Single point of entry (POE) model: A model of long-term care in which patients can obtain all the services they need through a single agency or organization.

Skilled nursing facilities: Facilities that provide medical, nursing, or rehabilitative services on an inpatient basis.

Social Health Maintenance Organizations (SHMOs) or Lifecare: Organizations that provide healthcare and long-term care services, with a special emphasis on home care services. SHMOs are funded by Medicare.

Social media marketing: A form of Internet marketing that seeks to achieve branding and marketing communication goals through participation in various social media networks (MySpace, Facebook, LinkedIn), social bookmarking (Digg, StumbleUpon), social media sharing (Flickr, YouTube), review/ratings sites (ePinions, BizRate), blogs, forums, news aggregators, and virtual 3D networks (SecondLife, ActiveWorlds). Each social media site can be optimized to generate awareness or traffic.

Social Security: A federal government program that pays benefits to senior citizens and certain other individuals. Social Security often serves as the primary source of retirement income for low income elderly persons.

Staffing: The recruitment and selection of qualified individuals, including performing job analyses, writing job descriptions, setting compensation levels, screening, and interviewing.

Strategic marketing: The process of developing a fit between an organization's goals and resources and changing market opportunities. It consists of the fundamental business planning tools of market research, a marketing plan, and its implementation.

Strategic planning: The long-term planning process by key stakeholders in which the organization's goals, measurable objectives, and direction for the immediate future are determined.

Strike: An organized work stoppage orchestrated by a union.

Sundowning: A symptom exhibited by some people with Alzheimer's or other dementias characterized by confusion, anxiety, and agitation in the early evening or into the night.

Systems development life cycle: A cyclical, iterative approach to designing an information system that consists of four phases: analysis, design, implementation, and maintenance.

Taft-Hartley Act: A 1947 act that defines and prohibits unfair labor practices by unions. Formally called the Labor Management Relations Act.

Telehealth: The delivery of health-related services and information via telecommunications technology.

Telemedicine: The practice of using technology, such as a telephone or computer, to monitor the medical condition of a patient from a long distance or consult with colleagues in different locations.

Theory of supportive design: A theory formulated by Roger Ulrich (1995) that promotes wellness in long-term care by encouraging designers to incorporate psychologically supportive physical surroundings that encourage: (1) a sense of control over physical/social surroundings and access to privacy; (2) access to social support from family and friends; and (3) access to nature and other positive distractions in one's physical surroundings.

Three-legged stool of economic security: A concept used by financial planners to describe the three most common sources of retirement income: Social Security retirement benefits, employee pensions, and personal savings.

Title XX: A block grant program under the Social Security Act that provides community-based care for the elderly and disabled, as well as funding for child care and child abuse prevention programs.

Tort: A civil case for money damages.

Total pain: A concept developed by Dame Cicely Saunders that recognizes that a patient's pain has more than just a physical component, and also includes suffering due to spiritual, psychological, and social aspects.

Turnover: The termination of employment, which can be either voluntary or involuntary.

Uniform Health Care Decisions Act (UHCDA): A 1993 model statute that facilitates and encourages the making of advance directives.

Universal design: A resident-centered approach to the design of the environment that focuses on the needs of the users regardless of functional impairments or disabilities.

Wandering: The act by a person with dementia of walking, riding, or driving off unsupervised, leading to a potentially dangerous situation.

Waterfall method: A traditional approach to information systems development in which each phase is completed before the next phase begins.

Workers' compensation: Insurance that provides compensation for medical care and rehabilitation for, and provides settlements to, employees who are injured during the course of employment.

Wrongful termination: Firing or laying off an employee for illegal reasons in violation of existing civil law.

References

AARP. 2005a. *Beyond 50.05: A Report to the Nation on Livable Communities: Creating Environments for Successful Aging.* Washington, DC: AARP.

———. 2005b. *State of 50+America Survey.* Washington, DC: AARP.

Abrahm, J. L. 2011. "Advances in Palliative Medicine and End of Life Care." *Annual Review of Medicine* 62 (February): 187–99.

Acorn, J. 2010. "A Security/Safety Survey of Long-term Care Facilities." *Journal of Healthcare Protection Management: Publication of the International Association for Hospital Security* 26 (2): 43–46.

Ader, R., and N. Cohen. 1975. "Behaviorally Conditioned Immunosuppression." *Psychosomatic Medicine* 37 (4): 333–40.

Administration on Aging (AoA). 2009. *A Statistical Profile of Black Older Americans Aged 65+.* Washington, DC: US Government Printing Office.

———. 2003. "A Profile of Older Americans: 2003." Accessed November 1, 2009. www .aoa.gov/AoAroot/Aging_Statistics/Profile/2003/index.aspx.

Agich, G. 2009. "Respecting the Autonomy of Old People Living in Nursing Homes." In *Healthcare Ethics: Critical Issues for the 21st Century,* 2nd ed., edited by E. Morrison, 184–200. Sudbury, MA: Jones & Bartlett.

AHIP Center for Research and Policy. 2007. "Long Term Care Insurance Partnerships: New Choices for Consumers—Potential Savings for Federal and State Governments." *AHIP.* Published January 24. www.ahipresearch.org/PDFs/IssueBriefSavingsfrom ExpandedLTCPartnerships1-24-2007.pdf.

Alden, A. L., and G. D. Weisman. 2004. "Closing the Circle: The Evaluation of Brewster Village." *Nursing Homes* 53 (6): 29–37.

Allgov.com. 2009. "Department of Veterans Affairs." Accessed February 10, 2012. www .allgov.com/Agency/Department_of_Veterans_Affairs.

Alzheimer's Association. 2012. "Three out of Five People with Alzheimer's Disease Will Wander." *Northern California Chapter Newsletter.* www.alz.org/norcal/in_my_ community_18411.asp.

———. 2011. "2011 Alzheimer's Disease Facts and Figures." *Alzheimer's & Dementia* 7 (2): 208–44.

Alzheimer's Foundation of America. 2011. "About Alzheimer's Disease." *Alzheimer's Prevention.* Accessed February 10, 2012. www.alzprevention.org/about-alzheimers-disease .php.

American Academy of Hospice and Palliative Medicine (AAHPM). 2006. "Position Statement: Statement on Palliative Sedation." Published September 15. www.aahpm.org/ positions/default/sedation.html.

American Association of Homes and Services for the Aging. 2008. *Overview of Continuing Care Retirement Communities.*

American Association on Mental Retardation (AAMR). 1992. *Mental Retardation: Definition, Classification, and Systems of Support,* 9th ed. Washington, DC: AAMR.

American Board of Medical Specialties (ABMS). 2006. "News Releases." *American Board of Medical Specialties.* Accessed August 24, 2008. www.abms.org/News_and_Events/ Media_Newsroom/news_releases.aspx.

American College of Health Care Administrators (ACHCA). 2007. "Code of Ethics." www.achca.org/content/pdf/Code%20of%20Ethics_Member_Redesign%20 Draft_100721%5B1%5D.pdf.

American College of Surgeons (ACS). 2006. "The 1919 'Minimum Standard' Document." *American College of Surgeons.* Published May 25. www.facs.org/archives/ minimumhighlight.html.

American Geriatrics Society (AGS). 2005. "The Aging Process." *Aging in the Know*. Accessed February 10, 2012. www.healthinaging.org/agingintheknow/chapters_ch_trial .asp?ch=1#Changes in Weight.

American Health Care Association (AHCA). 2012. "Research on Staffing and Workforce." Accessed February 1. www.ahcancal.org/research_data/staffing/Pages/default.aspx.

———. "Report of Findings: Nursing Facility Staffing Survey 2010." Published October 1. www.ahcancal.org/research_data/staffing/Pages/default.aspx.

———. 2011b. "Report of Findings: 2009 Nursing Facility Staff Retention and Turnover Survey." Published May 1. www.ahcancal.org/research_data/staffing/ Pages/default.aspx.

———. 2008. "Report of Findings: 2007 AHCA Survey—Nursing Staff Vacancy and Turnover in Nursing Facilities." Published July 21. www.ahcancal.org/research_data/ staffing/Documents/Vacancy_Turnover_Survey2007.pdf.

———. 2010. "Report of Findings: 2008 Nursing Facility Staff Vacancy, Retention and Turnover Survey." Published October 1. www.ahcancal.org/research_data/staffing/ Pages/default.aspx.

American Health Care Association (AHCA) and National Center for Assisted Living (NCAL). 2010. "US Long-Term Care Workforce at a Glance." Accessed February 10, 2012. www.ahcancal.org/research_data/staffing/Documents/WorkforceAtAGlance.pdf.

American Medical Association (AMA). 2009. "AMA Code of Medical Ethics." *AMA*. Published August 18. www.ama-assn.org/ama/pub/physician-resources/medical-ethics/ code-medical-ethics.page?.

American Nurses Association. 2001. "Code of Ethics for Nurses with Interpretive Statements." *Nursing World*. Published August 18. http://nursingworld.org/MainMenu Categories/EthicsStandards/CodeofEthicsforNurses/Code-of-Ethics.aspx.

American Pain Society. 2006. "Treatment of Pain at the End of Life: A Position Statement from the American Pain Society: 2006 Update." *American Pain Society*. Accessed September 21, 2008. www.ampainsoc.org/advocacy/statements.htm.

Anderzhon, J. W., I. L. Fraley, and M. Green. 2007. *Design for Aging Post-occupancy Evaluations*. New York: John Wiley & Sons, Inc.

Andrews, E. 2005. "GOP Courts Blacks and Hispanics on Social Security." *New York Times,* March 20, A15.

Angel, R., and J. Angel. 2006. "Diversity and Aging in the United States." In *Handbook of Aging and the Social Sciences,* 6th ed., edited by R. Binstock and L. George. Boston: Academic Press.

———. 1999. *Who Will Care for Us?: Aging and Long-Term Care in a Multicultural America.* New York, NY: New York Press.

Aranda, M. P. 2006. "Older Latinos: A Mental Health Perspective." In *Handbook of Social Work in Health and Aging,* edited by B. Berkman and S. D'Ambruoso. New York: Oxford University Press.

Arling, G. 2007. "Improving Quality Assessment Through Multilevel Modeling: The Case of Nursing Home Compare." *Health Services Research* 42 (3): 1177–99.

Assisted Living Facilities of America (ALFA). 2008. *2008 Overview of Assisted Living.* Alexandria, VA: ALFA.

———. 2009. "About Assisted Living Federation of America." Accessed Feburary 2. www.alfa.org.

AssistedLivingFacilities.org. 2011. "California Assisted Living Facilities." Accessed March 9. www.assistedlivingfacilities.org/directory/ca.

Assisted Living Quality Coalition (ALQC). 1998. *Assisted Living Quality Initiative: Building a Structure That Promotes Quality.* Washington, DC: ALQC.

Associated Press. 2009. "Florida Medicaid Patients Settle Lawsuit with State." *Miami Herald.* Published September 18. http://psychrights.org/states/Florida/090918FlaMedi caidPtsSettleLawsuitWithState.htm.

Association of American Medical Colleges (AAMC) Task Force: Medical School Objectives Project. 1999. *Report III: Contemporary Issues in Medicine: Communication in Medicine.* Washington, DC: AAMC.

Aultman Hospital. 2007. "Annual Report 2007." Accessed July 29, 2008. www.aultman .org.

Baker, L. C., S. J. Johnson, D. Macaulay, and H. Birnbaum. 2011. "Integrated Telehealth and Care Management Program for Medicare Beneficiaries with Chronic Disease Linked to Savings." *Health Affairs* 30 (9): 1689–97.

Baldwin, D. 2003. "Disparities in Health and Health Care: Focusing Efforts to Eliminate Unequal Burdens." *Online Journal of Issues in Nursing* 8 (1). Published January 31. www.nursingworld.org/MainMenuCategories/ANAMarketplace/ANAPeriodicals/

OJIN/TableofContents/Volume82003/No1Jan2003/DisparitiesinHealthandHealth-Care.aspx.

Ball State University. 2005. "Study Finds Negative Advertising Stereotypes of Elderly Are Unpopular." *Ball State University*. Published November 1. www.bsu.edu/news/article/0,1370,-1019-37652,00.html.

Barba, B., A. Tesh, and N. Courts. 2002. "Promoting Thriving in Nursing Homes: The Eden Alternative." *Journal of Gerontological Nursing* 28 (3): 7–13.

Barranti, C. C. R., and H. Cohen. 2000. "Lesbian and Gay Elders: An Invisible Minority." In *Gerontological Social Work: Knowledge, Service Settings, and Special Populations*, 2nd ed., edited by R. L. Schneider, N. P. Kropf, and A. J. Kisor, 343–67. Belmont, CA: Brooks/Cole.

Bedney, B. J., and R. Goldberg. 2009. "Health Care Cost Containment and NORC Supportive Service Programs: An Overview and Literature Review." *NORCs*. Published April 22. www.norcs.org/page.aspx?id=198924.

Bell, C. 2002. *Managers as Mentors: Building Partnerships for Learning*, 2nd ed. San Francisco: Berrett-Koehler.

Bennis, W. 2003. *On Becoming a Leader: The Leadership Classic*. Cambridge, MA: Perseus.

———. 1999. "The Leadership Advantage." *Leader to Leader Journal* 12 (Spring): 18–23.

Bergman-Evans, B. 2004. "Beyond the Basics: Effects of the Eden Alternative Model on Quality of Life Issues." *Journal of Gerontological Nursing* 30 (6): 27–34.

Berkowitz, E. 2010. *Essentials of Health Care Marketing*, 2nd ed. Burlington, MA: Jones and Bartlett.

Betancourt, J., A. Green, J. Carrillo, and E. Park. 2005. "Cultural Competence and Health Care Disparities: Key Perspectives and Trends." *Health Affairs* 24 (2): 499–505.

Better Jobs Better Care (BJBC). 2008. *A Crisis with a Solution*. www.leadingage.org/uploadedFiles/Content/About/Center_for_Applied_Research/Center_for_Applied_Research_Initiatives/Better_Jobs_Better_Care_Catalogue.pdf.

———. 2005. "Linking Payment to Long-Term Care Quality: Can Direct Care Staffing Measures Build the Foundation?" Washington, DC: Institute for the Future of Aging Services.

Billings, J. A. 2000. "Recent Advances: Palliative Care." *British Medical Journal* 321 (7260): 555–58.

Billings, J. A., F. D. Ferris, N. Macdonald, and C. Von Gunten. 2001. "The Role of Palliative Care in the Home in Medical Education: Report from a National Consensus Conference." *Journal of Palliative Medicine* 4 (3): 361–71.

Bilmes, L. 2007. "Soldiers Returning from Iraq and Afghanistan: The Long-term Costs of Providing Veterans Medical Care and Disability Benefits." Faculty Research Working Paper Series RWP07-001, Kennedy School of Government, Harvard University, Cambridge, MA.

Bishop, C. E., D. B. Weinberg, W. Leutz, A. Dossa, S. G. Pfefferle and R. M. Zincavage. 2008. "Nursing Assistants' Job Commitment: Effect of Nursing Home Organizational Factors and Impact on Resident Well-Being." *The Gerontologist* Special Issue I (48): 36–45.

Blechman, A. D. 2008. *Leisureville: Adventures in America's Retirement Utopias.* New York: Atlantic Monthly Press.

Bodell, J., and M. Weng, 2000. "The Jewish Patient and Terminal Dehydration: A Hospice Ethical Dilemma." *American Journal of Hospice & Palliative Care* 17 (3): 185–88.

Bogutz, A. D., R. N. Brown, J. M. Krauskopf, and K. L. Tokarz. 2005. *Elder Law Advocacy for the Aging,* 2nd ed. Eagan, MN: West Publishing.

Borrell, L., F. Dallo, and K. White. 2006. "Education and Diabetes in a Racially and Ethnically Diverse Population." *American Journal of Public Health* 96 (9): 1637–42.

Bowers, B., S. Esmond, and N. Jacobson. 2003. "Turnover Reinterpreted: CNAs Talk About Why They Leave." *Journal of Gerontological Nursing* 29 (3): 36–43.

Branch, J. 2008. Strategic Marketing Seminar. Presented at Zagreb School of Economics and Management, Zagreb, Croatia, March 28.

Brawley, E. C. 2006. *Design Innovations for Aging and Alzheimer's: Creating Caring Environments.* New York: John Wiley & Sons.

Brody, J. 2009. "A Personal, Coordinated Approach to Care." *New York Times,* June 22.

Brown, J., and J. Hillam. 2004. *Your Questions Answered: Dementia,* 79. New York: Churchill-Livingstone.

Brown, J. R., and A. Finkelstein. 2009. "The Private Market for Long-Term Care Insurance in the United States: A Review of the Evidence." *Journal of Risk and Insurance* 76 (1): 5–29.

———. 2008. "The Interaction of Public and Private Insurance: Medicaid and the Long-term Care Insurance Market." *American Economic Review* 98 (3): 1083–1102.

Brown University, Alpert Medical School. 2012. "Long-Term Care: Facts on Care in the US." *LTCfocUS.org*. Accessed February 10. www.ltcfocus.org/About.aspx.

Brown University, Center for Gerontology and Healthcare Research. 2005. "Step by Step Guide to Responding to a Deficiency." Updated March 30. www.chcr.brown.edu/pain/stepguide.htm.

Budwell, B. O., and B. Jackson. 1994. "The Disabled Elderly and Their Use of Long-Term Care." *US Deptartment of Health and Human Services*. Published July 1. http://aspe.hhs.gov/daltcp/reports/html.

Buchbinder, S. B., and D. Buchbinder. 2007. "Managing Healthcare Professionals." In *Introduction to Health Care Management*, edited by S. Buchbinder and N. Shanks. Sudbury, MA: Jones and Bartlett.

Buchbinder, S. B., and J. M. Thompson. 2007. "Teamwork." In *Introduction to Health Care Management*, edited by S. Buchbinder and N. Shanks. Sudbury, MA: Jones and Bartlett.

Butler, S. S. 2006. "Older Gays, Lesbians, Bisexuals, and Transgender Persons." In *Handbook of Social Work in Health and Aging*, edited by B. Berkman and S. D'Ambruoso, 273–82. New York: Oxford University Press.

Byrd, L., A. Fletcher, and C. Menifield. 2007. "Disparities in Health Care: Minority Elders at Risk." *ABNF Journal* 18 (2): 51–55.

Caffrey, C., M. Sengupta, A. Moss, L. Harris-Kojetin, and R. Valverde. 2011. "Home Health Care and Discharged Hospice Care Patients: United States, 2000 and 2007." *National Health Statistics Reports* (38).

California Association of Adult Day Services (CAADS). 2010. "A Brief History of Adult Day Health." *CAADS*. Accessed March 12, 2011. Published February 1. www.caads.org/pdf/pdf/adhc_brief_history_30_yrs_of_service_rev2010_03_05_web_format_2010_03_16.pdf.

Calkins, M. 1988. *Design for Dementia: Planning Environments for the Elderly and Confused.* Owings Mills, MD: National Health Press.

Campbell, J. C., N. Ikegami, and M. J. Gibson. 2010. "Lessons from Public Long-Term Care Insurance in Germany and Japan." *Health Affairs* 29 (1): 87–95.

CARF International. 2012. "List of CARF-CCAC Accredited Continuing Care Retirement Communities." Accessed February 10. www.carf.org/ccrcListing.aspx.

———. 2009. "Provider List." Accessed February 2. www.carf.org/consumer.aspx?Content=content/about/providerlist.htm&ID=6.

Casarett, D., J. Karlawish, K. Morales, R. Crowley, T. Mirsch, and D. A. Asch. 2005. "Improving the Use of Hospice Services in Nursing Homes." *JAMA* 294 (2): 211–17.

Castle, N. G., and J. Engberg. 2007. "The Influence of Staffing Characteristics on Quality of Care in Nursing Homes." *Health Services Research* 42 (5): 1822–47.

Cavanaugh, G. 2010. *American Business Values: A Global Perspective*, 6th ed. Upper Saddle River, NJ: Prentice-Hall.

Center for Gerontology and Health Care Research. 2005. "Brown Atlas of Dying." Updated April 15. www.chcr.brown.edu/dying/brownatlas.htm.

Center to Advance Palliative Care. 2012. "Palliative Care Tools, Training & Technical Assistance." Accessed November 23, 2008. www.capc.org.

Centers for Disease Control and Prevention (CDC). 2009. "Prevalence and Most Common Causes of Disability Among Adults—United States, 2005." Published May 1. www.cdc.gov/mmwr/preview/mmwrhtml/mm5816a2.html.

Centers for Medicare & Medicaid Services (CMS). 2011a. "HIPAA Overview." Updated July 19. www.cms.gov/hipaageninfo.

———. 2011b. "Medicare Enrollment: Hospital Insurance and/or Supplementary Medical Insurance Programs for Total, Fee-for-Service and Managed Care Enrollees as of July 1, 2010: Selected Calendar Years 1966–2010." Accessed September 28. www.cms.gov/MedicareMedicaidStatSupp/08_2011.asp.

———. 2009. "CMS Manual System: Section 483.65 Infection Control." Published December 2. www.cms.gov/transmittals/downloads/R55SOMA.pdf.

———. 2008a. "Chapter 4: Centers for Medicare and Medicaid Services Department of Health and Human Services, Volume 2. Parts 400 to 429 Hospice Care." In *The Code of Federal Regulations: Title 42: Public Health*. Revised June 5. www.gpoaccess.gov/cfr.

———. 2008b. "Home page." Accessed November 23. www.cms.hhs.gov.

———. 2008c. "Medicare and Medicaid Programs: Hospice Conditions of Participation. Final Rule." *Federal Register* 73 (109): 32087–220.

———. 2002. "Evaluation Results for the Social/Health Maintenance Organization II Demonstration." Accessed February 10, 2012. www.cms.gov/DemoProjectsEvalRpts/downloads/SHMO_Report.pdf.

Cerquone, J. 2001. "Administrating Eden." *Balance* 5 (6): 4–6.

Certo, S. C., and S. T. Certo. 2009. *Modern Management*, 11th ed. Upper Saddle River, NJ: Prentice-Hall.

Chambers, C. 2004. *No Need to Fear, No Need to Hide: A Training Program About Inclusion and Understanding of Lesbian, Gay, Bisexual, and Transgendered Elders for Long-Term Care and Assisted Living Facilities.* New York: SAGE and Brookdale Center on Aging.

Chen, P. 2009. "Bridging the Culture Gap." *New York Times.* Published July 16. www.nytimes.com/2009/07/16/health/16chen.html.

Chin, A. E., K. Hedberg, G. K. Higginson, and D. W. Fleming. 1999. "Oregon's Death with Dignity Act: The First Year's Experience." *Oregon Health Authority.* Published February 18. www.oregon.gov/DHS/ph/pas/docs/year1.pdf.

Choi, N. G. 2001. "Relationship Between Life Satisfaction and Postretirement Employment Among Older Women." *International Journal of Aging and Human Development* 52 (1): 45–70.

Ciemins, E. L., L. Blum, M. Nunley, A. Lasher, and J. M. Newman. 2007. "The Economic and Clinical Impact of an Inpatient Palliative Care Consultative Service: A Multifaceted Approach." *Journal of Palliative Medicine* 10 (6): 1347–55.

Clark, D. 2006. *Cicely Saunders: Selected Writings 1958–2004.* Oxford, UK: Oxford University Press.

Clark, R. L., R. V. Burkhauser, M. Moon, J. F. Quinn, and T. M. Smeeding. 2004. *The Economics of an Aging Society.* Malden, MA: Blackwell.

Code of Federal Regulations. 42 C.F.R. § 483.70 Physical environment. Title 42—Public Health PART 483—REQUIREMENTS FOR STATES AND LONG TERM CARE FACILITIES Subpart B—Requirements for Long Term Care Facilities § 483.70 Physical environment.

Cohen, L. L. 2008. "Racial/Ethnic Disparities in Hospice Care: A Systematic Review." *Journal of Palliative Medicine* 11 (5): 763–68.

Cohen-Mansfield, J. 2001. "Nonpharmacological Interventions for Inappropriate Behaviors in Dementia: A Summary, Review, and Critique." *American Journal of Geriatric Psychiatry* 9 (4): 361–81.

Coile, R. 2002. "Health Care's New Consumers: Boomers, Bobos, Health Seekers, and the Wired Retired." *Russ Coile's Health Trends* 14 (5): 1.

Committee on Nursing Home Regulation. 1986. *Improving the Quality of Care in Nursing Homes.* Washington, DC: National Academies Press.

Congressional Budget Office (CBO). 2005. *An Analysis of the President's Budgetary Proposals for Fiscal Year 2006.* Washington, DC: CBO.

Connole, P. 2010a. "EMRs Enhance Retention, Recruitment." *Provider Magazine* (March): 45–50.

———. 2010b. "Providers Agree: HIT Beats Paper." *Provider Magazine* (January): 44–45.

Cooke, M., D. M. Irby, W. Sullivan, and K. M. Ludmerer. 2006. "American Medical Education 100 Years After the Flexner Report." *New England Journal of Medicine* 355 (13): 1339–44.

Cooper, J., and J. Cronin. 2000. "Internal Marketing: A Comprehensive Strategy for the Long-Term Care Industry." *Journal of Business Research* 48 (3): 177–81.

Covey, S. 1989. *The Seven Habits of Highly Effective People.* New York: Free Press.

Crawley Lavera, M. 2005. "Racial, Cultural and Ethnic Factors Influencing End-of-Life Care." *Journal of Palliative Medicine* 8 (Suppl.): 58–69.

Cruzan v. Director, Missouri Dept. of Health, 497 U.S. 261at 279 (1990).

Cummings, J. L., and D. L. Benson. 1992. *Dementia: A Clinical Approach,* 2nd ed. Stoneham, MA: Butterworth-Heinemann.

Curtis, E. F., and J. L. Dreachslin. 2008. "Diversity Management Interventions and Organizational Performance: A Synthesis of Current Literature." *Human Resource Development Review* 7 (1): 107–34.

Daft, R. 2004. "Theory Z: Opening the Corporate Door for Participative Management." *Academy of Management Executive* 18 (4): 117–21.

Dawson, S. 2007. "Recruitment and Retention of Paraprofessionals." Paraprofessional Healthcare Institute presentation. Published June 28. www.directcareclearinghouse.org/download/Dawson_IOM_6-28-07.pdf.

Day, J. C. 1993. "Population Projections of the United States, by Age, Sex, Race, and Hispanic Origin: 1993 to 2050." US Census Bureau, *Current Population Reports*, P25-1104. Accessed March 19, 2011. www.census.gov/population/www/pop-profile/natproj.html.

Deaton, G., P. Winn, R. Johnson, and C. Johnson. 1998. "The Eden Alternative: An Evolving Paradigm for Long Term Care." *Southwest Journal on Aging* 14 (2): 133–36.

Delgado-Guay, M. O., H. A. Parsons, L. J. Palmer, and E. Bruera. 2009. "Symptom Distress, Interventions, and Outcomes of Intensive Care Unit Cancer Patients Referred to a Palliative Care Team." *Cancer* 115 (2): 437–45.

Deming, W. E. 1982. *Out of the Crisis*. Cambridge, MA: MIT Press.

Dillon, C. 2005. "Critical Cleaning in LTC Settings." *Nursing Homes* 54 (3): 66–68.

Dolan, G. 2009. "Respect for Seniors: Environmental Services and Long-Term Care." *Health Facilities Management* 22 (8): 36–37.

Donoghue, C., and N. G. Castle. 2009. "Leadership Styles of Nursing Home Administrators and Their Association with Staff Turnover." *Gerontologist* 49 (2): 166–74.

Dorr, W. R. 1912. "Regulation of Hospitals." *California State Journal of Medicine* 10 (6): 262–67.

Dougherty, M. 2010. "Long-Term, Post-Acute Care Advocate for Attention." *Advance for Health Information Professionals* (July 14): 29.

Dreachslin, J., and F. Hobby. 2008. "Racial and Ethnic Disparities: Why Diversity Leadership Matters." *Journal of Healthcare Management* 53 (1): 1–12.

Dunn, R. T. 2007. *Haimann's Healthcare Management*, 8th ed. Chicago: Health Administration Press.

Dychtwald, K. 1990. *Age Wave: How the Most Important Trend of Our Time Will Change Your Future*. New York: Bantam Books.

Eckroth-Bucher, M., and J. Siberski. 2009. "Preserving Cognition Through an Integrated Cognitive Stimulation and Training Program." *American Journal of Alzheimer's Disease & Other Dementias* 24 (3): 1–12.

Edelman, P., and S. Hughes. 1990. "The Impact of Community Care on Provision of Informal Care to Homebound Elderly Persons." *Journal of Gerontology* 45: S74–S84.

Eden Alternative. 2009. "Our Ten Principles." Accessed February 1, 2012. www.edenalt.org/about/our-10-principles.html.

Elliott, S. 2005. "No More Same Old." *New York Times*, May 23.

Enyeart, S. 2008. "The LTC Training Dilemma: Finding the Right Training Company: All Vendors Are Not the Same; Understand How They Can Help You, Specifically." *Long Term Living* 57 (11): 23–26.

Equal Employment Opportunity Commission (EEOC). 2012. "The Law." Accessed February 11. www.eeoc.gov/eeoc/history/35th/thelaw/index.html.

———. 2011a. "Pregnancy Discrimination." Accessed May 4. www.eeoc.gov//laws/types/pregnancy.html.

———. 2011b. "The Age Discrimination in Employment Act of 1967." Accessed May 4. www.eeoc.gov/laws/statutes/adea.cfm.

———. 2011c. "The Equal Pay Act of 1963." Accessed May 4. www.eeoc.gov/laws/statutes/epa.cfm.

———. 2011d. "Title VII of the Civil Rights Act of 1964." Accessed May 4. www.eeoc.gov/laws/statutes/titlevii.cfm.

Estes, C. L., D. M. Zulman, S. C. Goldberg, and D. D. Ogawa. 2004. "State Long-Term Care Ombudsman Programs: Factors Associated with Perceived Effectiveness." *Gerontologist* 44 (1): 104–15.

Evans, D. A., D. A. Bennett, R. S. Wilson, J. L. Bienias, M. C. Morris, P. A. Scherr, L. E. Hebert, E. Aggarwal, L. A. Beckett, R. Joglekar, E. Berry-Kravis, and J. Schneider. 2003. "Incidence of Alzheimer Disease in a Biracial Urban Community: Relation to Apolipoprotein E Allele Status." *Archives of Neurology* 60 (2): 185–89.

Evashwick, C. 2007. *The Continuum of Long-Term Care*, 3rd ed. New York: Delmar Publishing.

Evashwick, C., and J. Riedel. 2004. *Managing Long-Term Care.* Chicago: Health Administration Press.

Farr, B. 2006. "What to Think if the Results of the National Institutes of Health Randomized Trial of Methicillin-Resistant Staphylococcus Aureus and Vancomycin-Resistant Enterococcus Control Measures are Negative (And Other Advice to Young Epidemiologists): A Review and an Au Revoir." *Infection Control & Hospital Epidemiology* 27 (10): 1096–1106.

Fazzi Associates. 2008. *Philips National Study on the Future of Technology and Telehealth in Home Care.* Andover, MA: Philips Consumer Health Solutions.

Federal Interagency Forum on Aging Related Statistics. 2010 *Older Americans 2010: Key Indicators of Well-Being.* Washington, DC: Federal Interagency Forum on Aging Related Statistics.

————. 2008. *Older Americans 2008: Key Indicators of Well-Being.* Washington, DC: US Government Printing Office.

————. 2004. *Older Americans 2004: Key Indicators of Well-Being.* Hyattsville, MD: National Center for Health Statistics.

————. 2000. *Older Americans 2000: Key Indicators of Well-Being.* Washington, DC: Federal Interagency Forum on Aging Related Statistics.

Ferris, F. D. 2005. *Palliative Care Within the Experience of Illness, Bereavement, and Risk.* San Diego, CA: San Diego Hospice.

Fogel, R. W. 2004. "Changes in the Process of Aging During the Twentieth Century: Findings and Procedures from the Early Indicators Project." *Population and Development Review* (30): 19–47.

Follwell, M., D. Burman, L. W. Le, K. Wakimoto, D. Seccareccia, J. Bryson, G. Rodin, and C. Zimmermann. 2009. "Phase II Study of an Outpatient Palliative Care Intervention in Patients with Metastatic Cancer." *Journal of Clinical Oncology* 27 (2): 206–13.

Ford, S. 2008. "Avoid Baby Talk in Dementia Care." *Nursing Times* 104 (31): 8.

Fox, S., and S. Jones. 2009. "The Social Life of Health Information." *Pew Internet.* Published June 11. www.pewinternet.org/Reports/2009/8-The-Social-Life-of-Health-Information.aspx.

Gehlert, S., D. Sohmer, T. Sachs, C. Mininger, M. McClintock, and O. Olopade. 2008. "Targeting Health Disparities: A Model Linking Upstream Determinants to Downstream Interventions." *Health Affairs* 27 (2): 339–49.

Gelfand, D. E. 2006. *The Aging Network: Programs and Services,* 6th ed. New York: Springer.

Gelhaus, L. 2010. "GE, Intel Create a Global Aging Venture." *Provider Magazine* (October): 15.

Gellatly, D. L. 2007. "Human Resources Management Along the Continuum of Care." In *Managing Human Resources in Health Care Organizations,* edited by L. Shi, 225–72. Boston: Jones and Bartlett.

Geneva Association. 2012. "Four Pillars." Accessed February 11. www.genevaassociation .org/Research_Programme/Four_Pillars_Pensions.aspx.

Genworth Financial. 2009. *Genworth 2009 Cost of Care Survey*. Richmond, VA: Genworth Financial.

Ghent, J. S. 1994. "Childbirth Education: A Natural Approach to Assessing Healthcare Clients." *Healthcare Marketing Report* 12 (5): 14–15.

Gibson, M. J., and A. Houser. 2007. *AARP Issue Brief: Valuing the Invaluable—A New Look at the Economic Value of Family Caregiving*. Washington, DC: AARP.

Gilmer, T., L. J. Schneider, H. Teetzel, J. Blustein, K. Briggs, F. Cohn, R. Cranford, D. Dugan, G. Komatsu, and E. Young. 2005. "The Costs of Nonbeneficial Treatment in the Intensive Care Setting." *Health Affairs* 24 (4): 961–71.

Gilster, S. D. 2005. *Changing Culture, Changing Care: S.E.R.V.I.C.E. First*. Cincinnati, OH: Cincinnati Book Publishing.

Gilster, S. D., and J. Dalessandro. 2010. "The Business Case for Developing Assistant Administrators." Presented at the 44th Annual Convocation and Exposition of the American College of Health Care Administrators, Philadelphia.

Ginzler, E. 2006. *Statement Before the Senate Committee on Health, Education, Labor and Pensions, Subcommittee on Retirement Security and Aging, on Aging in Place and Naturally Occurring Retirement Communities*. Washington, DC: AARP.

Gleckman, H. 2009. "A New Model for Aging in Place." *Kiplinger's Retirement Report*, January.

Goh, R. 2011. "What Is a Smart Home?" *Ehow Health*. Accessed March 18. www.ehow .com/about_6122442_smart-medical-home_.html.

Golding, G. 1981. "A Protohospice at the Turn of the Century: St. Luke's House, London from 1893 to 1921." *Journal of the History of Medicine and Allied Sciences* 36 (4): 383–415.

Goldsmith, B., J. Dietrich, D. Quingling, and R. S. Morrison. 2008. "Variability in Access to Hospital Palliative Care in the United States." *Journal of Palliative Medicine* 11 (8): 1094–102.

Goleman, D. 2004. "What Makes a Leader?" *Harvard Business Review* 82 (1): 82–91.

Government Accountability Office (GAO). 2010. "Older Americans: Continuing Care Retirement Communities Can Provide Benefits, but Not Without Some Risk." Published June 1. www.gao.gov/new.items/d10611.pdf.

———. 2008. *Veterans' Affairs: Improved Management Would Enhance VA's Pension Program.* GAO Report #08-112. Washington, DC: US Government Accountability Office.

Gozalo, P., and S. Miller. 2007. "Hospice Enrollment and Evaluation of Its Causal Effect on Hospitalization of Dying Nursing Home Patients." *Health Services Research* 42 (2): 587–610.

Grandal, K. 2008. "An MDS 3.0 Overview for Activity Professionals and Recreation Therapists." *Re-Creative Resources.* Accessed June 1, 2009. www.recreativeresources.com/documents/MDS3.0News.pdf.

Green, R. 2005. *Diagnosis and Management of Alzheimer's Disease,* 2nd ed. West Islip, NY: Professional Communications, Inc.

Green, C. R., K. O. Anderson, T. A. Baker, L. C. Campbell, S. Decker, R. B. Fillingim, D. L. Kalauokalani, K. E. Lasch, C. Myers, R. C. Tait, K. H. Todd, and A. H. Vallerand. 2003. "The Unequal Burden of Pain: Confronting Racial and Ethnic Disparities in Pain." *Pain Medicine* 4 (3): 277–94.

Haag, S., and M. Cummings. 2008. *Management Information Systems for the Information Age,* 7th ed. New York: McGraw-Hill Irwin.

Haley, B., and R. W. Grey. 2008. *Section 202 Supportive Housing for the Elderly: Program Status and Performance Measurement.* Washington, DC: US Department of Housing and Urban Development, Office of Policy Development and Research.

Hallberg, I. R., and A. Norberg. 1993. "Strain Among Nurses and Their Emotional Reactions During One Year of Systematic Clinical Supervision Combined with the Implementation of Individualized Care in Dementia Nursing." *Journal of Advanced Nursing* 18 (12): 1860–75.

Hallowell, E. M. 2005. "Overloaded Circuits: Why Smart People Underperform." *Harvard Business Review* 83 (1): 54–62.

Harrington, C., T. Tsoukalas, C. Rudder, R. J. Mollot, and H. Carrillo. 2008. "Variation in the Use of Federal and State Civil Money Penalties for Nursing Homes." *Gerontologist* 48 (5): 679–91.

Hartman, M., A. Martin, O. Nuccio, A. Catlin, and the National Health Expenditure Accounts Team. 2010. "Health Spending Growth at a Historic Low in 2008." *Health Affairs* 29 (1): 147–55.

Hawes, C., C. D. Phillips, M. Rose, S. Holan, and M. Sherman. 2003. "A National Survey of Assisted Living Facilities. *Gerontologist* 43 (6): 875–82.

He, W., M. Sengupta, V. A. Velkoff, and K. A. DeBarros. 2005. "65+ in the United States: 2005." US Census Bureau, *Current Population Reports*, P23-209. Washington, DC: US Government Printing Office. www.census.gov/prod/2006pubs/p23-209.pdf.

Health Care and Education Reconciliation Act of 2010. 2010. HR 4872. Accessed May 1. http://thomas.loc.gov/cgi-bin/query/z?c111:H.R.4872.

Health Resources and Services Administration (HRSA), Bureau of Health Professions. 2004. "Nursing Aides, Home Health Aides, and Related Health Care Occupations—National and Local Workforce Shortages and Associated Data Needs." Published February 1. http://bhpr.hrsa.gov/healthworkforce/reports/rnhomeaides.pdf.

Health Resources Online. 2011. "Hospice Management Resources." Accessed November 12, 2008. www.healthresourcesonline.com/hospice.

Henry J. Kaiser Family Foundation. 2012. "Medicaid and CHIP." *State Health Facts*. Accessed February 11. www.statehealthfacts.org/comparecat.jsp?cat=4_Medicaid & Chip.

———. 2001. "National Survey on Nursing Homes." *Public Broadcasting Service*. Published October 1. www.pbs.org/newshour/health/nursinghomes/highlightsand chartpack.pdf.

Higginson, I. J. 1999. "Evidence Based Palliative Care." *British Medical Journal* (International Edition) 319 (7208): 462–63.

Hillier, R. L. 2009. *Medicaid and Medicare Reimbursement*. Columbus, OH: RLH Consulting.

Hindman, S. 2009. "Adult Day Care More Than Just a Place to Go During the Day." *Silver Planet*. Published December 3. www.silverplanet.com/silver-planet-aging/adult-day-care-more-just-place-go-during-day/55981.

Hollinger-Smith, L., A. Ortigara, and D. Lindeman. 2001. "Developing a Comprehensive Long-Term Care Workforce Initiative." *Alzheimer's Care Quarterly* 2 (3): 33–40.

Holmes, H. M., D. C. Hayley, G. C. Alexander, and G. A. Sachs. "Reconsidering Medication Appropriateness for Patients Late in Life." *Archives of Internal Medicine* 166 (21): 605–9.

Hooyman, N., and H. A. Kiyak. 2011. *Social Gerontology*, 9th ed. Boston: Allyn and Bacon.

Hoskins, A. B. 2006. "Occupational Injuries, Illnesses, and Fatalities among Nursing, Psychiatric, and Home Health Aides, 1995–2004." *US Bureau of Labor Statistics*. Published June 30. www.bls.gov/opub/cwc/sh20060628ar01p1.htm.

Houser, A., and M. J. Gibson. 2009. *Valuing the Invaluable: The Economic Value of Family Caregiving, 2008 Update.* Washington, DC: AARP Public Policy Institute.

Huber, M., R. Rodrigues, F. Hoffmann, K. Gasior, and B. Marin. 2009. *Facts and Figures on Long-Term Care: Europe and North America.* Vienna, Austria: European Centre for Social Welfare Policy and Research.

Hurley, B. 2008. "Outstanding Customer Service Pays Personal, Bottom Line Dividends." *Colorado Springs Business Journal*, June 13.

Hwalek, M., V. Straub, and K. Kosniewski. 2008. "Older Workers: Opportunities to Expand the Long-Term Care/Direct Care Labor Force." *Gerontologist* 48 (1): 90–103.

Iowa CareGivers Association (2000). *Certified Nursing Assistant Recruitment and Retention Project: Final Report Summary.* Published December 2000. www.iowacaregivers.org/uploads/pdf/finalsummary.pdf.

Illinois Department of Health and Human Services. 2011. "Title XX Social Service Reports." *Illinois Department of Health and Human Services.* Accessed March 12. www.dhs.state.il.us/page.aspx?item=31680.

Improving Chronic Illness Care. 2011. "The Chronic Care Model." Accessed March 22. www.improvingchroniccare.org/index.php?p=The_Chronic_Care_Model&s=2.

Institute of Medicine. 2002. *Unequal Treatment: Confronting Racial and Ethnic Disparities in Health Care.* Washington, DC: National Academies Press.

Iwasaki, J. 2008. "State Second in Nation to Allow Lethal Prescriptions." *Seattle PI*. Published November 4. www.seattlepi.com/local/article/State-second-in-nation-to-allow-lethal-1290516.php.

Janicki, M. P., T. Heller, G. B. Seltzer, and J. Hogg. 1996. "Practice Guidelines for the Clinical Assessment and Care Management of Alzheimer's Disease and Other Dementias

Among Adults with Intellectual Disability." *Journal of Intellectual Disability Research* 40 (4): 374–82.

Jedrziewski, M. K., V. M. Lee, and J. Q. Trojanowski. 2007. "Physical Activity and Cognitive Health." *Alzheimer's & Dementia: The Journal of the Alzheimer's Association* 3 (2): 98–108.

John, R. 2004. "Health Status and Health Disparities." In *Closing the Gap: Improving the Health of Minority Elders in the New Millennium,* edited by K. Whitfield. Washington, DC: Gerontological Society of America.

Johns Hopkins University. 2004. *Chronic Care in America: A 21st Century Challenge. A Study of the Robert Wood Johnson Foundation and Partnership for Solutions.* Baltimore, MD: Johns Hopkins University.

Johnson, C. 1998. "A Proposal for Minimum Standards for Low Stimulus Alzheimer's Wings in Nursing Facilities." In *Annual Editions: Aging*, 12th ed., edited by Harold Cox, 184–86. New York: McGraw-Hill.

Johnson, R. W., D. Toohey, and J. M. Wiener. 2007. "Meeting the Long Term Care Needs of the Baby Boomers: How Changing Families Will Affect Paid Helpers and Institutions." *The Urban Institute*. Published May 1. www.urban.org/Uploaded PDF/311451_Meeting_Care.pdf.

Jones, A. L., L. L. Dwyer, A. R. Bercovitz, and G. W. Strahan. 2009. *The National Nursing Home Survey 2004*. Washington, DC: Center for Disease Control and Prevention.

Joseph, A. 2006. "Health Promotion by Design in Long-Term Care Settings." *The Center for Health Design*. Published August 1. www.healthdesign.org/sites/default/files/Health Promotion by Design in LTC Settings_0.pdf.

Kane, R., and L. Cutler. 2008. "Sustainability and Expansion of Small-House Nursing Homes: Lessons from the Green Houses® in Tupelo, MS." *University of Minnesota School of Public Health*. Accessed February 11, 2012. www.sph.umn.edu/hpm/ltcresourcecenter/research/greenhouse/attachments/GreenHouseSustainabilityand ExpansionSeptember2008.pdf.

Kane, R., L. Cutler, T. Lum, and A. Yu. 2005. "Results from the Green House Evaluation in Tupelo, MS." Presentation at the AcademyHealth Annual Meeting, Honolulu, HI, June 26.

Kane, R., T. Lum, L. Cutler, H. Degenholtz, and T. Yu. 2007. "Resident Outcomes in Small-House Nursing Homes: A Longitudinal Evaluation of the Initial Green House Program." *Journal of the American Geriatric Society* 55 (6): 832–39.

Kauffman, J. A. 2002. "American Indian and Alaska Native Roundtable on Long-Term Care." *National Indian Council on Aging.* Accessed March 19, 2011. www.nicoa.org/ PDFs/2002 NICOA LTC Roundtable Report.pdf.

Kaye, H. S., C. Harrington, and M. P. LaPlante. 2010. "Long-Term Care: Who Gets It, Who Provides It, Who Pays and How Much?" *Health Affairs* 29 (1): 11–21.

Kaye, H. S., M. P. LaPlante, and C. Harrington. 2009. "Do Non-institutional Long-Term Care Services Reduce Medicaid Spending?" *Health Affairs* 28 (1): 262–72.

King, D. E., and B. Bushwick. 1994. "Beliefs and Attitudes of Hospital Inpatients About Faith Healing and Prayer." *Journal of Family Practice* 39 (4): 349–52.

Kinsella, K., and W. He. 2009. *An Aging World: 2008.* Washington, DC: US Health and Human Services (National Institute on Aging) and US Department of Commerce (US Census Bureau).

Konetzka, T., S. C. Stearns, R. Konrad, J. Magainzer, and S. Zimmerman. 2005. "Personal Care Aide Turnover in Residential Care Settings: An Assessment of Ownership, Economic, and Environmental Factors." *Journal of Applied Gerontology* 24 (2): 87–107.

Koo, W. L., and T. V. Hoy. 2003. "Determining the Economic Value of Preventive Maintenance." Accessed February 2, 2010. www.sitemason.com/files/b2tJra/Preventive%20 Maintenance.pdf.

Koren, M. 2010. "Person-Centered Care for Nursing Home Residents: The Culture-Change Movement." *Health Affairs* 29 (2): 312–18.

Kotler, P., and K. L. Keller. 2006. *Marketing Management,* 12th ed. Toronto: Pearson Prentice Hall.

Kovner, C. T., M. Mezey, and C. Harrington. 2002. "Who Cares for Older Adults? Workforce Implications of an Aging Society." *Health Affairs* 21 (5): 78–89.

Kübler-Ross, E. 1969. *On Death and Dying: What the Dying Have to Teach Doctors, Nurses, Clergy and Their Own Families.* New York: Macmillan.

Kurdek, L. 2005. "What Do We Know About Gay and Lesbian Couples?" *Current Directions in Psychological Science* 14 (5): 251–54.

Lakdawalla, D., J. Bhattacharya, D. P. Goldman, M. Hurd, G. Joyce, and C. Panis. "Forecasting the Nursing Home Population." *Medical Care* 41 (1): 8–20.

Lambert, S. 2005. "Gay and Lesbian Families: What We Know and Where to Go from Here?" *Family Journal* 13 (1): 43–51.

Lang, F., and T. Quill. 2004. "Making Decisions with Families at the End of Life." *American Family Physician* 70 (4): 719–23.

LaPorte, M. 2009. "Recognition and Gratitude Make Big Impact." *Provider* 35 (11): 21–35.

Larson, D. G., and D. R. Tobin. 2000. "End-of-Life Conversations: Evolving Practice and Theory." *JAMA* 284 (12): 1573–78.

LaTour, K. M., and S. Eichenwald-Maki (eds.). 2006. *Health Information Management*, 2nd ed. Chicago: American Health Information Management Association.

Lee, R. H., B. J. Gajewski, and S. Thompson. 2006. "Reliability of the Nursing Home Survey Process: A Simultaneous Survey Approach." *Gerontologist* 46 (6): 772–79.

Lee v. Harclerod, 522 U.S. 927 (1997).

Lee v. State of Oregon, 107 F.3d 1382 (9th Cir., 1995).

Leland, J. 2009. "Helping Elderly Leave Nursing Homes for a Home." *New York Times*, September 18.

LeRoy, L., K. Treanor, and E. Art. 2010. "Foundation Work in Long-Term Care." *Health Affairs* 29 (1): 207–12.

Levine, C., D. Halper, A. Peist, and D. A. Gould. 2010. "Bridging Troubled Waters: Family Caregivers, Transitions, and Long-Term Care." *Health Affairs* 29 (1): 116–24.

Lewin Group. 2006. *Office of the Assistant Secretary for Planning and Evaluation Ensuring a Qualified Long-Term Care Workforce: From Pre-Employment Screens to On-the-Job Monitoring*. Falls Church, VA: Lewin Group.

LifePlans, Inc. 2007. *Who Buys Long-Term Care Insurance: A 15 Year Study of Buyers and Non-Buyers, 1990–2005. A Study Prepared for America's Health Insurance Plans*. Washington, DC: America's Health Insurance Plans.

Likert, R. 1932. "A Technique for the Measurement of Attitudes." *Archives of Psychology* 22 (140): 1–55.

Livermore, G., D. C. Stapleton, and M. O'Toole. 2011. "Growth in Federal and State Assistance to Working Age People with Disabilities." *Health Affairs* 30 (9): 1664–72.

Longest, B. B., Jr., and K. Darr. 2008. *Managing Health Services Organizations and Systems*, 5th ed. Baltimore, MD: Health Professions Press.

Louisiana Department of Health and Hospitals. 2004. "Long-Term Care for the Elderly and Disabled." Accessed October 24, 2009. www.dhh.louisiana.gov.

Lourde, K. 2009. "Facing Discrimination Issues." *Provider* 35 (7): 20–32.

Lovelock, C., and J. Wirtz. 2007. *Instructor's Resource Manual for Services Marketing: People, Technology, Strategy*, 6th ed. New York: Prentice Hall.

Maag, S. 2012. "CCRCs Today: How to Respond to Media Inquiries." *LeadingAge*. Published January 17. www.leadingage.org/How_to_Respond_to_Media_Inquiries.aspx.

MacLean, C. D., B. Susi, N. Phifer, L. Schultz, D. Bynum, M. Franco, A. Klioze, M. Monroe, J. Garrett, and S. Cykert. 2003. "Patient Preference for Physician Discussion and Practice of Spirituality." *Journal of General Internal Medicine* 18 (1): 38–43.

Magee, M. 2005. *Health Politics: Power, Populism and Health.* New York: Spencer.

Maheu, M. M., P. Whitten, and A. Allen. 2001. *E-Health, Telehealth and Telemedicine: A Guide to Start-Up and Success.* San Francisco: Jossey-Bass.

Mara, C. M., and L. K. Olson (eds.). 2008. *Handbook of Long-Term Care Administration and Policy.* Boca Raton, FL: Taylor and Francis Group.

Marsh, J. 2002. "House Calls." *Rochester Review* 64 (3). www.rochester.edu/pr/Review/V64N3/feature2.html.

Mashburn, S. 2011. "Aging Services: What You Need to Know About CCRCs." *Leading Age*. Published March 22. www.leadingage.org/Article.aspx?id=205.

Massachusetts Advocates for Nursing Home Reform. 2008. "Culture Change FAQ." Accessed February 1, 2012. www.manhr.org/culture_chng_faq.aspx.

Matter of the Application of Phillip K. Eichner, on Behalf of Joseph C. Fox, 73 AD2d 431, 456 (1980).

Maugans, T. A., and W. C. Wadland. 1991. "Religion and Family Medicine: A Survey of Physicians and Patients." *Journal of Family Practice* 32 (2): 210–13.

McCormick, W., C. Ohata, J. Uomoto, H. M. Young, A. B. Graves, W. Kukull, and E. B. Larson. 2002. "Similarities and Differences in Attitudes Toward Long-Term Care Between Japanese Americans and Caucasian Americans." *Journal of the American Geriatrics Society* 50 (6): 1149–55.

McCormick, W., J. Uomoto, H. Young, A. B. Graves, P. Vitaliano, J. A. Mortimer, and E. B. Larson. 1996. "Attitudes Toward Use of Nursing Homes and Home Care in Older Japanese-Americans." *Journal of the American Geriatrics Society* 44 (7): 769–77.

McDonald, P., M. Wykle, M. Kiley, and C. Burant. 2004. "Depressive Symptoms in Persons with Type 2 Diabetes: A Faith-Based Clinical Trial." *Gerontologist* 44 (Special Issue 1): 417.

McGregor, D. 1960. *The Human Side of Enterprise.* New York: McGraw-Hill.

McLaughlin, C. P., and A. D. Kaluzny. 2006. *Continuous Quality Improvement in Healthcare,* 3rd ed. Sudbury, MA: Jones and Bartlett.

Medley, B. D., A. Y. Stith, and A. R. Nelson. 2003. *Unequal Treatment: Confronting Racial and Ethnic Disparities in Health Care.* Washington, DC: National Academies Press.

Melzack, R. 1975. "The McGill Pain Questionnaire: Major Properties and Scoring Methods." *Pain* 1 (3): 277–99.

MetLife Mature Market Institute. 2011. *The 2011 MetLife Market Survey of Nursing Home, Assisted Living, Adult Day Services, and Home Care Costs.* Westport, CT: MetLife Mature Market Institute.

———. 2010. *The 2010 MetLife Market Survey of Nursing Home, Assisted Living, Adult Day Services, and Home Care Costs.* Westport, CT: MetLife Mature Market Institute.

———. 2006. *Out and Aging: The MetLife Study of Lesbian and Gay Baby Boomers.* New York: MetLife Mature Market Institute.

Mickan, S. M. 2005. "Evaluating the Effectiveness of Health Care Teams." *Australian Health Review* 29 (2): 211–17.

Miller, E. A., M. Booth, and V. Mor. 2008. "Assessing Experts' Views of the Future of Long-Term Care." *Research on Aging* 30 (4): 450–73.

Miller, S. C., V. Mor, N. Wu, P. Gozalo, and K. Lapane. 2002. "Does Receipt of Hospice Care in Nursing Homes Improve the Management of Pain at the End of Life?" *Journal of the American Geriatric Society* 50 (3): 507–15.

Min, J., and A. Moon. 2006. "Older Asian Americans." In *Handbook of Social Work in Health and Aging,* edited by B. Berkman and S. D'Ambruoso. New York: Oxford University Press.

Miñino, A. M., M. P. Heron, S. L. Murphy, and K. D. Kochankek. 2007. "Deaths: Final Data for 2004." *National Vital Statistics Report* 55 (19): 1–119.

Mintzberg, H. 1973. *The Nature of Managerial Work.* New York: HarperCollins.

Moen, P., and K. Chermack. 2005. "Gender Disparities in Health: Strategic Selection, Careers, and Cycles of Control." *Journals of Gerontology Series B: Psychological Sciences & Social Sciences* 60 (Special Issue 2): S99–S108.

Mollot, R. J., and C. Rudder. 2008. *New York's Single Point of Entry for Long-Term Care: A First Year Assessment of Consumer Experience with Recommendations for the Future.* New York: Long-Term Care Community Coalition.

Montgomery, R., L. Holley, J. Deichert, and K. Kosloski. 2005. "A Profile of Home Care Workers from the 2000 Census: How It Changes What We Know." *Gerontologist* 45 (5): 593–600.

Morrison, R. S., and D. E. Meier. 2004. "Clinical Practice: Palliative Care." *New England Journal of Medicine* 350 (25): 2582–90.

Morrison, R. S., J. D. Penrod, J. B. Cassel, M. Caust-Ellenbogen, A. Litke, L. Spragens, and D. E. Meier. 2008. "Cost Savings Associated with US Hospital Palliative Care Consultation Programs." *Archives of Internal Medicine* 168 (16): 1783–90.

Moschis, G. P., and A. Mathur. 1993. "How They Are Acting Their Age." *Marketing Management Chicago* 2 (2): 40–51.

Munet-Vilaro, F. 2004. "Health Promotion for Older Adults: Latino Elders." *Northwest Geriatric Education Center.* Accessed March 19, 2011. http://coa.kumc.edu/gecresource/samples/Northwest/LatinoElders.pdf.

MySeniorCare. 2010. "Veterans' Benefits and Senior Housing." Published April 14. www.myseniorcare.com/senior-housing/insurance-payment/veterans-benefits-and-senior-housing-article.

National Adult Day Services Association (NADSA). 2011. "About Adult Day Services." Accessed March 12. www.nadsa.org/?page_id=118.

National Association for Home Care and Hospice (NAHC). 2010. "Basic Statistics about Home Care." *NAHC.* Accessed February 11, 2012. www.nahc.org/facts/10hc_stats.pdf.

National Center for Health Statistics (NCHS). 2004. "National Nursing Home Survey Overview." Washington, DC: NCHS.

———. 1989. "The National Nursing Home Survey: 1985 Summary for the US." *Vital and Health Statistics* Series 13, No. 97, DHHS Pub 89-1758. Washington, DC: NCHS.

National Clearinghouse on the Direct Care Workforce. 2011. "Who Are Direct-Care Workers?" Published February 1. www.directcareclearinghouse.org/download/NCDCW Fact Sheet-1.pdf.

National Council on Aging. 2012. "Senior Centers: Fact Sheet." *National Council on Aging.* Accessed February 11, 2012. www.ncoa.org/press-room/fact-sheets/senior-centers-fact-sheet.html.

National Health Policy Forum. 2011. *The Basics: National Spending for Long-Term Care Services and Supports.* Washington, DC: George Washington University.

National Hospice and Palliative Care Organization (NHPCO). 2012. "2011 Edition: NHPCO Facts and Figures: Hospice Care in America." Accessed July 25, 2011. www.nhpco.org/files/public/Statistics_Research/2011_Facts_Figures.pdf.

———. 2007. "National Data Set." *NHPCO.* Accessed November 23, 2008. www.nhpco.org/i4a/pages/index.cfm?pageid=3378.

National Institute of Neurological Disorders and Stroke (NINDS). 2007. "Disorder Index." Accessed December 4. www.ninds.nih.gov/disorders/disorder_index.htm.

National Institute on Aging. 2012. "About Alzheimer's Disease: Alzheimer's Basics." *National Institutes of Health.* www.nia.nih.gov/alzheimers/topics/alzheimers-basics.

National PACE Association. 2012. "Research." Accessed February 11. www.npaonline.org/website/article.asp?id=30.

Nelson, H. W., K. Hooker, K. DeHart, J. A. Edwards, and K. Lanning. 2004. "Factors Important to Success in the Volunteer Long-Term Care Ombudsman Role." *Gerontologist* 44 (1): 116–20.

Neuborne, E. 1997. "Companies Save, but Workers Pay." *USA Today*, February 25, 2B.

New York Times. 2009. "The New Old Age: A Nighttime Program for Alzheimer's Care." *New York Times.* Published June 12. http://newoldage.blogs.nytimes.com/2009/06/12/a-nighttime-program-for-patients-with-alzheimers.

New York v. United States, 505 U.S. 144 (1992).

Ng, T., C. Harrington, and M. Kitchener. 2010. "Medicare and Medicaid in Long-Term Care." *Health Affairs* 29 (1): 22–28.

Ng, T., C. Harrington, and M. O'Malley. 2009. *Medicaid Home and Community-Based Services Programs: Data Update.* Washington, DC: Henry F. Kaiser Family Foundation.

Niles-Yokum, K., and D. Wagner. 2011. *The Aging Networks: A Guide to Programs and Services.* New York: Springer Publishing Company.

Novak, M., and C. Guest. 1989. "Application of a Multidimensional Caregiver Burden Inventory." *Gerontologist* 20 (6): 798–803.

Oetjen, D., and R. Oetjen. 2006. "The Moral and Ethical Implications of Elder Abuse." In *Elder Abuse: A Public Health Perspective*, edited by A. M. Hoffman and R. W. Summers, 77–96. Thousand Oaks, CA: Sage Publications.

Office of Minority Health. 2001. *National Standards on Culturally and Linguistically Appropriate Services.* Washington, DC: US Government Printing Office.

Ogden, L. L., and K. Adams. 2009. "Poorhouse to Warehouse: Institutional Long-Term Care in the United States." *Publius* 39 (1): 138–63.

Oliver, D. P., D. Porock, and S. Zweig. 2005. "End-of-life Care in US Nursing Homes: A Review of the Evidence." *Journal of the American Medical Directors Association* 6 (3): S21–S30.

Omnibus Budget Reconciliation Act of 1990, P.L. 101-508, § 4206 and 4751, codified at 42 U.S.C. § 1395cc (a)(1)(Q), 1395mm (c)(8), 1395cc (f), 1396a (57), (58), 1396a (w).

O'Reilly, K. B. 2010. "Physician-Assisted Suicide Legal in Montana, Court Rules." *American Medical News.* Published January 18. www.ama-assn.org/amednews/2010/01/18/prsb0118.htm.

O'Shaughnessy, C. V. 2008. "The Aging Services Network: Accomplishments and Challenges in Serving a Growing Elderly Population." *National Health Policy Forum.* Published April 11. www.nhpf.org/library/details.cfm/2625.

Pandya, S. M. 2005. "Racial and Ethnic Differences Among Older Adults in Long-Term Care Service Use." Fact Sheet No. 119. *AARP Public Policy Institute.* Published June 2005. http://assets.aarp.org/rgcenter/il/fs119_ltc.pdf.

Paraprofessional Healthcare Institute. 2011. "Who Are Direct Care Workers?" *National Clearinghouse on the Direct Care Workforce.* Published February 2011. www.directcare clearinghouse.org/download/NCDCW Fact Sheet-1.pdf.

———. 2002. *Recruiting Quality Health Care Paraprofessionals.* South Bronx, NY: Paraprofessional Healthcare Institute.

Partners in Caregiving. 2002. "National Study of Adult Day Services, 2001–2002." www.rwjf.org/pr/product.jsp?id=16996.

Partnership to Fight Chronic Disease. 2011. "About the Crisis." Accessed May 8. www.fightchronicdisease.org/facing-issues/about-crisis.

Peacock, J. 1995. "Redefining the Nurse's Station." *Nursing Homes* 444 (7): 32–34.

Pearce, B. W. 2007. *Senior Living Communities: Operations Management and Marketing for Assisted Living, Congregate and Continuing Care Retirement Communities,* 2nd ed. Baltimore, MD: Johns Hopkins University Press.

Phillips, C. D., A.-M. Kimbell, C. Hawes, J. Wells, J. Badalamenti, and M. J. Koren. 2008. "It's a Family Affair: Consumer Advocacy for Nursing Home Residents in the United States." *Ageing & Society* 28 (1): 67–84.

Pillemer, K., R. Meador, C. Henderson, Jr., J. Robison, C. Hegeman, E. Graham, and L. Schultz. 2008. "A Facility Specialist Model for Improving Retention of Nursing Home Staff: Results from a Randomized, Controlled Study." *Gerontologist* 48 (Special Issue): 80–89.

Pratt, J. R. 2010. *Long-Term Care: Managing Across the Continuum,* 3rd ed. Sudbury, MA: Jones and Bartlett.

———. 2004. *Long-Term Care: Managing Across the Continuum,* 2nd ed. Sudbury, MA: Jones and Bartlett.

President's Commission for the Study of Ethical Problems in Medicine and Biomedical and Behavioral Research. 1983. "Deciding to Forego Life-Sustaining Treatment: Ethical, Medical, and Legal Issues in Treatment Decisions." *Bioethics Research Library at Georgetown University.* Published March 1983. http://bioethics.georgetown.edu/pcbe/reports/past_commissions/deciding_to_forego_tx.pdf.

Printz v. United States, 521 U.S. 898 (1997).

Project Management Institute. 2004. *The Project Management Body of Knowledge,* 4th ed. Philadelphia, PA: Project Management Institute.

ProximityOne. 2011. "Population Age 65 & Over Estimates & Projections." Accessed September 30. www.proximityone.com/st003065.htm.

Rahman, A., and J. Schnelle. 2008. "The Nursing Home Culture-Change Movement: Recent Past, Present, and Future Directions for Research." *Gerontologist* 48 (2): 142–48.

Randall, D. A. 2008. "The New Hospice Conditions of Participation: Changes in Compliance Focus." *Health Care Compliance Association* 27: 30–35.

Ratliff, D. 1999. "Maintenance: The Assisted Living Difference." *Nursing Homes* 48 (3): 44.

Rauma, P. 1992. "Surviving with the ADA: Environmental Modification." *Nursing Homes* 41 (4): 28–29.

Raymond, B., and C. Dold. 2002. *Clinical Information Systems: Achieving the Vision.* Oakland, CA: Kaiser Permanente Institute for Health Policy.

Redfoot, D. 2008. *Overview of Assisted Living.* Washington, DC: Center for Excellence in Assisted Living.

Regnier, V. 2002. *Design for Assisted Living: Guidelines for Housing the Physically and Mentally Frail.* New York: John Wiley & Sons.

Relethford, J. 2007. *The Human Species: An Introduction to Biological Anthropology*, 7th ed. New York: McGraw-Hill.

———. 1990. *The Human Species: An Introduction to Biological Anthropology.* Mountain View, CA: Mayfield.

Resnick, H. E., B. B. Manard, R. I. Stone, and M. Alwan. 2008. "Use of Electronic Information Systems in Nursing Homes, 2004." *Journal of the American Medical Informatics Association* 16 (2): 179–86.

Rice, K. N., E. A. Coleman, R. Fish, C. Levy, and J. S. Kutner. 2004. "Factors Influencing Models of End of Life Care in Nursing Homes: Results of a Survey of Nursing Home Administrators." *Journal of Palliative Medicine* 7 (5): 668–75.

Ricketts, T. C. 1999. *Rural Health in the United States.* New York: Oxford University Press.

Rittenhouse, D. R., L. P. Casalino, R. R. Gillies, and S. M. Shortell. 2009. "The Patient-Centered Medical Home: Will It Stand the Test of Healthcare Reform?" *JAMA* 301 (19): 2038–40.

Roberts, D. C. 2007. *Deeper Learning in Leadership: Helping College Students Find the Potential Within.* San Francisco: Jossey-Bass.

Rodriguez, K. L., J. T. Hanlon, S. Perera, E. J. Jaffe, and M. A. Sevick. 2010. "A Cross-Sectional Analysis of the Prevalence of Undertreatment of Nonpain Symptoms and Factors Associated with Undertreatment in Older Nursing Home Hospice/Palliative Care Patients." *American Journal of Geriatric Pharmacotherapy* 8 (3): 225–32.

Rogers, C. C. 1999. *Changes in the Older Population and Implications for Rural Areas.* Washington, DC: US Department of Agriculture.

Rollins, G. 2000. "Preventing the Fall." *Safety & Health* 162 (3): 38–42.

Rollow, W., T. R. Lied, P. McGann, J. Poyer, L. LaVoie, R. Kambic, D. W. Bratzler, A. Ma, E. D. Huff, and L. D. Ramunno. 2006. "Assessment of the Medicare Quality Improvement Organization Program." *Annals of Internal Medicine* 145 (5): 342–53.

Rosenfeld, J. P., and W. Chapman. 2008. *Design in an Aging World.* New York: Fairchild Books, Inc.

Ross, K., and C. Bing. 2007. "Emergency Management: Expanding the Disaster Plan." *Home Healthcare Nurse* 25 (6): 370–77.

Rural Long-Term Care Workgroup. 2008. *Expanding Rural Elder Care Options: Models That Work. Proceedings from the 2008 Rural Long Term Care Access and Options Workshop.* Alexandria, VA: National PACE Association.

Sasse, R. 2007. "Facility Condition Assessment in Nursing Homes." *Nursing Homes* 56 (6): 22–28.

Satzinger, J., R. B. Jackson, and S. D. Burd. 2007. *Systems Analysis and Design,* 4th ed. Boston, MA: Course Technology.

Saunders, C. 1976. "The Challenges of Terminal Care." In *Scientific Foundations of Oncology,* edited by T. Syminton and R. I. Carter, 673–79. London: Heinemann.

Scherzer, T., S. Chapman, and R. Newcomer. 2004. "Lost-Worktime Injuries and Illnesses of Nursing Aides, Orderlies, and Attendants." *Center for Personal Assistance Services.* Published June 10. http://pascenter.org/documents/Lost_workdays_and_NA.pdf.

Schuler, R. S. 1987. *Personnel and Human Resource Management.* New York: West.

Schwarz, B., and R. Brent. 1999. *Aging, Autonomy, and Architecture: Advances in Assisted Living.* Baltimore, MD: Johns Hopkins Press.

Sclar, D. 2006. "US Supreme Court Ruling in *Gonzales v. Oregon* Upholds the Oregon Death with Dignity Act." *Journal of Law, Medicine & Ethics* 34 (3): 639.

Seale, G. 2010. "Emergency Preparedness as a Continuous Improvement Cycle: Perspectives from a Postacute Rehabilitation Facility." *Rehabilitation Psychology* 55 (3): 247–54.

Seavey, D. 2004. "The Cost of Frontline Turnover in Long-Term Care." *Better Jobs Better Care*. Published October 1. www.directcareclearinghouse.org/download/TO CostReport.pdf.

SeniorHomes.com. 2012. "CCRC Costs: How Much Will You Pay?" Accessed February 1. www.seniorhomes.com/p/ccrc-costs.

Senior Journal. 2006. "Professor Says Much of New Technology Should Be Known as Nana Technology." *Senior Journal*. Published August 16. http://seniorjournal.com/NEWS/Features/6-08-16-ProfessorSays.htm.

Senior Veterans Service Alliance. 2012a. "About Compensation and Other Related Benefits." Accessed February 12. www.veteransaidbenefit.org/service_conected_disabilities.htm.

———. 2012b. "Long Term Care Benefits for Veterans." Accessed February 12. www.veteransaidbenefit.org/va_healthcare_for_long_term_care.htm.

———. 2012c. "State Veterans Homes." Accessed February 12. www.veteransaidbenefit.org/state_veterans_nursing_homes.htm.

Shanks, N. H. 2007. "Management and Motivation." In *Introduction to Health Care Management*, edited by S. Buchbinder and N. Shanks. Sudbury, MA: Jones and Bartlett.

Shi, L., and G. D. Stevens. 2005. *Vulnerable Populations in the United States*. San Francisco: Jossey-Bass.

Shih, A., D. M. Dewar, and T. Hartman. 2007. "Medicare's Quality Improvement Organization Program Value in Nursing Homes." *Health Care Financing Review* 28 (3): 109–16.

Shin, D. 2008. "Residential and Caregiver Preferences of Older Korean Americans." *Journal of Gerontological Nursing* 34 (6): 48–54.

Shuster, G., D. Clough, P. Grant Higgins, and B. Klein. 2009. "Health and Health Behaviors Among Elderly Hispanic Women." *Geriatric Nursing* 30 (1): 18–27.

Silverstein, N. M., G. Flaherty, and T. S. Tobin. 2002. *Dementia and Wandering Behavior: Concern for the Lost Elder*. Ney York: Springer.

Sim, J. 1999. "Improving Return-to-Work Strategies in the United States Disability Programs, with Analysis of Program Practices in Germany and Sweden." *Social Security Bulletin* 62 (3): 41–50.

Singh, D. A. 2005. *Effective Management of Long-Term Care Facilities*. Sudbury, MA: Jones and Bartlett.

Smedley, B. D., A. Y. Stith, and A. R. Nelson (eds.). 2003. *Unequal Treatment: Confronting Racial and Ethnic Disparities in Health Care*. Washington, DC: National Academies Press.

Smith, D. B., and Z. Feng. 2010. "The Accumulated Challenges of Long-Term Care." *Health Affairs* 29 (1): 29–34.

Smith, D. G., and J. D. Moore. 2008. *Medicaid Politics and Policy, 1965–2007*. New Brunswick, NJ: Transaction Publishers.

Smith, G., J. O'Keefe, L. Carpenter, P. Doty, G. Kennedy, B. Burwell, R. Mollica, and L. Williams. 2000. "Understanding Medicaid Home and Community Services: A Primer." *US Department of Health and Human Services*. Accessed February 12, 2012. http://aspe .hhs.gov/daltcp/reports/primer.htm.

Smith, M., G. R. Hall, L. A. Gerdner, and K. C. Buckwalter. 2006. "Application of the Progressively Lowered Stress Threshold (PLST) Model Across the Continuum of Care." *Nursing Clinics of North America* 41 (1): 57–81.

Smith, P. C., and L. M. Kendall. 1963. "Retranslation of Expectations: An Approach to the Construction of Unambiguous Anchors for Rating Scales." *Journal of Applied Psychology* 47: 149–55.

St. Christopher's Hospice. 2011. "Hospice Overview." Accessed November 23, 2008. www.stchristophers.org.uk/hospiceoverview.

Stanley, S., N. Zane, G. C. Nagayama Hall, and L. K. Berger. 2009. "The Case for Cultural Competency in Psychotherapeutic Interventions." *Annual Review of Psychology* 60: 525–48.

Starr, P. 1982. *The Social Transformation of American Medicine*. New York: Basic Books.

State of Louisiana Department of Health and Hospitals. 2012. "September 2004 Health Care Reform Panel Reference Materials." Accessed February 11, 2012. www.dhh.louisiana .gov/offices/page.asp?ID=157&Detail=4640.

Stewart-Pollack, J., and R. Menconi. 2005. *Designing for Privacy and Related Needs.* New York: Fairchild Publications.

Stevenson, D. G., M. A. Cohen, E. J. Tell, and B. Burwell. 2010. "The Complementarity of Public and Private Long-Term Care Insurance." *Health Affairs* 29 (1): 96–101.

Stone, R. I. 2000. *Long-Term Care for the Elderly with Disabilities: Current Policy, Emerging Trends, and Implications for the Twenty-First Century.* New York: Millbank Memorial Fund.

Stone, R., and M. Harahan. 2010. "Improving the Long-Term Care Workforce Serving Older Adults." *Health Affairs* 29 (1): 109–15.

Stross, R. 2011. "Digital Domain: Tracking Vital Signs, Without the Wires." *New York Times*, September 3.

Sutton, E., and H. L. Sterns. 1990. "A Competency Based Matrix of Knowledge and Skills for Specialists in Developmental Disabilities and Aging." Washington, DC: US Department of Education, Office of Special Education and Rehabilitative Services.

Tabloski, P. A. 2010. *Gerontological Nursing*, 2nd ed. Mahwah, NJ: Pearson Publishers.

Taft-Hartley Act. LMRA; 29 U.S.C. Sec. Sec. 141-197 [Title 29, Chapter 7, United States Code].

Tan, J., with F. C. Payton. 2010. *Adaptive Health Management Information Systems.* Boston: Jones and Bartlett.

Tate, H. 2009. "Cultural Competence Counts." *Provider* 35 (12): 37–40.

Taylor, D. H., Jr., J. Ostermann, C. H. Van Houtven, J. A. Tulsky, and K. Steinhauser. 2007. "What Use of Hospice Maximizes Reduction in Medical Expenditures Near Death in the US Medicare Program?" *Social Science and Medicine* 65 (7): 1466–78.

Thomas, W. 2004. *What Are Old People For? How Elders Will Save the World.* Acton, MA: VanderWyk & Burnham.

———. 2003. "The Evolution of Eden." *Journal of Social Work in Long-Term Care* 2 (1/2): 141–57.

———. 1996. *Life Worth Living.* Acton, MA: VanderWyk & Burnham.

Thompson, J. M. 2007. "The Strategic Management of Human Resources." In *Introduction to Health Care Management*, edited by S. Buchbinder and N. Shanks. Sudbury, MA: Jones and Bartlett.

Thornton, P. 1994. "Surviving the 1990s Through Integrated Marketing." *Nursing Homes* 43 (3): 38–40.

Torres-Gil, F., and K. Moga. 2002. "Multiculturalism, Social Policy and the New Aging." *Journal of Gerontological Social Work* 36 (3): 12–32.

Tracey, B. J., and A. E. Nathan. 2002. "The Strategic and Operational Roles of Human Resources: An Emerging Model." *Cornell Hotel and Restaurant Administration Quarterly* 43 (4): 17–26.

Tucker, K. 2004. "Medico-Legal Case Report and Commentary: Inadequate Pain Management in the Context of Terminal Cancer." *Pain Medicine* 5 (2): 214–18.

Ulrich, R. 1997. "A Theory of Supportive Design for Healthcare Facilities." *Journal of Healthcare Design: Proceedings From The ... Symposium On Healthcare Design. Symposium On Healthcare Design*, 93–7.

US Bureau of Health Professions, Division of Nursing. 2001. "The Registered Nurse Population: National Sample Survey of Registered Nurses—March 2000." Rockville, MD: Health Resources and Services Administration.

US Bureau of Labor Statistics (BLS). 2012. "Economic News Release: Union Members Summary." Published January 27. www.bls.gov/news.release/union2.nr0.htm.

———. 2008. "Workplace Injuries and Illnesses in 2007." Published October 23. www.bls.gov/iif/oshsum.htm.

———. 2003–04. "Occupational Employment." *Occupational Outlook Quarterly* Winter. www.bls.gov/opub/ooq/2003/winter/art02.pdf.

US Bureau of Labor Statistics and US Department of Labor. 2009. "Occupational Employment Statistics, 2009." www.bls.gov/oes.

———. 2003. "Workplace Injuries and Illnesses in 2002." Published December 18. www.bls.gov/iif/oshwc/osh/os/osnr0018.txt.

US Census Bureau. 2011a. *Profile America: Facts for Features—Older Americans Month May 2011.* Report CB11-FF.08. Washington, DC: US Census Bureau.

———. 2011b. *2011 Statistical Abstract of the United States.* Washington, DC: US Census Bureau.

———. 2008a. *An Older and More Diverse Nation by Midcentury.* Washington, DC: US Department of Commerce.

————. 2008b. "National Population Projections: Released 2008 (Based on Census 2000)." Published November 1. www.census.gov/population/www/projections/downloadablefiles.html.

————. 2008c. *Projections of the Population by Age and Sex for the United States: 2010 to 2050.* Washington, DC: US Census Bureau.

————. 2004. *Survey of Income and Program Participation.* Washington, DC: US Census Bureau.

US Department of Health and Human Services (HHS), Office of Inspector General. 2006. "Nursing Home Emergency Preparedness and Response During Recent Hurricanes." *Published August 1.* http://oig.hhs.gov/oei/reports/oei-06-06-00020.pdf.

US Department of Justice. 2011. "ADA Enforcement." Published December 8. www.ada.gov/enforce.htm.

————. 2009. "Americans with Disabilities Act of 1990, as Amended." Updated March 25. www.ada.gov/pubs/ada.htm.

US Department of Labor. 2011. "Workers' Compensation." Accessed May 4. www.dol.gov/dol/topic/workcomp/index.htm.

US Department of Labor, Employment and Training Administration. 2012. "Registered Apprenticeship." Updated March 16. www.doleta.gov/oa.

US Department of Labor, Wage and Hour Division. 2012. "Family and Medical Leave Act." Accessed February 12. www.dol.gov/whd/fmla.

————. 2008. "Face Sheet #17A: Exemption for Executive, Administrative, Professional, Computer and Outside Sales Employees under the Fair Labor Standards Act (FLSA)." Published July 1. www.dol.gov/whd/regs/compliance/fairpay/fs17a_overview.pdf.

US Department of Veterans Affairs, Office of Patient Care Services, Technology Assessment Program (VA). 2010. "Bibliography: Home Telehealth." *Veterans Administration.* Published June 1. www.va.gov/VATAP/docs/Hometelehealth2010.pdf.

University of Minnesota. 2011. "Nursing Services: Staffing Ratios." *NHRegsPlus.* Updated November 22. www.hpm.umn.edu/nhregsplus/NH%20Regs%20by%20Topic/Topic%20Nursing%20Services%20-%20Staffing%20Ratios.html.

Vicari, S., U. Nocentini, and C. Caltagirone. 1994. "Neuropsychological Diagnosis of Aging in Adults with Down Syndrome." *Developmental Brain Dysfunction* 7 (6): 340–48.

Vincent, G. K., and V. A. Velkoff. 2010. "The Next Four Decades: The Older Population in the United States: 2010 to 2050." *US Census Bureau*. Published May 1. www.census.gov/prod/2010pubs/p25-1138.pdf.

Vladeck, B. C. 2005. "Economic and Policy Implications of Improving Longevity." *Journal of the American Geriatric Society* 53 (9): S304–S307.

Wager, K. A., F. W. Lee, and J. P. Glaser. 2009. *Managing Healthcare Information Systems*, 2nd ed. San Francisco: Jossey-Bass.

Wagner, E. H. 1998. "Chronic Disease Management: What Will It Take to Improve Care for Chronic Illness?" *Effective Clinical Practice* 1 (Aug-Sep): 2–4.

Wagner, L. 2010. "Collaborative Seeks Federal Funds." *Provider Magazine* (October): 16.

Wallace, S. P., and V. M. Villa. 2003. "Equitable Health Systems: Cultural and Structural Issues for Latino Elders." *American Journal of Law and Medicine* 29 (2–3): 247–67.

Walshe, K., and C. Harrington. 2002. "Regulation of Nursing Facilities in the United States: An Analysis of Resources and Performance of State Survey Agencies." *Gerontologist* 42 (4): 475–86.

Weiss, R. 1994. "Market Response Systems: A Community Interface." *Health Progress* 75 (61): 68–69.

Wen, M., K. A. Cagney, and N. A. Christakis. 2005. "Effect of Community Social Environment on the Mortality of Individuals Diagnosed with Serious Illness." *Social Science and Medicine* 61 (6): 1119–34.

Williams, K. N., R. Herman, B. Gajewski, and K. Wilson. 2009. "Elderspeak Communication: Impact on Dementia Care." *American Journal of Alzheimer's Disease and Other Dementias* 24 (1): 11–20.

Williams, P. 2009. "Senate Committee Adopts Senior Related Amendments to Healthcare Reform Legislation." Assisted Living Federation of America, News Release, September 25. Alexandria, VA: Assisted Living Federation of America.

Wilson, A. M. 2001. "Mystery Shopping: Using Deception to Evaluate Service Performance." *Psychology and Marketing* 18 (7): 721–34.

Wilson, K. B. 2007. "Historical Evolution of Assisted Living in the United States, 1979 to the Present." *Gerontologist* 47 (Suppl. 1): 8–22.

Wilson, K. P. 2009. "Culture Change: Definition and Models." *Gerontology Special Interest Section Quarterly /American Occupational Therapy Association* 32 (3): 1–2.

Wiscott, R., K. Kopera-Frye, and L. Seifert. 2000. "Issues in Neuropsychological Assessment: Older Adults with Mental Retardation." *Clinical Gerontologist* 22 (3/4): 71–86.

Wolff, J., J. Kasper, and A. Shore. 2008. "Long-Term Care Preferences Among Older Adults: A Moving Target?" *Journal of Aging & Social Policy* 20 (2): 182–200.

World Health Organization (WHO). 2011. "What Do We Mean by Sex and Gender?" Accessed March 19. www.who.int/gender/whatisgender/en.

Wright, A. A., B. Zhang, A. Ray, J. W. Mack, E. Trice, T. Balboni, S. L. Mitchell, V. A. Jackson, S. D. Block, P. K. Maciejewski, and H. G. Prigerson. 2008. "Associations Between End-of-Life Discussions, Patient Mental Health, Medical Care Near Death, and Caregiver Bereavement Adjustment." *JAMA* 300 (14): 1665–73.

Wunderlich, G., F. Sloan, and C. K. Davis. 1996. *Nursing Staff in Hospital and Nursing Homes: Is It Adequate?* Washington, DC: National Academies Press.

Yale Medical Group. 2010. "Hospice Care Services." Accessed March 25. www.yalemedicalgroup.org/stw/Page.asp?PageID=STW023255.

Yale University. 2008. "In Memoriam: YSN Dean, Florence Wald, Founder of Hospice in the US." *Yale News*. Published November 21. http://news.yale.edu/2008/11/21/memoriam-ysn-dean-florence-wald-founder-hospice-care-us.

Yancu, C. N., D. F. Farmer, and D. Leahman. 2009. "Barriers to Hospice Use and Palliative Care Services Use by African American Adults." *American Journal of Hospice Palliative Care* 27 (4): 248–53.

Zarem, J. E. (ed.). 2010. "Today's Continuing Care Retirement Community (CCRC)." *CCRC Task Force*. Published July 2010. www.seniorshousing.org/filephotos/research/CCRC_whitepaper.pdf.

Zarit, S. H., and J. M. Zarit. 1998. *Mental Disorders in Older Adults*. New York: Guilford.

Zeisel, J., N. Silverstein, J. Hyde, S. Levkoff, M. P. Lawton, and W. Holmes. 2003. "Environmental Correlates to Behavioral Health Outcomes in Alzheimer's Special Care Units." *Gerontologist* 43 (5): 697–711.

Zhang, B., A. A. Wright, H. A. Huskamp, M. E. Nilsson, M. L. Maciejewski, C. C. Earle, S. D. Block, P. K. Maciejewski, and H. G. Prigerson. 2009. "Health Care Costs in the

Last Week of Life Associations with End-of-Life Conversations." *Archives of Internal Medicine* 169 (5): 480–88.

Ziegler Capital Markets. 2009. *Ziegler National CCRC Listing and Profile.* Milwaukee, WI: Ziegler Capital Markets.

Zimmerman, S., A. L. Gruber-Baldini, P. D. Sloane, J. Eckert, J. R. Hebel, L. A. Morgan, S. C. Stearns, J. Wildfire, J. Magaziner, C. Chen, and T. R. Konrad. 2003. "Assisted Living and Nursing Homes: Apples and Oranges?" *Gerontologist* 43 (Suppl. 2): 107–17.

Index

ABOUT THE CONTRIBUTORS

Jullet A. Davis holds an MHA and a PhD from Pennsylvania State University and a BS in health services administration from Herbert H. Lehman College. Prior to receiving her academic degrees, she worked as a healthcare practitioner in the nursing home and public health fields. Her primary research interests are organizational theory, long-term care, and gerontology.

Suzanne Discenza, PhD, is an associate professor and director of the master of healthcare leadership program in the Hauptmann School for Public Affairs at Park University. She completed her PhD in public affairs, with an emphasis in health and social policy, at the University of Colorado. She also holds a master's in communication disorders from the University of Oklahoma. Dr. Discenza previously was director of the interdisciplinary Gerontology Program at the Metropolitan State College of Denver, served on the board of directors of the Colorado Culture Change Coalition, and owned and managed her own rehabilitation business in Colorado Springs. She currently serves as president of the Greater Kansas City Chapter of the American Society for Public Administration and on numerous healthcare-related boards and committees in the Kansas City area. Her research publications have focused on healthcare management issues, hospital ER diversion initiatives, and healthcare concerns for disadvantaged populations, including aging adults, the homeless, the disabled, and the uninsured.

Margie Eckroth-Bucher, PhD, RN, is professor of nursing at Bloomsburg University in Bloomsburg, Pennsylvania. She has more than 29 years of experience in the field of mental health and holds board certification and licensure as a clinical nurse specialist in adult psychiatric and mental health. She has published in the area of gerontology, and her research focus is cognitive issues affecting the elderly.

Barbara H. Edington, PMP, MBA, DPS, is an associate professor at St. Francis College in Brooklyn Heights, New York, where she is also the director of the Center of Excellence in Project Management. Prior to her career in academics, she worked in the financial services industry and managed products and projects in the United States and abroad.

Karen Kopera-Frye, PhD, is the Joseph A. Biedenharn Endowed Chair and professor in gerontology in the Department of Gerontology, Sociology, and Political Science at the University of Louisiana at Monroe. She received all of her degrees (BA, MA, PhD) in lifespan developmental and clinical psychology, with specialization in gerontology, from Wayne State University in Detroit. Her current research interests include promoting healthy aging, healthcare delivery among ethnically diverse elders and rural-dwelling elders, and caregiving of loved ones with dementia. She has published extensively on research with older adults and has expertise in grantsmanship. She currently cares for her 87-year-old mother, who has vascular dementia.

Peter Gomori, PhD, is professor of management and IT at St. Francis College in New York, where he has been a faculty member since 1983. He earned a BS in economics from the City College of New York, an MBA in finance from Baruch College, and a PhD in economics from the CUNY Graduate Center. His present research interests are the current European financial crisis and the integration of the Central and East European countries.

Reetu Grewal, MD, obtained her medical degree from the University of Medicine and Dentistry of New Jersey–Robert Wood Johnson Medical School in 2001. She completed her residency in family medicine at Spartanburg Regional Medical Center in Spartanburg, South Carolina, where she also served as chief resident. She then pursued a fellowship in hospice and palliative medicine at Mayo Clinic in Jacksonville, Florida. Currently she serves as a clinical assistant professor in the Department of Community Health and Family Medicine at the University of Florida, Jacksonville campus.

Christopher Johnson holds a PhD in sociology with a major in aging–family and a minor in social psychology from Iowa State University. He is also a licensed marriage and family therapist. He is a retired Endowed Professor of Gerontology and Sociology from the University of Louisiana at Monroe. He has published widely in sociology, gerontology, and dementia. Currently he is an instructor in the Department of Applied Social Sciences at Stirling University in Scotland. He and his wife, Roxann, run a long-term care consulting agency, Aging Consultants Incorporated.

Edward L. King, RN, JD, EdD, is an attorney admitted to practice law in New York and Connecticut and is also a certified hospice and palliative care nurse. He teaches in the Allied Health Department–Nursing Unit at Hostos Community College, CUNY. His research interest is in the bioethical area concerning end-of-life care.

Patricia R. Loubeau, DrPH, has taught a variety of strategic planning and marketing courses at the undergraduate, graduate, and executive levels in the Marketing and International Business Department of the Hagan School of Business at Iona College, New Rochelle, New York. Prior to joining the faculty of Iona College, Professor Loubeau was a senior executive in hospital management in one of New York City's largest healthcare systems and has had operational responsibility for strategic planning and marketing in various settings.

Carol Molinari, PhD, is an associate professor of health systems management at the University of Baltimore. For more than three decades Dr. Molinari has worked as a healthcare educator, director, researcher, trustee, and consultant. Assessing cultural diversity and developing cultural competence are current areas of her pedagogy and research.

JoAnn Nolin, JD, RN, is an associate professor and chair of the Department of Public Health at the University of North Florida. She is a nurse attorney with extensive experience in the area of health facility and practitioner regulation. She teaches in the areas of health law and long-term care administration.

Judith Jopling Sayre, PhD, an adjunct professor at the University of North Florida, also is a research consultant and visiting scientist at the Mayo Medical School, Mayo Clinic Florida, where she serves on the hospice and palliative care team. She has taught classes and workshops on communication in healthcare to undergraduate and graduate students and to medical interns and residents. Her research interests focus on the specific communication needs of the elderly and patients and caregivers in end-of-life communication, including initiating the palliative care discussion and incorporating communication skills training into the medical school curriculum.

James Siberski, MS, CMC, is an assistant professor, coordinator of gerontological education, and director of geriatric care management at Misericordia University, Dallas, Pennsylvania. He is an affiliate member of the American Association for Geriatric Psychiatry and is certified in gerontology by the National Academy of Certified Care Managers. He is an editorial advisory board member of *Aging Well* magazine, a member of the National Association of Professional Geriatric Care Managers, and a prior member of the board of directors of the Greater PA Alzheimer's Association. He has multiple publications, lectures, and consults on geriatric/psychiatric/intellectual disability populations.

Robert Spinelli, DBA, is an assistant professor in the Department of Health Administration and Human Resources at the University of Scranton in Scranton, Pennsylvania. Dr. Spinelli serves as director of the undergraduate program in health administration and teaches courses in healthcare finance, administration, leadership, planning, and other health administration concentrations. He has been employed in the healthcare field all of his professional career and spent 26 years as a hospital/healthcare system CEO.

MAJ Lawanda D. Warthen, PhD, is a major in the United States Army, Medical Service Corps, and has worked as an administrative officer for 15 years. During her time in the service, she has been stationed in Korea, Kuwait, Germany, and Washington, DC. She is presently Commander of the Army Health Clinic–Kaiserslautern in Kaiserslautern, Germany. Her education includes a bachelor's in psychology from North Carolina Wesleyan, a master's in public administration with an emphasis on healthcare from Columbus State University, and a PhD in health services from Walden University.

G. Dale Welch has an MA and a PhD in sociology from Louisiana State University. Dr. Welch served as department head and taught half-time at the University of Louisiana, Monroe, for 33 years and taught full-time online for the last two years before retiring in 2008. Currently, he serves as education coordinator for the Louisiana Geriatrics Society, standing member of the Education Committee for the National Association of Long Term Care Administrator Boards (NAB), and accreditation site visitor for NAB. Dr. Welch was editor of the fifth edition of NAB's *Nursing Home Administrators' Examination Study Guide* (2009).

ABOUT THE EDITORS

Mary Helen McSweeney-Feld, PhD, is an associate professor in the Office of Collaborative Programs and a research associate in the Center for Productive Aging at Towson University in Towson, Maryland. A native of New York City, Dr. McSweeney-Feld earned a bachelor of arts in English and political science from Wellesley College, a master of philosophy in economics and master's in international affairs from Columbia University, and a doctorate in economics from the Graduate Center of the City University of New York. Prior to her academic career, Dr. McSweeney-Feld was a human resources director and economist for Equitable Life Assurance Society in New York City. She has numerous publications in the healthcare and human resources fields, with an emphasis in healthcare finance and long-term care issues. She has been involved in a variety of grant and demonstration programs for Alzheimer's disease and direct care worker issues and is a founding member of the Northeastern Pennsylvania End of Life Coalition sponsored by the Greater Pennsylvania Chapter of the Alzheimer's Association.

As an active member of the Association of University Programs in Health Administration, Dr. McSweeney-Feld has been the co-chair of the Long-Term Care Faculty Forum and a member of the Undergraduate Program Committee and has served on numerous self-study teams for AUPHA's undergraduate full membership certification. She is a member of the Education Committee of the National Association of Long Term Care Administrator Boards and a member of the Academy of Long Term Care Leadership and Development of the American College of Health Care Administrators.

Reid Oetjen, PhD, is an associate professor and program director for the University of Central Florida's graduate programs in health services administration in Orlando. Dr. Oetjen teaches courses at both the graduate and undergraduate levels in the Department of Health Management and Informatics. Dr. Oetjen focuses his teaching on long-term care administration, healthcare quality management, human resources management, leadership, and the aging of the population.

Dr. Oetjen has numerous peer-reviewed publications and regularly presents his research at academic and practitioner conferences. His research foci are long-term care quality, developing tools for healthcare practitioners, and the scholarship of teaching and learning. In addition to his academic experience, Dr. Oetjen served as an assistant administrator for a national skilled nursing facility chain and spent ten years as an operations manager for a major international airline.

Contents

Introduction

These papers emerged from a series of lectures given by the staff of the School of Hebrew, Biblical and Theological Studies at Trinity College, Dublin in the Spring of 1990. They are presented now to a wider audience because the lively discussion which they generated when first delivered suggests that the issues raised are ongoing and critical ones not only in Irish society today.

It is fair to say that the two constitutional referenda of the nineteen eighties had brought sharply into focus for thinking Irish people the tension between a personal moral stance and ethical norms imposed from outside and enshrined in law. Irrespective of which position one adopted on the questions being put to the people, one could not be unaware that there was abroad a new climate of opinion in which people sought to make up their own minds on serious issues of both private and public morality.

In a society such as Ireland where traditionally the church has played the role of guardian of faith and morals, the danger is that a vacuum is created once external authority, especially in morals, begins to collapse. Important and enduring human values can easily be lost sight of and a climate of hostility to any serious discussion of morality may quickly take over.

The fact is, as Vincent MacNamara points out in a pivotal paper in this collection, that moral questions arose as human questions before Christianity, and morality retains its independent structure today. Yet the Judaeo-Christian religious tradition has a strong ethical bent that sometimes has been able to speak in a very similar voice to that of secular human ethics (as in the natural law tradition) and sometimes (particularly since the Enlightenment) has found itself in opposition to what has been proposed in the name of human freedom. The task for a theologically grounded, yet critical ethics today, is not to reject as ungodly and immoral all secularist human values. Rather, as Werner Jeanrond stresses, it must enter into a public and serious debate that is both critical and self-critical, that is at once challenging the adequacy for all human life in this world of what is often proposed as good liberal humanism, while at the same time being challenged to examine its own theory and praxis in terms of both foundations and performance.

The Bible has always been regarded as a repository of human wisdom and insight as well as of religious belief. Its continued role in shaping the moral values of Western civilisation is sometimes lost sight of, because of its religious use in the churches. Andrew Mayes and Seán Freyne approach two of the main biblical witnesses to distinctive moral insights – Moses and Jesus – with a view to retrieving something of the originality and radical nature of their ethical visions, while keeping a particular eye on the contemporary situation also. The treatment of foundational questions is completed by Gabriel Daly, who examines the notion of moral failure within a religious context (sin), evaluates the role that conscience has in the making of moral choices and perceptively explores the most troublesome of all issues surrounding ethical and moral failure, namely that of guilt.

The danger with all ethical discussion is that it remains abstracted from the real life and death choices that face us all – the dangerous dichotomy between theory and praxis to which we are all so prone. The final four papers address practical issues of immediate concern for contemporary life. Katherine Zappone adopts a narrative approach in her efforts to raise consciousness about the special problems facing women and poverty by outlining one highly imaginative proposal for addressing the question of justice for all in our society. Kenneth Kearon sensitively lays out for us the ethical issues surrounding the beginning and end of life, especially in the light of modern scientific developments, and explains the different emphases on these questions within the main Christian churches. Denis Carroll's paper is a timely reminder that responsibility for the environment is a serious ethical obligation for Christians in the light of their own foundational stories. Finally, Terence McCaughey addresses the question of how a prophetic theology, faithful to the story of Jesus, could challenge both our political and religious institutions here – a challenge that we often seem reluctant to address.

These papers are not intended as answers, but as questions which all thinking people, religious and otherwise, should be interested in exploring further. Each paper is intended as a statement, rather than a finished argument, that invites others to probe further and ask other questions that we all need to address. It is only in the asking of serious questions about our present in the light of our past but with a view to creating a better future, that justice can begin to flower for all in our society and in our world.

Seán Freyne

CHAPTER 1

Theory and Praxis: A New Career for Ethics?

Werner G. Jeanrond

Everybody is talking about ethics nowadays. Ethics committees are set up in all ways of life. In the past few years the traditional professions, such as health workers, lawyers, museum people and trade unionists, have been discussing ethical principles and guidelines for their particular work. Our political representatives have established ethics committees, and more recently even the parliaments in the formerly communist-ruled countries of Central and Eastern Europe have formed ethics committees. What does this move towards ethics mean? Has the world turned ethical at last? What lies behind this breathtaking career of ethics in recent years?

But not only the different professional and political realms have cried out for more and better ethics, even the theologians claim of late that ethics is in fact their basic discipline because it alone connects the theological discourse with real life. In other words, ethical reflection gives a practical focus to this otherwise very theoretical discipline. Already in the middle of the last century Karl Marx had postulated that the goal of human reflection must not be to interpret reality but to change it. And so it seems that finally even the theologians have woken up to their ultimate vocation, namely not only to interpret God's will but to transform this world accordingly. And the heading under which they respond to their practical calling is 'ethics'. Ethics has to do with praxis, whereas theology so far often meant only theory. Ethics, so it seems then, is the magic word for the theology of the nineties and provides the key not only for a better world but also for a more relevant theology.

The nine essays in this book will explore critically and from different perspectives this new magic of ethics. In what follows I wish to examine first this new interest in ethics; in the second section of my essay I shall discuss some of the categories and methods of ethical thinking. Thirdly, I shall reflect upon the relationship between religion and ethics in general in order to prepare the ground for the more detailed discussion of Israelite and Christian ethics in subsequent essays. In my fourth and final section I shall discuss the new career of ethics in terms of the claim that it will solve the traditional conflict between theory and praxis in Christian theology.

1. The New Interest in Ethics

I think that the still increasing attention to ethical considerations in Western cultures has to do with at least two developments in European, Australian and Northern American societies. First, a vacuum of moral guidance has been experienced in these parts of the world, and secondly, there is an increasing suspicion against the ways in which the sciences have been operating, not only the natural sciences, but also the humanities. I would like to explain these two developments briefly. But before doing that I wish to define first of all what I understand by the term 'ethics'.

Generally speaking, 'ethics' means thinking about what is good and bad, about what is right and wrong, about what makes us happy and unhappy. More precisely, 'ethics' reflects upon the values, interests, motivations and norms which inform and direct our human activity. Thus, 'ethics' concerns not only the concrete nature of our human activity in this universe, but also the principles of human decision-making. In that sense there cannot be any non-ethical situation because every human activity is, consciously or unconsciously, informed, structured and guided by some motivations, interests, values and norms, and thus ethically determined, hence by either good or bad ethics.

In the past, at least in our part of the world, one spoke of 'morality' and of 'moral' or 'immoral' decisions, acts, structures and situations. But since the direct influence of religion in general and of Christianity in particular has begun to decrease in Europe due to the developments which we are going to consider in a moment, in the context of a general discussion, it appears to be more appropriate to speak of 'ethics' instead of 'morality', even though both terms overlap very significantly. However, for a great number of people 'morality' smells clerical and suggests a set of firm dogmatic convictions which are to tell us what is sinful or not. Thus, while the term morality is still used in inner-religious discourse, particularly within the Roman Catholic church, the term ethics is a more philosophical and religiously neutral term, and as such promises a better entry into the wider discussion about what is good and bad, right and wrong, and what makes us happy and unhappy.

May I stress once more that ethics concerns all aspects of human existence. More precisely, ethical thinking considers all aspects of human activity which are characterised by a choice.

For example, even such a trivial decision as the one whether or not to use the car on one's way to work is ethically significant, because it confronts the car-owner with a choice. Should he or she use the car and thus add to the level of dangerous smokes clouding the Dublin sky already, or should he or she use public transport and thus minimise the effect of human movement on the environment and so forth? What is better? How should we balance the goods, i.e. the good of public health and the good of private comfort? This example also demonstrates that not all of our decisions which have to be made in the course of our daily life are necessarily resulting from an explicit ethical reflection. But all decisions, even those which arise in our daily existence, can become the object of ethical reflection since every human decision is ethically significant.

One of the problems with regard to ethical thinking is that not everybody can afford to take a lot of time every morning or evening to consider carefully all the possible principles in order to come to a decision as to what is the best possible transport. Therefore, everybody needs some ethical guidelines or an ethical system which allows him or her to make quicker decisions in everyday domestic, professional and political circumstances.

In past centuries, especially in Europe, Christianity and Judaism provided such systems of ethics. These religions have offered the foundations for particular ethical decisions which has made it relatively easy for the members of such religious traditions to know in a given situation how best to act, what best to decide for and against. But as I have indicated already, these religions have lost some of their attraction so that many people today do not avail any longer of explicitly religious principles in order to structure their world and develop ethical strategies. The medieval consensus in ethical matters supported and facilitated by a detailed canon law has long broken down. Decisions are now based more on individual insight than on moral laws handed down from above.

Nevertheless, we all search for ethical principles which can direct our lives and free us from the impossible task of balancing all aspects of a decision every time we are making a choice. Before we discuss how we may develop such principles for decision-making in our modern – or if you prefer 'post-modern' – context we ought to look briefly at the reasons which have caused the new confusion in contemporary ethical thinking.

The Protestant Reformation in the sixteenth century and the resulting religious discord on the one hand and the Enlightenment since the eighteenth century on the other hand have radically changed the traditional foundations of ethics not only here in Western Europe. The immediate consequence of the Reformation was that there was no longer only one church in the West that claimed to provide authentic guidance to its followers, but two. Moreover, the religious ethos of the Protestant church differed from the traditional Catholic ethos, insofar as it concentrated much more on the direct experience of the individual believer with his or her God while the Catholic ethos continued to emphasise the role of the individual within the boundaries of the church and of those states which were sanctioned by the church. Not enough that there were now two Christian institutions with somewhat different individual and social orientations, the emerging Enlightenment challenged the absolute claims of both of these and of any other religious institution by demanding that every human being was called to live his or her own life by following his or her own best insights into morality.

The philosopher Immanuel Kant provided the most famous formulation of this new foundation of human morality in his book *Foundations of the Metaphysic of Morals* (1785). Here he formulated his well-known categorical imperative: You ought to act in such a way that the maxim of your own action could well become the maxim of everybody's action. In other words, morality was now based primarily on the considered and self-critical action of the individual. The individual was to remain the focus of ethical reflection for quite some time. And the subsequent theories of the state or of society including those provided by the French revolutionaries as well as by Marx and Engels, and those discussed by contemporary social theorists, such as Jürgen Habermas, are all based primarily on the rights of the individual. The declaration of Human Rights (1789), whose bicentenary we have just celebrated and to which all the recent revolutions in Central and Eastern Europe have appealed so forcefully, this declaration documents most strongly the change in the focus of ethical thinking since the Enlightenment.

Parallel to the emergence of the individual as the ultimate focus of ethical thinking, we can observe a growing belief in the scientific progress as guarantor of the individual's existence in this world. That means, since the nineteenth, but especially in the twentieth century, for many people the belief in science and its development has replaced the traditional order of life and decision-making which in the past had been provided mainly by religious systems. However, as we know today, although on the whole our daily life has been made much easier as a result of scientific progress, our ethical situation has not been made easier at all. Instead it has become much more complex: new ethical dilemmas have arisen, such as, for example, the need to know if and when to switch off a machine which is capable of prolonging human life beyond the traditional point of death; or the question whether or not to attend to an AIDS-victim given the danger of becoming infected oneself while helping such a person. Questions of the actual extension, of the value and quality of life, old life, injured life, unborn life, handicapped life etc. have arisen and complicated the ordinary daily business not only of the health worker. On a more global level, many of us experience the distribution of wealth in this world as problematic, and we search for ways of transforming this unjust situation for the better.

In trying to cope with all of these questions which concern ethical awareness and knowledge, we are faced with decisions which previous generations have not known, yet unlike previous generations we no longer recognise the traditional ordering factors and systems which had promised to guide human decision-making. The price both of the newly-won freedom of the individual since the Enlightenment on the one hand, and of the scientific progress on the other hand is a much more delicate and complex ethical situation which calls for a continuous and critical process of reflection on ethical principles. As far as I see there are only two options: either we give up our personal freedom and adopt any antiquated moral system which pretends to know answers for every conceivable situation, or we enter into the ongoing and laborious discussion on ethical principles. The first option has been tried by a number of fundamentalist movements in different cultures, the second option includes the demand that the culture be based on the acknowledgement of human rights and enlightened critical and self-critical thinking.

This is the situation in which all forms of ethical thinking including Christian ethics must be developed today. Thus, no approach to ethics which deserves to be called critical can escape from participating in the public discussion of ethical principles. Of course, such a willingness to participate must not be misunderstood as a readiness to agree with everything proposed in such a wider public dialogue on ethical principles. Rather this wider dialogue lives from the critical participation of different ethical approaches, of adequate principles, categories and methods of ethical thinking. What are categories and methods of ethical thinking?

2. Categories and Methods of Ethical Thinking
In order to develop any principle for appropriate decision-making it is first of all necessary to consider those categories which condition ethical thinking in a particular culture. Secondly, those philosophical methods of ethical reflection need to be discussed critically which have emerged in recent centuries and which claim to offer an adequate procedure of ethical thinking. Assuming here that a phenomenon such as a 'European culture' exists, I shall now attempt to list some of the major categories which have an impact on decision-making in this European culture.

1) In Europe there is a consensus on the need to respect, protect and sustain *human life* and to improve its quality as much as possible. However, questions of the boundaries and the quality of human life are discussed in often different ways.

2) This respect for human life finds expression not only in the recognition of the *individual person* but also in a strife to enhance the *common good*. Although in Europe there is a radical plurality of opinions as to what constitutes the common good, no European culture would deny that the common good represents a necessary category in decision-making.

3) Every decision must arrive at some kind of a *balance between its individual and its social aspects*.

4) In all European societies we find legal codes which attempt to order the relationship between individual citizens on the one hand and between the individual and the state on the other hand. Ethical reflection has to respect these codes, but such respect must include

the possibility of a *critical discourse* on such codes in order to review the actual ethical foundation of these codes.

5) Such a critical discourse must also respect the *conscience of the individual*. But in turn, the development of individual conscience must respect the challenge presented by such critical discourse.

6) Both the individual conscience and the ethical discourse in a culture are informed to some extent by existing ethical systems, such as are provided by *religious faiths and non-religious humanist worldviews*.

7) Thus, in every European culture we encounter a *principle of tradition* in ethical thinking and a *set of ethical authorities*. These authorities may be persons, texts or institutions. For an example of such a personal ethical authority you may think of the late Ayatollah Khomeini in Iran; for an example of a textual authority you may recall the power which the Roman Catechism used to exert in Roman Catholic families; for examples of institutional authority you may think of the churches and their officers, of the socialist or communist parties in some European countries, or of the Red Cross organisation. Of course, such authorities can increase or lose their ethical authority. As we all know, the churches are currently battling to stabilise or regain their ethical authority, as do with much less success at this point in time the communist parties in most European countries.

When we look at this list of categories which are operative in every act of decision-making and which therefore are themselves objects of ethical reflection, we must conclude that there is not one such category which could claim to be on top of a possible hierarchy of ethical categories. Even the emphasis on critical and self-critical discourse would be meaningless without the presence of traditional ethical systems which are always in need of being reviewed critically. Thus, instead of organising some form of a hierarchy of ethical categories we ought to recognise their mutual interdependence. That, however, means that we always have to reckon with the complex nature of any human search for ethical principles and we need to reject any mono-causal ethics which has derived all ethical principles from only one of these categories.

For example, if we accept some form of an enlightened paradigm of ethical thinking as I am advocating here, then we must reject any ethical system which is built exclusively on the rights of only one section of a society and which has no regard for the common good. We must also reject the claims of any ethical system that attempts to speak for all without allowing the participation of all in its development. An example for the latter would be the introduction of a particular religious system of values and norms into an entire society even though only a section of that society was actively supporting this religious system. Another form of ethical reflection must be rejected, namely that kind of reflection which is undertaken by an elite in strictly private discourse, even by an academic or clerical elite. As soon as ethical discourse is not open to the entire public it is in danger of becoming sectarian and thus finally tyrannical.

I have so far discussed the human need for ethical principles and the complexity of ethical categories. Now I would like to move on to a brief reflection on some of the different ways of ethical thinking in the West which have been proposed and established since philosophers in ancient Greece have triggered off the sort of ethical discussion which concerns us in these essays. May I just list some of these classical approaches and comment on their viability for us today.

It has become a general custom to distinguish between an ethics which looks at the end and/or consequences of actions themselves and an ethics which tries to follow a particular code of do's and don'ts. The first ethics is called *teleological* (referring to the Greek word 'telos' for goal), and the second ethics is called *deontic* or *deontological* (referring to the particular concepts of what ought to be done in order to lead a happy life). In this sense the tradition of grounding an ethics on 'natural law' is teleological insofar as it wishes to make decisions on the basis of what constitutes an end in nature, and deontological insofar as it claims also to know exactly what nature is and what it demands. Two further approaches to ethics which are related to the two already mentioned need to be named here: the *utilitarian* ethics and the ethics aiming at the consensus within an enquiring community, i.e. the *ethics by argumentation or discourse*. A utilitarian ethics is interested in creating the greatest possible happiness of an individual or a particular group of people, while an ethics based on rational argumentation aims at creating a consensus among all those who participate in the particular ethical discourse. Thus, ethics by argumentation is a modern version of deontological ethics: it too wishes to follow the canon of generally accepted values and norms, whereas utilitarian ethics is basically another version of teleological ethics because it is motivated by the pursuit of the good of an individual or a particular group.

How should we relate to these four options in ethical reflection? First of all, we must realise that these approaches do not exclude one another, rather they represent different ways of dealing with the same problem, namely the problem of decision-making. Moreover, we can see that the ancient need for ethical orientation – or, if you prefer, moral guidance – is taken seriously in the modern version of deontological ethics, namely in the effort of grounding ethical decisions in a mutually critical conversation rather than in a canon of doctrines. But there is no guarantee that the democratic form of arriving at an ethical consensus through open and unrepressed discourse will always be able to reveal what is ultimately good and therefore ought to be done or what is ultimately bad and therefore ought to be avoided. Similarly, no form of teleological ethics or of utilitarian ethics can ever define once and for all what is the good or the bad inherent in an action or situation. Such decisions are always conditioned by a whole network of presuppositions, interests and interpretations of our reality.

Examples which can illustrate our human dilemma of establishing the right way for making decisions are found very easily. Take for instance the Roman Catholic prohibition of all means of birth control. That is a prohibition based on a particular version of deontological ethics. A system of doctrines which has been portrayed to be always right yields the moral norm: you shall never use condoms etc. What is not considered in such an ethical system is the consequence of such a norm. Over against such a purely deontological foundation, a teleologically based ethics would look at the effects which arise from the act of birth control: will there be no more children so as to endanger the human species or will there be fewer children so as to make life on this earth possible for all who are living on it instead of allowing the current trend of overcrowding to continue etc. Thus, while deontological ethics can be accused of neglecting the consequences arising from its ethical demands, teleological ethics can be accused of neglecting the question of the essence of things and actions, i.e. whether or not birth control or something else is right or wrong in itself.

This analysis of only one ethical dilemma demonstrates already that every ethically conscious decision is drawn between on the one hand the need to reflect on the nature of the goods about which one decides and on the other hand the need to consider the consequences which arise from such a decision.

Ethics in the natural sciences, insofar as it has existed as a conscious activity at all until now, was usually teleological, that means it operated on the basis of looking at the likely effect of a certain action, let us say of a particular scientific experiment. The unreflected law was that whatever could be made should be made or ought at least to be tried. This insufficient level of ethical awareness, however, has led the natural sciences into deep crisis and confusion, as soon namely as people questioned the acceptability of certain consequences and wanted to know the criteria which would justify the acceptance of certain consequences of scientific actions over against others.

For example, the question of nuclear energy: very few people would wish to question the legitimacy of a radiological examination as part of a medical check-up. But particularly since the accident at Chernobyl, many people have questioned the legitimacy of a nuclear power station because they weigh the risk arising from such a station to human life higher than the benefit of cheaper electricity. This example shows that as long as a basic core of human values is not put into question, we seem quite prepared to argue teleologically, but as soon as human life is one of the goods to be considered in competition with other goods (such as economical benefit) we are becoming suspicious of teleological procedures and wish to resort to normative value structures, which means we wish to define our ethical principles in a deontological way.

In this context it is interesting to observe that many religious and ideological systems have, at particular occasions, ranked human life lower than a supposedly important common good and thus at times accepted the lethal result of military actions to human life. These are instances where deontological approaches were overrun by purely teleological concerns.

These examples have clarified sufficiently that there is no single approach to ethics which one could recommend without important qualifications. Moreover, I hope to have demonstrated that ethical consideration is one way of facing up both to the general uncertainty of human life and to reflecting on the purpose of human existence. There are no absolute methods, rules or norms which one could *always* trust and follow. However, this insight does not mean that one should abandon the search for such absolutes. It seems to me that the mystery of our human existence demands such a search, but our human freedom refuses to accept absolute answers. Some may regret this paradox; I for my part welcome it and like it, because it safeguards that we keep on seeking for better insights into the mystery of this universe and of our human existence in it and, at the same time, remain open to learn from each other's tentative answers and approaches without surrendering our critical faculties. As soon as we stop being critical we will become victims of other people's theories and actions. As soon as we stop searching for ethical absolutes we will limit ourselves to the level of mere sceptics who nevertheless have to live and thus will be dominated eventually by norms and rules which they can no longer influence. Again, the option is either to participate in the ongoing ethical reflection or to be dominated by it.

3. Religion and Ethics

Today there is a debate among philosophers on the question whether one should engage in a formal and theoretical discussion of ethics or rather concentrate on interpreting the actual relationships between individual human beings and their natural and social environment. But there can be no debate about the point that whatever way one follows one will encounter the influence of religion. Already in so-called primitive cultures we can observe the ordering function of religion. These 'primitive people' divided their world into sacred and profane spheres and thus established a first principle of order which was able to provide guidance for people seeking the right or good life. On reflection, our situation today reveals the same basic structure, even though the particular mode of defining what counts as sacred or profane has changed. But the need for a basic principle of orientation in the midst of a confusing universe has remained stable throughout the history of culture. Depending on one's particular definition of what counts as 'religion' one may conclude either that all human beings are by nature religious, or that in a post-religious culture one can detect at least some pseudo-religious phenomena. Rituals, cults, myths and sacred texts can be identified in all human cultures. They function as signals of our human purpose and also as basic guides through the confusions which arise both from our individual development and from our place in the natural and social dimensions of our cosmos. Not all of these religious or related systems of orientation include an element of transcendence beyond the visible spheres of our lives, as for instance Christianity, Judaism, Islam and various Hindu religions do. But even Buddhism and the different strands of Marxist ideology which do not recognise the presence of a God do acknowledge the need to think beyond the requirements of only the individual human being. For them as for the theistic religious traditions some kind of balance must be achieved between individual hope or strive for personal salvation on the one hand and the perfecting of human society as a whole on the other hand.

In Europe today we encounter a serious challenge to our particular ethical traditions, namely the phenomenon of an increasingly pluricultural or multi-cultural society in which different religions, world-views and ideological systems are informing their respective following. This phenomenon leads to the question how a society can arrive at a consensus on ethical principles at all given the conflicting claims about ethical categories, categories such as the nature of human life, the nature of nature, the limits of scientific research, the understanding of education, the balance between individual life and the welfare of the community, and the understanding of the state and of its laws as either secular or theocratic in nature. In view of this conflict of basic orientations about the status and ranking of the different ethical categories it will always be difficult to determine what shall count as right or wrong in a given European society or in an integrated Europe. Therefore it would appear to be naïve to say that we do not need some kind of explicit discussion on ethics. Rather it seems to me that such an explicit and public discussion of ethical principles, categories and approaches is needed more than ever so as to help us to become better aware of the particularities of ethical convictions and to focus more sharply on the requirements of a viable consensus in these matters.

This all too brief general hint at the impact of religious systems or other systems of meaning on human thinking and acting will at least serve to emphasise that every ethical consideration in a future Europe will always be embedded in such a context of religious and humanist world-views. The aim of a critical approach to ethics must be, therefore, first of all to recognise the particular religious or ideological context, and secondly to review it critically. And that is precisely what this series of essays wishes to achieve with particular respect to the Jewish-Christian religious traditions. Such a critical examination, however, will itself be influenced by some kind of religious or ideological presupposition. We can never reach a neutral vantage-point from which we could review our action and thought. We can only try to gain insight into the network of aspects which determine our thinking and doing, and then establish criteria for decision-making in the future and for an assessment of our human decision-making in the past.

4. Ethics and the Theory-Praxis-Dilemma in Theology

The significance of ethical reflection for our life is beyond question. What has to be questioned, however, in the light of our considerations here, is the hope that ethics will offer a quasi-magical solution to one perennial problem of theology, namely its distance from practical concerns of human life. As we have seen ethics itself is first and foremost a theory, ethical reflection is theoretical by nature. But it is a theoretical reflection which is moved by concrete human situations, problems and dilemmas. As such it has an eminently practical focus. Theological ethics responds critically to our practical needs, at least good ethics ought to do so. But the actual response to our concrete needs must not be dictated by these needs alone, rather the critical reflection upon these needs ought to happen in the wider search for adequate approaches to life in this universe.

That brings us back to the problem mentioned earlier in this essay when I referred to the necessity of searching for ethical absolutes without ever being satisfied with any particular answer. With regard to Christian ethics that means that we theologians have to interpret again and again both the Jewish-Christian tradition and all aspects of the universe in which we live in order to search for more adequate general approaches to the problems of our life. In other words, theological ethics acknowledges the basic human need for orientation in this universe and considers this need within the context of the wisdom of our particular religious tradition. This wisdom might not only enlighten or even alter our understanding of our particular human needs, but it might also help us to reassess our overall approach to our life and to our life's context. In this sense, the theoretical nature of our theological reflection on ethics represents a major opportunity for us to see our human needs in a much wider horizon and then possibly arrive at a response to our needs which may be far more intriguing and rewarding than any answer suggested directly by whatever might appear to us as required by a specific situation.

Take for example the use of force to combat violence in our society. The recent increase in armed robberies in Ireland has demonstrated the acuteness of this ethical dilemma. What contribution could a theological voice make to the public ethical discourse on this topic in our society? Following our immediate needs and instincts we may demand that any kind of force necessary should be used to free our society from criminal threats. Following a purely deonto-logical model we could state that life is sacred; therefore nobody should use the force of a gun against any human being. Following a purely teleological model we could state: it is better to eliminate the few criminals in our society and thus achieve a good end through the regrettable use of force. However, a Christian reflection on this problem would first of all point to the universal love of God for all human beings as the context in which we ought to consider pos-sible moves to protect the lives of all members of our society. On this principal basis, however, we would need to enter into a discussion of circumstances and strategies which would allow us to qualify this general respect for the God-given life. But whatever answer we may come to in weighing particular circumstances, as Christians we should never be forgetful of the God-given dignity of all human life. That is not to say that an armed police force was out of the question according to Christian wisdom. But it is to say that from a Christian perspective one would need to lobby for the general respect of all human life in the public ethical discussion, including the life of the potential or actual criminal.

5. Conclusion

Let us, then, welcome the recent increase in ethical reflection. It has helped us to focus more sharply on the complexity of the process of decision-making, but also on the wisdom given to us through our religious traditions which we ought to explore more fully. It has also helped to show us that we must overcome any purely one-sided approach to human decision-making. Instead we all ought to participate in the development of yet more adequate principles of decision-making. But the development of such principles does not free us from the act of decision-making itself. No ethical principle will ever be able to address all the dimensions of a specific human situation. The task of applying ethical principles is ours alone in our concrete circumstances. Of course, we may enlighten and support one another in our decision-making and in our acting, and we may accept the guidance of religious traditions in this process, but we should never take away from anybody the freedom and at the same time the burden of deciding for herself or himself.

It was the German Reformer Martin Luther who reminded us that our faith does provide us with general guidelines, that is with principles for our human praxis, but not with automatic answers to all situations. Instead Luther urged that on the basis of our Christian faith we should participate even in the most difficult process of human decision-making while constantly praying to God for enlightenment, wisdom and forgiveness. It is this risky participation which makes us experience the sweet and the bitter taste of human freedom: we are free to decide, but ultimately we are always insecure and vulnerable when we make decisions. Luther saw clearly that religious faith is no substitute for ethical reflection, but provides a foundation for such reflection. Similarly, ethical reflection is no substitute for ethical action, but it may provide good principles for human praxis.

[In this essay I have incorporated an edited version of some parts of a paper which I delivered at the Fifteenth Annual Meeting of the Association for Dental Education in Europe (ADEE) in Brussels, Belgium, in September 1989, and which appeared in Proceedings of the Fifteenth Annual Meeting of the Association For Dental Education in Europe. *79-92. Brussels: Dental Institute, Vrije Universiteit Brussel, 1990.]*

Further Reading

Alasdair MacIntyre, *A Short History of Ethics*, New York: Collier Books, 1966.

David Tracy, *Plurality and Ambiguity: Hermeneutics, Religion, Hope*, London: SCM, 1988.

A New Dictionary of Christian Ethics, eds, John Macquarrie and James Childress, London: SCM, 1986. [*Reference work*]

CHAPTER 2

The Decalogue of Moses:
An Enduring Ethical Programme?

A.D.H. Mayes

The liturgy for the baptism of children in the Anglican tradition includes this charge to the godparents of the newly baptised child: 'You are to take care that this child be brought to the bishop to be confirmed by him so soon as he can say the creed, the Lord's prayer and the ten commandments, and be further instructed in the church catechism set forth for that purpose.' The presupposed function of the ten commandments in this context is clearly that of the definition of the Christian life, a function which has a long history in Christian tradition. On the other hand, the ten commandments also appear in the Anglican tradition in the order for the Administration of the Lord's Supper or Holy Communion with a different function. Near the beginning of that service there is provision for the recitation of each commandment by the celebrant, following which the people respond 'Lord, have mercy upon us, and incline our hearts to keep this law.' Here there is perhaps reflected that especially strong tradition in the church that the law performs the negative function of revealing sin.

Both of these functions of the law, and indeed perhaps of the decalogue in particular, are to be traced back into the New Testament. The response of Jesus to the rich man who asked him 'What must I do to inherit eternal life?' was in the first instance 'You know the commandments: do not kill, do not commit adultery, do not steal, do not bear false witness, do not defraud, honour your father and mother' (Mark 10:19); the rich man's continuing dissatisfaction, reflected in his protest 'Teacher, all these I have observed from my youth', may indicate that it was only in its negative function that the decalogue had meaning for him. Certainly, for Paul the decalogue, with the other Old Testament law, performed that negative function of producing a sense of sin and guilt (Rom 1:29-31), although even for Paul within the context of faith in Christ the decalogue has a positive function: 'the commandments, you shall not commit adultery, you shall not kill, you shall not steal, you shall not covet, and any other commandment, are summed up in this sentence "You shall love your neighbour as yourself"' (Rom 13:9).

Whether negatively or positively understood, the decalogue has had a fundamental significance, a significance which, of course, is highlighted in different ways within the Hebrew Bible itself. It stands at the very foundation of Israel at Sinai; it is not directed to any special group, priests, judges, or whatever, but to the whole undifferentiated people of God; it is the direct and unmediated communication of God himself to Israel while the rest of the law is mediated through Moses; it is given its own special name 'the ten words'; it is repeated in Ex 20 and Deut 5.

Despite this fundamental significance, however, it is perhaps the case that the decalogue no longer has that centrality and foundational significance with which the tradition invests it. It maintains at least a formal place in the liturgy, but it is rarely, if ever, recited; insofar as people still have a knowledge of it, it is more a knowledge of the idea of it than of the decalogue itself; within the framework of a general discouragement of learning by rote the decalogue, like much else in religious tradition, has perhaps been marginalised to the edge of consciousness; within the context of a general distrust and suspicion of all authority as more or less arbitrary restraint on individual freedom, the decalogue is seen, like the Bible as a whole, as just another authority, our relationship with which is highly problematic.

Our task, then, seems to be a dual one: on the one hand, to seek out the ground and nature of the central significance which the decalogue has traditionally enjoyed; on the other hand, to ask with what continuing significance we may regard it. I think that these questions are by no means unrelated, and even if as a biblical scholar of a historical sort I concentrate on the first aspect of our task, the understanding of the decalogue to which that may lead us has, I believe, something to say in response to the question that defines the second aspect of our task.

II

In our consideration of the decalogue I would like to start with a brief discussion of some general formal issues, then to move on to some general questions of substance, before focusing in on more particular issues associated with the decalogue. Our formal considerations relate first to the decalogue as a series of ten commandments, and, secondly, to the way in which these commandments are brought to expression.

Everybody used to know the ten commandments; at least, those of us brought up by the traditional rote learning methods knew the ten commandments. Or did we? The fact of the matter is that the ten commandments are not the same for everyone. This apparently single collection of ten commandments bearing the title, the decalogue, comprises slightly but significantly different content for different religious traditions. The Hebrew Bible speaks of ten 'words', rather than commandments, and it finds one 'word' in the following: 'You shall have no other gods before me. You shall not make yourself a graven image, or any likeness of anything that is in heaven above, or that is in the earth beneath or that is in the water under the earth; you shall not bow down to them or serve them.' This is followed also by the Catholic and Lutheran religious traditions, but not by the Reformed tradition. According to the latter there are two commandments here: 'You shall have no other gods before me', and 'You shall not make yourself a graven image', and these are in fact reckoned as the first two commandments of the decalogue. The Hebrew Bible takes as its first 'word' 'I am the Lord your God who brought you out of the land of Egypt, out of the house of bondage'; the Catholic and Lutheran traditions, on the other hand, maintain the number ten for the total by finding two commandments in 'You shall not covet your neighbour's house; you shall not covet your neighbour's wife, or his manservant or his maidservant, or his ox, or his ass, or anything that is your neighbour's'; all of this, on the other hand, is taken as one 'word' in the Hebrew Bible and as one commandment in the Reformed tradition.

All of this seems a bit nit-picking, and perhaps we should not make too much of it; in any case, surely it is quite unrelated to what is certainly the really significant thing: the decalogue is a fundamental rule of life understood to have divine origin. In one way or another surely the same substance is there whatever esoteric differences there might be in the organisation of it. In fact, however, these formal points do suggest an important consideration of substance: the decalogue is not a fixed entity, a clearly defined text, but is rather something more fluid. We cannot simply take the decalogue for granted, as something known, and then go on to discuss the question of its meaning and application; rather, the questions of meaning, understanding and application belong right at the heart of the decalogue, right at the point of the very definition of the decalogue, and are not secondary questions which we bring to it as to a given accepted entity.

Maybe I exaggerate the problem, for surely there is a decalogue, a fixed single entity, a quite definite text, and the differences I have been speaking of are themselves secondary differences, differences in the way in which this once-fixed text has been interpreted and transmitted in the various religious traditions. It is, however, more complicated than that. The term 'ten commandments', or, to use the terminology of the Hebrew Bible, 'ten words', is not used in Ex 20 where the decalogue first appears; rather, this chapter refers simply to 'all these words'. The term 'ten words' first appears in Ex 34:28 (where it is used in relation to a quite different collection of commandments) and then next, with reference to our more familiar decalogue, in Deut 4:13; 10:4. In fact, the term 'ten commandments' or 'ten words' never appears in immediate connection with the decalogue, but belongs rather in secondary contexts which make reference to this collection of commandments. If we relate this to the difficulty there most evidently is in finding here ten words or commandments then the conclusion to which we seem to be pointed is that the use of the term 'ten words' appears to be an attempt to impose order and uniformity on what was essentially a much more fluid and unstable collection which could be looked at in different ways. It seems almost to be an attempt to bring canonical order to what was by origin and nature much less fixed and determined. It represents an attempt to create a recognisable and memorable statement by imposing order on existing material which was essentially much less ordered and defined. There is, if you like, a process of finding meaning and order going on right at the heart of the decalogue. The decalogue is a statement of meaning, almost a statement of intention, rather than an immediately clearly defined set of regulations.

This seems almost to undermine or contradict what we understand by the term commandment. Surely this, of all forms of speech, must embody clarity and precision, and yet just this quality seems to be questioned by the uncertainty over what is meant by the decalogue. This brings me to the second aspect of our formal considerations, the way in which these commandments are brought to expression, for it seems to me that the customary use of the term commandments itself introduces implications which are not necessarily present.

Even a superficial perusal of those parts of Exodus and Deuteronomy which contain laws will reveal the variety of forms of expression which these laws use. Here are two of these. Ex 21:18-19 reads: 'When men quarrel and one strikes the other with a stone or with his fist and the man does not die but keeps his bed, then if the man rises again and walks abroad with his staff, he that struck him shall be clear; only he shall pay for the loss of his time and shall have him thoroughly healed'; Ex 23:9 reads: 'You shall not oppress a stranger; you know the heart of a stranger, for you were strangers in the land of Egypt.' On the one hand, there is a law which in an impersonal way describes a particular case in some detail and then prescribes an appropriate punishment. This is case law and we can understand how it could well have been used in the administration of justice in the concrete conditions of daily life in ancient Israel; collections of such laws would have constituted the precedents by which order and uniformity would have been brought to judicial administration. On the other hand, however, there is a prohibition which is direct and personal; it gives no detailed description of a case and it does not prescribe any punishment. Indeed, whereas in the first instance an offence is presupposed as having been committed and a punishment is then provided for it, in the second instance no offence is presupposed as having been committed. This is a prohibition directed to future behaviour rather than a law which attempts to deal with past behaviour.

The decalogue clearly belongs with the type of the prohibition rather than the type of case law. Even in the case of those two commandments which have a positive formulation rather than a negative ('Remember the Sabbath day to keep it holy', and 'Honour your father and your mother'), the address is still direct and future oriented and no punishment is prescribed. There is in the decalogue no case law; there is no precedent here on which a judge in a court situation could rely. Not only is no punishment prescribed for any breach of the prohibition, but the prohibition is expressed in such general and all inclusive terms as to be virtually useless in the concrete circumstances of any given situation. 'You shall not kill': does this include the slaughter of animals; does it apply in a situation of war; does it have any relevance to capital punishment? These prohibitions and commands are not laws; they give expression to the most general directions for life in the context of one person instructing another.

Our formal considerations thus lead to the conclusion that the decalogue is teaching rather than law, into which a certain order and uniformity has been brought by the attempt to mark out ten words or ten commandments in this teaching.

III

Let us try to lead this on a little further by gradually introducing issues relating more to the general substance of this teaching. We cannot immediately terminate our more formal considerations, however, for these are inextricably connected with the questions of substance. Formally, the decalogue commandments have been seen to be teaching rather than law, instruction appropriate to a setting different from the law court situation to which case law belongs. What is this setting for the teaching of the decalogue?

The Old Testament context within which the decalogue is set is that of God proclaiming the law of the covenant on Mount Sinai. The decalogue is the only part of this law that is given directly by God to Israel. Insofar as the decalogue contains direct, personal prohibitions and commands, it is presupposed that God is the speaker and Israel is the addressee, and this, indeed, has sometimes been considered to be the explanation of this particular expression of Israel's law. The direct form of address presupposes a speaking authority and an immediate addressee; so the setting of the decalogue, and indeed of all direct prohibitions and commands in the Old Testament, was always that of God addressing Israel and declaring the terms of his covenant with his people. 'You shall have no other gods before me' could never have been uttered in any other context than that of God addressing his people and declaring to them the terms of his covenant relationship with them. This form of law has, therefore, a religious context of origin: it originated in and belongs to a religious festival of covenant making and covenant renewal in the course of which the decalogue was proclaimed by a priest uttering the direct word of God to the assembled people.

This understanding of the decalogue is correct so far as it goes, but it seems to me that a lot more can be said which can lead to a better appreciation of the nature of the decalogue. In the first place, while the decalogue as such may always have been presented as the direct speech of God, this is not true of all the commands and prohibitions of the Old Testament which have the direct form of address. In other words, as a form of speech, the commands and prohibitions are not necessarily rooted in this religious context. A closely analogous form is to be found in the book of Proverbs, as in Prov 22:22ff: 'Do not rob the poor ... make no friendship with a man given to anger ... remove not the ancient landmark', and here the setting is explicitly that of the father instructing his son or the wise man his pupil. This more secular setting of instruction is presupposed also in Jer 35:6ff. Here, we read, the conservative clan of the Rechabites lived according to the teaching of their ancestor Jonadab, who prescribed: 'You shall not drink wine, neither you nor your sons for ever; you shall not build a house; you shall not sow seed; you shall not plant or have a vineyard.' This last context of use is particularly significant for it clearly suggests a setting for this form of instruction which is old and original, viz. that of the clan elder instructing his followers, or those being initiated into the way of life he represented. The speaking authority which the form presupposes is that of the clan elder with the whole weight of clan tradition behind him; those addressed are the members of the clan, those responsible for the maintenance and transmission of that way of life. The instruction comprises the basic principles, the fundamental truths, which have traditionally defined and constituted that way of life.

Now this suggests a much more comprehensive framework within which to examine the decalogue once more. The form in which the decalogue is expressed is the form used in order to express the fundamental principles which traditionally characterise a particular life context. Thus, it is the form used for the clan ethic of the Rechabites; it is also the form used in a series of prohibitions in Ex 23:1-3, 6-9 'You shall not utter a false report; you shall not follow a multitude to do evil; you shall not be partial to a poor man in his suit; you shall not pervert the justice due to the poor; you shall take no bribe; you shall not oppress a stranger', all of which are related to the administration of justice and constitute a kind of *vade mecum* for judges. The basic purpose behind these prohibitions is to make explicit the constitutional rules of conduct, the limiting principles,

within the framework of which the one who adheres to the life context addressed by these principles is to work out his way of living.
The teaching enshrined in these principles does not cover every issue; it sets the external limits, the boundaries beyond which one
may not pass and still remain a member of the particular community
addressed by that teaching.

One cannot set the decalogue apart from considerations such as
these and simply claim it as the word of God to Israel. At the very
least, it uses human speech forms, and, moreover, human speech
forms which carry over with them into the decalogue context quite
particular implications. But the connection between the decalogue
and those other uses of prohibitions and commands is even closer
than that suggests, for it is clear that the decalogue cannot be understood independently simply as the original and founding word
of God to Israel. It is not consistently formulated as the word of
God; rather, it speaks of God in the third person in three commandments ('You shall not take the name of the Lord your God in vain';
'the seventh day is a Sabbath to the Lord your God'; 'Honour your
father and your mother, that your days may be long in the land
which the Lord your God gives you'), and so presupposes a setting
other than one in which God himself is speaker. What this suggests
is that the decalogue is a mixed composition in which existing
speech forms, existing commands and prohibitions, have been sec-
ondarily brought together into a collection. Many of these commands and prohibitions already existed before they were brought
into this decalogue context.

Like the commands and prohibitions in general, so also the decalogue seeks to formulate a set of basic principles, a constitution,
within the framework of which those addressed by it must live. Unlike many of these other commands and prohibitions, however, the
decalogue is not addressed to a specific group, Rechabites, judges
or whatever; rather, it is addressed to a total community which
may comprise all of these or none of these.

The community addressed by the decalogue is defined neither by
socio-economic life-style, like the Rechabites, nor by professional
occupation, like the judges; it is a community defined by its common adherence to 'the Lord your God who brought you out of the
land of Egypt' and by its adherence to a principle of respect for the

integrity of the other which is understood to flow from that; it is a community which finds its unity not on the basis of particular common social, economic or professional interests, but on the basis of a unity of faith which both transcends and also holds in check the ultimately selfish divisions characteristic of social, economic and professional life.

IV

Our general considerations relating to the form and substance of the decalogue have led to the following conclusions: that the decalogue is teaching rather than law; that the notion of ten specific commandments may be a secondary attempt to bring clarity and order to a more fluid collection; that the decalogue in the wider context of commands and prohibitions expresses the fundamental and traditional rules of life in community, defining its boundaries; and that the community addressed by the decalogue is one that is not restricted by social, economic and professional interests. Now, let us turn our attention finally to the decalogue much more specifically with some quite definite historical, literary and religious questions in mind. There are two concluding issues which I wish to discuss: first, the general context of origin of the decalogue and what this means for our understanding of it; and, secondly, the ongoing significance of the decalogue.

The decalogue is presented to us in Ex 20 as the word of God to Israel at Sinai, at the time of the foundation of Israel. It is a founding document serving to call the people of God into existence. Is this historically verifiable? Attempts to provide a critical justification for deriving the decalogue from the beginning of Israel's history have not been lacking, but they have never coped successfully with the following points. First, from a literary point of view, the decalogue in Ex 20 is quite isolated: its context makes no reference to it and does not presuppose its presence. Secondly, the early history of Israel, insofar as it is known from the traditional material in Joshua, Judges, Samuel and Kings, makes no reference to the decalogue, and, indeed, in that a story such as Jg17f presupposes the use of images in Israelite worship, it might be argued that this history excludes the decalogue. Thirdly, although an early prophet, Hosea, castigates behaviour which is prohibited by the decalogue ('There is swearing, lying, killing, stealing, and committing adultery; they break all bounds and murder follows murder' 4:2), it is much more likely that this prophet is anticipating the decalogue prohibitions rather than depending on them. Fourthly, the particular corpus of Israelite literature with which the decalogue has its closest links is the deuteronomic corpus, and that corpus belongs at the end of Israel's pre-exilic history rather than at the beginning.

Such a late dating for the decalogue implies that it is a distillation of Israel's ongoing tradition and teaching rather than that it is the basic text which was foundational to that tradition and teaching; it represents a breakthrough to a recognition of what constituted the people of God which was won only at the cost of painful experience, it is not a divine gift which came independent of history and experience. In fact, it is almost a summary expression of two prophetic traditions in Israel: on the one hand, the tradition represented by Hosea and Jeremiah which emphasised the absolute demand for the worship of God alone; and, on the other hand, the tradition represented by Amos and Isaiah which is so strongly characterised by its ethical demand. As the concise distillation of so much that stands in the earlier Israelite religious and literary tradition, the decalogue takes on the character of a classic expression of faith, which, like the creeds and like the biblical canon in general, has behind it theological dispute and confirming experience. It grew out of the thinking and reflection of different religious and cultural streams in Israel, and is, then, a point of arrival rather than a point of departure. It represents a breakthrough to an expression of basic religious and ethical teaching, which is at a level of generality sufficient for it to transcend cultural distinctiveness and historical particularity.

Now, I am very much aware that by describing the decalogue in these terms I imply that it is something very different from the revealed word of God to Moses at Mount Sinai; it is, rather, an insight which was formulated in deuteronomic circles only at the cost of experience and dispute. This experience and this dispute includes prophetic preaching, and insofar as one thinks of the prophets as messengers of God, then the preaching which found its deposit in the decalogue may be considered the word of God. Such a description must, however, be defined more closely.

The preaching of the prophets cannot be understood as the impart-

ing of divine revelation in the sense that the prophets were privileged recipients of private and esoteric knowledge. Their condemnations of Israel arise, not from private revelation of something
new but rather from their insight into and recognition of what is
known to be wrong behaviour. The first two chapters of Amos, for
example, contain a series of oracles in which the activities of the nations around Israel are held up for condemnation. It is a condemnation uttered in the name of God and the crimes mentioned are understood as violations of the will of God. These crimes did not
necessarily involve Israel in any way, so it is not because of this that
Amos condemned them. Rather, the focus is on the crimes themselves, which are understood to violate the will of God. But on
what grounds can Amos condemn Edom, Moab, Damascus, the
Philistines and others? These are non-Israelite peoples; they had received no revelation of law from God. Surely, the very foundation
of the condemnations of Amos must be what can be called 'natural
law'. There is a way of behaviour built into the created order,
which is there to be perceived by all peoples, and by this all men
must live; it is the foundation of all life and integral to all life; it is
not something additional to creation but flows from creation.
Amos appeals not to Moses but to fundamental ethical standards to
which all men are bound.

Indeed, this must be the basis also of his comprehensive denunci-
ation of Israel. Again, no Mosaic revelation, and no private prophetic
revelation, forms the foundation of his preaching; rather, it is
norms of behaviour which people know to be right. Psalm 19 declares that 'the law of the Lord is perfect, reviving the soul; the testi-
mony of the Lord is sure, making wise the simple; the precepts of
the Lord are right, rejoicing the heart; the commandment of the
Lord is pure, enlightening the eyes; the fear of the Lord is clean, enduring for ever; the ordinances of the Lord are true, and righteous
altogether ... Moreover, by them is thy servant warned; in keeping
them there is great reward.' Again, however, it is most unlikely
that it is a Mosaic revelation on which the psalmist is reflecting.
There is no reference to Moses or Sinai, no reference to God's making
a covenant with his people, to his coming down on the mountain to
deliver his law. In fact, the most appropriate way to interpret it is
by reference to the beginning of the same psalm: 'The heavens are
telling the glory of God; and the firmament proclaims his handi-

work. Day to day pours forth speech and night to night declares knowledge. There is no speech, nor are there words; their voice is not heard; yet their voice goes out through all the earth, and their words to the end of the world.' This law is the law of the natural order; it is the way of life to which human beings as part of that natural order are bound; it is the fundamental principles of behaviour which are to be discerned through experience and reflection.

Amos and the other prophets do not represent an isolated tradition within Israel in this respect. Their appeal to known fundamental principles of behaviour has a close relationship to Israel's wisdom tradition. The proverbs of wisdom are the literary expression of the basic assertion that there is a moral order in creation, and that violation of that moral order is destructive of order in creation. There is no appeal here to a revealed law backed up by the authority of a punishing God; rather, the consequences of violation of the moral order are immediate and direct, forming an integral part of that violation: 'These men lie in wait for their own blood, they set an ambush for their own lives. Such are the ways of all who get gain by violence; it takes away the life of its possessors' (Prov 1:18f); 'The integrity of the upright guides them, but the crookedness of the treacherous destroys them ... The righteousness of the blameless keeps his way straight, but the wicked falls by his own wickedness. The righteousness of the upright delivers them, but the treacherous are taken captive by their lust' (11:3, 5f); 'He who closes his ear to the cry of the poor will himself cry out and not be heard' (21:13); 'He who digs a pit will fall into it, and a stone will come back upon him who starts it rolling' (26:27). This proverbial wisdom, with its characteristic understanding of the synthetic nature of human action, in which act and consequence together form a single whole, is the background of prophetic preaching. Its particular expression reflects a particular historical and cultural context, and stands in considerable conflict with the later reflections of Job and Ecclesiastes. Yet, its presupposed assertion of a moral order in creation remains as the ultimate foundation of the decalogue: 'You shall not kill' is not a law requiring the judicial execution or life imprisonment of murderers, but a prohibition which warns against the destructive violation of what is recognised to be a basic element of that moral order.

This brings me to the second of my two concluding concerns: the ongoing significance of the decalogue. The decalogue is a point of arrival, a breakthrough to what is generally valid; it emerged as a statement of meaning and intent which was to a limited extent fluid and changeable in itself, but which certainly always had to be interpreted for changing religious and historical situations. That it was to some extent a fluid rather than a permanently fixed statement is indicated by a number of points which I have already hinted at, and which have considerable intrinsic interest. First, there is some indication that individual commandments have experienced modification within the framework of the decalogue. Near the beginning of the decalogue the prohibition 'You shall not make for yourself a graven image' was probably originally an independent prohibition referring specifically to images of Israel's God, Yahweh; as a reference to images of other gods it would be superfluous after the immediately preceding prohibition of the worship of these other gods. Yet it is clear that at a very early stage the image prohibited was understood to be that of another god. The elaboration of that prohibition in the words 'or any likeness of anything that is in heaven above or that is in the earth beneath, or that is in the water under the earth' expands the application of the prohibition beyond the bounds of the worship of Yahweh; the further elaboration 'You shall not bow down to them or worship them' firmly links the prohibition of images with the prohibition of having other gods, binding the two together as one single prohibition of the worship of other gods. This unity of concern is then presupposed by the motivation 'for I the Lord your God am a jealous God', for the jealousy of Yahweh is always related to his exclusive claim on Israel and his absolute intolerance of her turning to other gods.

At the end of the decalogue, the commandment 'You shall not covet ...' seems originally to have referred not simply to feelings of envy but rather to the concrete steps taken in order to appropriate what belongs to another. This sense of the verb 'covet' is presupposed in Ex 34:24 which commands that all Israelite men should go to the sanctuary three times a year, and declares 'no man shall covet your land when you go up to appear before the Lord your God three times in the year'. If this is the older sense of the verb 'covet', however, it implies a major overlap with the prohibition 'You shall not steal', both meaning effectively the same thing. Since such duplication is unlikely in a summarising and generalising statement like the decalogue, it may be that the prohibition 'You shall not steal' originally had a specifying object, 'a man,' and that its concern was to prohibit not theft in general but kidnapping in particular. This is a concern of laws outside the decalogue, and is, in fact, an early Jewish interpretation of the commandment in its present form. If this does represent its original concern then a coherent sequence of topics results for the second half of the decalogue: they protect, in turn, the life of the individual, his marriage, his freedom, his reputation and his property, so including all the basic spheres of the individual's experience. It was when the meaning of the verb 'covet' eventually developed, as it did develop, to have reference only to feelings of envy and desire, that the general subject of theft then ceased to be covered by the decalogue; it was this loss that was made good by dropping the specifying object from the original commandment 'You shall not steal a man'.

Now this is quite obviously a fairly speculative reconstruction of part of the internal history of the decalogue; but much less speculation is involved in the second indication that the decalogue was open to internal modification. There are some important objective differences between the decalogue as it occurs in Ex 20 and its form in Deut 5. These differences illustrate the nature of the decalogue as a statement of meaning which was itself open to interpretative organisation and expression. The major differences are these: the motivation for the observance of the Sabbath in the Deuteronomy version, unlike that in Exodus, refers to the exodus from Egypt, and in so doing provides a catchword link with the reference to Egypt in the beginning of the decalogue; that same motivation adds a reference to the ox and ass, which should likewise benefit from the Sabbath rest, and this makes a catchword link with the final commandment of the decalogue; in the Deuteronomic decalogue the commandments 'You shall not kill, you shall not commit adultery, you shall not steal, you shall not bear false witness, you shall not covet', do not appear as separate commandments as in the Exodus version, but are all joined into a single literary unit by the use of the conjunction, and this provides a balance for the long literary unit found at the beginning of the decalogue. The result is a regular alternation of long and short literary units in which the central, long unit has catchword links with the beginning and end of the decalogue. The overall effect of these modifications is to create a new literary structure, known as a chiasm or ring pattern, which has the intended effect of pushing forward and emphasising the centre as the focal point: in the case of the version of the decalogue in Deut 5 it is the Sabbath commandment which receives this emphasis.

It is because the decalogue represents what we might call a charismatic breakthrough to a general interpretation of what it means to be a member of the people of one God that it maintained a general stability and uniformity while at the same time was open to some internal adaptation: its basic requirement of what might be called a practical monotheism, embracing both religious and ethical behaviour, remained constant even if its expression received now one new formulation and now another, now one new emphasis and now another. It is this openness to new understanding, within a constant basic framework, belonging to the very nature of the decalogue, which is the foundation for the radical reinterpretation of the demands of the decalogue in the Sermon on the Mount; it is that same openness which is the justification for the continued reinterpretation and extension of the demands of the decalogue in the history of the religious communities which valued it. The decalogue is a classic statement of the life of a community of faith; like the classic in any context it is a total statement in which now one part, now the other, may be highlighted. Ultimately, however, it is valued for the basic single insight which it reflects: that the worship of one God implies respect for the integrity of others, that respect for the integrity of others implies the worship of one God.

Further Reading:

A. Alt, 'The Origins of Israelite Law', *Essays on Old Testament History and Religion*, Blackwell, 1966.

B.S. Childs, *Exodus (Old Testament Library)*, SCM Press, 1974.

Interpretation Vol XLIII, No 3, July 1989.

W. Johnstone, 'The "Ten Commandments": some recent interpretations", *Expository Times 100*, 1988-89, 453ff.

A.D.H. Mayes, *Deuteronomy (New Century Bible)*, Marshall, Morgan & Scott, 1979.

E. Nielsen, *The Ten Commandments in New Perspective*, SCM Press, 1968.

A.C.J. Phillips, *Ancient Israel's Criminal Law*, Blackwell, 1970.

J.J. Stamm & M.E. Andrew, *The Ten Commandments in Recent Research*, SCM Press, 1967.

CHAPTER 3

The Ethic of Jesus:
The Sermon on the Mount Then and Now
Seán Freyne

The present situation in Society and Church
These are heady times for the idealists among us – those who like to think about the emerging world as one family, all living happily together in a single global village. For Europeans in particular the collapse of what from the outside appeared to be an immovable and impenetrable socialist block, has been a very strange, even weird experience. Nobody seems quite sure how to react, whether to rejoice or be scared. The demise of the old enemy, Communism, has left us somewhat breathless, unsure of the future and where we might all be headed. For those of us who operate under the liberal democratic philosophy of the west all these developments could easily be seen as a vindication of our dominant world-view – the success of the free-market economy and its myth of progress, leading to a better world for all.

I recall these political facts of our times merely to point up some of the ironies of our contemporary situation which apply not just to the political sphere, but to the religious and the ethical as well. In different ways, we are all faced with the question of how to subscribe to universal dreams while retaining the identity that is part of our particular experience – be it political, cultural or religious. The collapse of the universal dreams of a socialist Europe imposed by force is due in no small measure to the reassertion of much older ethnic and cultural differences that could not be wiped out or glossed over. It would be ironic indeed if such events should give rise to a different form of liberal universalism that would seek to ignore differences in human life as these express themselves in so many aspects of our experience – everything from language to the ways we think about the universe and its ultimate destiny. In many cases of resistance, religion played a significant role in ensuring the non-acceptance of a totalitarian regime. The question now is: will it be a divisive or a creative factor in the shaping of the new Europe, either by attempting to control and dominate, or by continuing to challenge some of the new ideologies of progress that are on offer?

For two centuries now, two opposing tendencies may be discerned in the way that Christians everywhere in the West have dealt with the problem of living within an increasingly secular environment. Either Christian values were assumed to correspond with universal human ones, and so there was nothing distinctive, at least in the domain of public morality, about being Christian, or alternatively, Christians so cut themselves off from the world and from each other that they developed highly individualistic, anti-world value-systems, which had little to say to the emerging secular ethos of the Enlightenment and modern humanism.

It was during the same centuries, and faced with that same secular-isation process, that 'the eclipse of biblical narrative' occurred, to use the title of Hans Frei's influential work. By this he means that in the wake of the changing scientific understanding of the universe and the emergence of the sense of the self as being wholly free and autonomous, people's self-understanding was no longer grounded in the biblical account of human and world origins. The story of Jesus, likewise, had to be shorn of the outdated mythological trappings in which it had been handed down in the gospels. In the many lives of Jesus that emerged in the nineteenth century he was made to represent the dominant value-system of the day, that of liberal humanism. Such lives were written for the best of motives, to salvage something from the wreckage that the Enlightenment was deemed to have caused to Christian faith through the apparent discrediting of its foundational documents. Thus, Jesus was seen as a wise teacher/philosopher whose life and teachings embodied the best liberal ideals in the pursuit of freedom and equality. Of course, both Catholic and Protestant orthodoxies in their different ways reacted to this liberal response. Within Roman Catholicism the anti-modernist crisis of the late nineteenth and early twentieth centuries represented a return to the medieval world-view as this had been defined in the Counter-Reformation period. Almost contempor-aneously the work of Karl Barth attempted to reaffirm the reform-ation principle of justification by faith, understood as a surrender of the self to God's saving action in Christ, as witnessed in scrip   ture.

Both positions can be seen as a reassertion of the quest for a timeless truth whereby Christian faith could ignore the vicissitudes of human history and culture. Though adopting very different starting points, both tend to ignore the changing historical and cultural circumstances within which human life is lived and human responses to God's call are fashioned. Neither takes seriously the subjective dimension of all truth claims, and the consequent need for careful attention to the linguistic, social, psychological and other conditioning that must be seen as substantive rather than purely accidental features of all human understanding in the world. In this paper, however, I propose to develop a different line of argument, because I am persuaded of the necessity for Christians, even in Ireland, to explore anew their own resources, spiritual and ethical, as a way of being challenged to enter into dialogue with other value systems.

Dr Jeanrond has suggested that a conversation model, in which competing truth-claims in ethics as in other spheres of life can be debated publicly, is a pressing need for our times. This demands that Christians can articulate their own distinctive vision, without on the one hand reducing it to a set of generalised truths, or on the other rejecting out of hand all other claims as false or unworthy. In the past, especially in Ireland, it has been a particular temptation for all the churches here to want to control the total ethos of the society in terms of its ethical values – for the best of reasons of course! In the changing culture that now obtains here, traditional norms are breaking down more rapidly than in societies that have for long been accustomed to questioning and change. We are threatened with a dangerous vacuum, in which the very question of values is likely to be dismissed, simply because the authority by which the traditional ones were imposed is now rejected. As Christians we must make more modest claims to universal truth, especially in ethics, while at the same time taking our own vision more seriously than heretofore.

Exploring the Ethical Vision of Jesus
But what have we got to offer? What particular insights from our tradition might be of special significance at the present juncture. That Jesus of Nazareth was one of the great 'classic' religious figures would be acknowledged by all thinking people, irrespective of their personal allegiance to him or to the religion that has emerged in his name. In the nineteenth century, as previously mentioned, it

was as a teacher of ethical truths that Jesus was seen by many 'enlightened' investigators. Certainly, the ethical teachings of Jesus have almost from the very beginning been singled out for attention, especially as they had been distilled to the early church through Matthew's gospel in the famous Sermon on the Mount (Mt chs 5-7), with some of the great early Christian fathers such as Origen and Augustine writing special commentaries on it. Luke, in his gospel has another, much shorter version, which he locates on a plain (Lk 6:19-49), something that reminds us that the career and teaching of Jesus have come to us through the interpretative activity of the early Christian community in often quite different circumstances. This already alerts us to an important aspect of Jesus' teaching, namely, that he was not a teacher of timeless moral truths of an unchanging and unchangeable character, but rather a prophetic figure who applied his particular vision of the kingdom of God to very specific and concrete situations and problems within everyday life of the Galilean country folk amongst whom his public ministry was conducted. If Jesus' life and teaching are to be accorded the status of the classic then he fulfills admirably the first condition for that epithet, namely, particularity of origins.

In view of the modern interest in Jesus as a teacher of ethics it may come as some surprise to hear that the role of teacher was not by any means the most obvious description of him by some at least of his contemporaries. True he is addressed in the gospels frequently as Rabbi/*didaskale*/teacher, but only by outsiders. Thus, Matthew at least would seem to want to distance Jesus from the role of the scribe, the official teachers within Judaism, who were a professional and elitist class according to one of their early representatives, Jesus son of Sirach from Jerusalem. By such standards Jesus did not rank. He had not studied, nor as a *tecton* or craftsman was he likely to have had the leisure to acquire the necessary knowledge to give him the status of a scribe (see Sir ch 38; Jn 7:15).

This observation points us in another direction in trying to identify the significance of Jesus for ethics. It is his life and ministry, his praxis, if you like, that distinguishes him, since as has often been observed many of his recorded sayings echo those of other great teachers, Jewish and Greek, emanating from that culture. His originality lay not so much in the sayings themselves but in the context within which they were uttered, a life that lived out the radical implications of these utterances, to the point that the sayings became a commentary on the one who spoke them.

The story of Jesus then is the important factor; it is a story of the one who in the name of God's kingly rule gathered around himself the messianic community that, according to the Israelite prophetic tradition, would be purified and restored, so that the great ideals of her communal life could at last be realised. Insofar as that vision was based on the restoration of right relations – with God, with the earth and its creatures and with fellow human beings – it was indeed a utopian vision; not utopian in the sense of being unrealisable, but as reflecting the most primordial longings of the human spirit faced with the reality of greed and selfishness distorting the way that things ought to be and could be, we are convinced, in our world. In the gospel stories about Jesus, therefore, we should hear again echoes of the stories of Paradise, not in terms of the mythological expressions of a lost Golden Age, but as realised historically in and through the career of Jesus of Galilee. We will never grasp the full meaning, and therefore, the full challenge of the sermon if we do not constantly remind ourselves that it is only in the setting of that story and all its implications that this particular ethical synthesis is intended to make full sense.

Mention has already been made of the contrasting settings – mountain and plain – that Matthew and Luke choose for the sermon. Like all good story-tellers they are seeking a suitable backdrop for their account, in order to stimulate, provoke and challenge their readers to be opened up to new possibilities, as they leave the everyday world (Matthew) or remain within it (Luke). Matthew's setting is particularly suggestive for our present purposes. Horizons of meaning as well as of vision change as we climb the mountain, and new and hitherto unexplored vistas are opened up before us. However, for the first readers of his work 'the mountain' and its association with 'city' and 'house' a few verses further on had other resonances emanating from the Hebrew Scriptures. According to Isaiah, at the end of days the mountain of the house of the Lord, that is, the new Jerusalem with its new temple, would raise itself higher than all other mountains and attract the nations there to learn the wisdom of the Lord (Is 2:2-4). That this futuristic imagery was intended to pervade the whole sermon is confirmed by the closing image of the wise person building a house on the rock, in contrast to that of the foolish person built on sand. Jesus, as Wisdom incarnate, builds himself a house on a rock, that is a community to which all are invited to enter and learn of wisdom.

As well as having imaginative evocations from the prophetic and wisdom traditions, houses and cities were also the places where the early Christians lived out their communal existence together. In such settings they undertook a radically alternative life-style that was subversive of the traditional value-systems of Greco-Roman culture, as we shall see. It was only within such caring communities that such ideals as turning the other cheek, loving one's enemies, sharing beyond the call of duty make sense. It is only when these extremes are undertaken within the context of communities bonded together in faith and love in the name of Jesus Christ, and thus providing a supportive ethos, that they become possible and viable, not foolhardy undertakings of a highly individualistic nature.

It is sometimes suggested that Matthew wanted to present Jesus as the giver of a second law to fulfil the Mosaic dispensation. While some of the utterances do indeed suggest such a contrast, it is clear from the overall tone and style that to interpret the whole in a legal fashion would be seriously to misconstrue the intention of Jesus, even as Matthew understands it. Unfortunately, that is what has happened in Christian history with some of the sayings such as those on divorce, whereas others like turning the other cheek have been largely ignored, even as possible ideals for Christians who have had no difficulties in fighting so-called just wars! General instruction is interspersed with personal address; warnings, exhortations and declarations of blessedness arising from the pursuit of certain values are to be found side by side with practical wisdom, rules, admonitions, examples of correct conduct in prayer, fasting and almsgiving, within this new vision. Here is neither the precision of a sustained law code nor the detached and abstract reflections of a philosophical ethician. Rather, it is the passionate, direct appeal of a charismatic preacher, the urgency of whose language betrays the sense of finality about the message.

Despite this very distinctive tone and language that marks the sermon as unmistakably Jewish, one can also detect an opening out to the larger world of discourse on ethical and other issues that was such a feature of the Mediterranean world generally, and which certainly marked Jesus' Galilean ministry. The golden rule – as you would that others should do to you do to them in like manner – was a commonplace among both Jewish teachers and pagan philosophers. Besides, such terms as justice (*dikaiosyne*) and perfection (*teleios*) were also much debated issues. In Matthew's account, however, the justice that Jesus talks about is that of the kingdom and the ideal of perfection that is proposed is that of the heavenly Father (6:53; 5:48). Even the golden rule is thoroughly Judaised, since after its citation, Matthew adds: 'for this is the law and the prophets' (7:10). Thus, the central ethical values of the culture were grounded theologically in Jesus' vision, but in such a way, however, that his life-style as an articulation of those values and their theological grounding, proved to be a severe threat, not just to the received understanding of justice and perfection, but to that of the kingdom of God, the law and the prophets and even the concept of God itself. It was because he was seen to be engaged in an attack both on the received value-system of the Roman world and the religious symbols of his own tradition that Rome and the Jewish religious establishment could join forces against this prophet from Galilee. Establishments, religious and political, can tolerate theoretical discussion as long as it remains isolated from so-called 'real life'. However, ethical stances always imply a particular belief-system and world-view, and it is in the resultant behaviour that these can be most easily identified, as every social reformer has learned, often to their cost, from Socrates in fifth-century Athens to Nelson Mandela in contemporary South Africa

As an experiment in identifying more precisely the distinctive ethic of Jesus we can attempt a comparison with the Greek ideal in regard to these two central categories of the sermon, justice and perfection.

Justice was an ideal that was particularly dear to the Greeks within the context of the *polis*, or city-state. For them it was a matter of fulfilling one's duties as these were defined within the particular social realms of the household or the city: 'giving to each its own in accordance with the laws' as Aristotle expresses it. The symbol of the scales was highly appropriate for such a notion since it was largely a matter of balancing the rights and duties of each, but in accordance with the structured patterns of rank within the particular setting. These ranged from males who were full citizens and who took precedence over all others, to women, children, slaves and aliens. According to the prevailing view it was those who were in a position to take on some *leitourgia* or service on behalf of the *polis* that were on the top rung of the ladder as far as justice was concerned. In the family hierarchy there was a similar structure with the paterfamilias as the first in terms of rights.

Jesus' vision was not based on abstract ideas of justice but on the prophetic ideal of *sedaqah*, which, as articulated by several prophets, entailed a radical social programme. In their view justice was first and foremost a righting of the social ills within Israel. This rather than worship of Yahweh in prayers, fasting and other religious and cultic practices was essential for a right relationship with Israel's God, who, unlike many other gods in her neighbourhood, had a strongly ethical character. 'I desire mercy (in the sense of deeds of loving kindness) not sacrifice' is Hosea's declaration, and this is twice quoted by the Matthean Jesus as the correct expression of his understanding of God's will also (Mt 9:13; 12:7). Later prophets such as Third Isaiah continue to spell out the same message after the restoration from the Babylonian exile. In a passage that touches on many topics developed in the Sermon on the Mount we read 'If you take away from the midst of you the yoke, the pointing of the finger and speaking wickedness, if you pour yourself out for the afflicted, then shall your light rise in the darkness ... and the Lord shall satisfy your desires with good things ... and your ancient ruins shall be rebuilt' (Is 58:1-12).

In this and other passages, the justice that is demanded is 'my justice'. God had entered into a partnership with Israel in slavery and thus justice was ongoing faithfulness to that relationship, no matter how badly Israel had failed. Justice as an ethical norm within Israel must always mirror God's justice, and that meant particular care for the poor, the needy and the socially outcast. Since God had not considered rank in the choice of a people, justice built on that memory had to be concerned with a radical reordering of all social relationships, including economic ones.

The realisation of such a justice had been long delayed. In the centuries between the Babylonian captivity and the first century c.e. the repressive experience of successive kingdoms, including for a time a Jewish national one, that of the Maccabeans, had only heightened the expectation among pious Jews of God's kingdom as opposed to all human kingdoms, when such a society could at last be realised. It was in the name of this kingdom that Jesus preached and lived his own ethical vision, not as some distant ideal, but as a reality now. Among his Jewish contemporaries others too proclaimed the dawning of the new era, but in terms very different from his. To take one example, not without its relevance for our world, the Zealots, or extreme nationalists, espoused a militant overthrowing of Roman rule and destruction of those who collaborated with the enemy. In Jesus' words they sought to force open the kingdom of heaven by violence. There is ample evidence from Josephus of the manner in which that particular ideology expressed itself throughout the first century, leading up to the revolt against Rome in the year 66 c.e. In God's name they espoused the annihilation, whereas Jesus called for love of the enemy, so startlingly portrayed in the images of turning the other cheek, or going an extra mile beyond that which one was constrained to do – a frequent form of harassment of a native population by an invading army.

As with justice, so also with perfection, the other general ethical category that Matthew's gospel shares with its larger environment. In the Greek ideal perfection was a matter of achieving the correct balance between the good and the beautiful, and therefore it had an aesthetic as well as an ethical dimension. Alternatively, in certain circles it had become an elitist ideal that separated 'the perfect' from society at large. Either way, it was a highly individualistic ideal achieved through self-restraint and training rather than in and through a life shared with others. The gods had achieved this inner harmony which expressed itself in detachment, and the individual could be exhorted to imitate god by living in accordance with nature (Stoics) or achieving an inner freedom from all passions and desires (Epicureans).

By contrast the perfect God of Jesus as Matthew portrays it is deeply involved with the world. This is emphasised by the fact that the same ideal, perfection, can be achieved through following Jesus. 'If you would be perfect', he tells the rich young man, 'Sell what you have, give to the poor and come follow me' (Mt 19:21). In the sermon itself the God of Jesus, 'the heavenly Father', is portrayed as totally involved with and in control of creation. In an extraordinarily evocative passage, Jesus contrasts the freedom of the animal and

plant life with the care-ridden existence of humans, expressed in terms of concern for food, drink and clothing. This passage expresses no romantic idealism about nature, however, but is rather deliberately provocative in terms of prevailing discussions about true and false cares. The Christian disciple is being challenged to let go, not just of daily cares, but of the care for existence itself, expressed under the metaphors of food, drink and clothing – the very basic necessities of life (Mt 6:25-34). In Paradise nakedness was natural, not because of the absence of sexual desires, but because total trust in and openness to God prevailed. Food and drink were present in abundance also. Against such a mythological background the God of Jesus is totally involved with creation, human anxiety has been taken care of and the possibility of a human community based on the sharing of God with the creation is once again a practical possibility. This is the perfection of God that the disciple is to imitate as it is defined in the ethic of Jesus.

We shall have to terminate at this point our exploration of the ethic of Jesus based on comparisons with similar ideals, pagan and Jewish. In this light its distinctive character, its radical demand and theological grounding stand out in clearer perspective. While it shared considerably with the other great traditions within which it was fashioned, its values, vision and communitarian character clearly differed from these in a very essential way. As Matthew views it, Christian disciples are to essay a more radical life-style than either Jewish or pagan standards; there was a 'more' demanded that was defined by Jesus himself. And yet this did not mean a 'holier than thou' attitude, since according to Isaiah, on whose vision it is based, all would want to ascend God's holy mountain and learn there the wisdom of Zion. Thus, the ethical vision of Jesus is not a perfectionist ideal for the few, but a radical statement of human possibility for all that will generate its own dynamism, if only it is attempted. 'People will see your good works and glorify (not you) but your Father who is in heaven' (Mt 5:16).

Fusing the Horizons: The Ethical Vision of Jesus in our Culture
Karl Marx has declared that the object of all human reflection should be, not to interpret reality, but to change it. This of course presumes that those who do the reflection are unhappy with the status quo and feel called on to do something about it. The reflection will both help to identify the problem and determine what one

ought to do. As Christians, we are pilgrim people, restless, struggling to ascend the mountain so that we get a clearer view of the farthest horizons and what lies between us and it. It is not however, as though we are struggling to ascend in order to catch a first glimpse, we have in fact already crossed over. As German theologian, Jürgen Moltmann declares, with reference to the liberation that Christians claim in Christ: 'When Freedom draws near, the chains begin to hurt; When Life has passed by Death becomes deadly.' We Christians cannot, or at least should not be satisfied with our world, or its *laissez-faire* attitudes, once we have been confronted with the ethical vision of Jesus and the possibilities for human transformation that it both envisages and proclaims as a possibility now.

We are, I submit, faced with two questions that are intimately related. Firstly, how are we as Christians to appropriate the ethical vision of Jesus today, and secondly, how might such an appropriation contribute to a more serious debate about ethics within contemporary life? This second question is all the more urgent, if, as I (and others) have suggested, the Christian churches have for the most part opted for the neo-conservative response of reasserting past orthodoxies, without listening to other voices in our culture that are also struggling with genuine ethical dilemmas.

First, however, we must begin to put our own house in order, taking seriously the advice of the sermon itself: do not seek to remove the speck from others' eyes, without removing first the log from our own. Interpreting the sermon has almost always in Christian history been seen as a task of negotiating its radical demands within the context of everyday life, either watering those demands down, choosing between them or seeing them as unattainable ideals. Thus, interpreting the ethics of Jesus is itself an ethical exercise, and for this, we are recommended, again by the sermon itself, to have our eye simple rather than evil, in order to hear its demands fully, and open ourselves up to the perspectives it unfolds before us (Mt 6:22f; 7:3-5).

Earlier, I stressed that as Christians we should not be tempted into the position of divorcing the ethic of Jesus from his story, which is the strange, paradoxical and profoundly disturbing story that in the life, death and resurrection of Jesus of Nazareth, God's ultimate purpose for this world has been disclosed. The fact that others ignore, dismiss or find this story unconvincing is ultimately not the point. It is our story and we are called on to affirm it by allowing our own personal and communal stories be judged by its radical demands and supported by its profound sense of hope in the midst of human failure and suffering. In practice this means that we feel called on to participate together in a radically new venture, called on, not as individuals, but in community, the messianic community that Jesus has gathered around him in order to live out his shared vision of human togetherness in the world.

We have already alluded more than once in passing to the image of climbing the mountain as an invitation to change our perspective. Useful as this image is, it is to the language of the sermon that we must look for its transformative effects, since language is not just descriptive of the way things are, but creative of the way things can and ought to be. As in all the utterances of Jesus, equally in his ethical statements, there is a strange, even paradoxical quality: the persecuted are declared blessed; disciples who are contrasted with hypocrites are themselves called hypocrites; birds and flowers can be used, not as romantic images of innocence, but as analogues for human activity – sowing, reaping, gathering into barns; logs of timber in the eye blocking one's vision are scarcely a normal occurrence! But then so much of the conduct that is enjoined is not 'normal' either – turning the other cheek, letting coat as well as cloak go, loving one's enemy. There is a strangeness about these demands, even hyperbole, but it is hyperbole that is not merely ornamental but which goes to the heart of the matter, literally as well as metaphorically. Here language is being used in a recklessly extravagant manner in order to shock us into seeing new and hitherto unperceived possibilities for human conduct. Their only logic is that of superabundance, as Paul Ricoeur puts it, a logic that gives rise to extravagance in doing and thinking. At crucial points we are directed to pay attention to the eye and the heart as focal points of vision and intention. We are invited to embark on a journey inwards as well as upwards. What would it be like if our eye were really simple, that is single minded, and we tried out this vision, but together, as a way of overcoming our self-centred and self-grounded super-egos, the product of both the Enlightenment's legacy of the totally free and autonomous self, and of the scientific revolution's myth of human self-sufficiency and control over our own destiny? The last enemy to be conquered is Death, declared one of the leaders of the French Revolution, and modern medicine seems hell-bent on taking him seriously!

Of course the sermon does not answer directly our specific ethical questions, since many of its examples are time-conditioned and are not (often at least) part of our culture. There is no substitute for the task of discerning, often painfully, what our detailed Christian response should be, but it does give us very clear directions if we really want to know. Justice, in terms of radical concern for human need wherever and in whatever form it is encountered, will be the keynote; concern with the other will increasingly define the self, and thus the values that will inform the life-style will often be in direct conflict with those that motivate the progressivist modern world, where 'greed is good' functions as the most fundamental principle of life. Our actions for and on behalf of others will always be anti-ideological, that is opposed to all forms of discrimination: sexism, racism, ageism, classism, monetarism. We will be deeply conscious that too often the Christian churches have been the propa-gators of these very ideologies, despite our most noble declarations that there is neither Jew nor Greek, slave nor free, male or female (Gal 3:24), and conscious also that ours is at best a highly ambiguous history in terms of the liberative praxis that we are called to as followers of Jesus, the prophet of liberation for all.

If Christians in Ireland, as elsewhere within western democracies, were to embark on such a messianic life-style, what difference would it make to our world? While each of our cultures has its own distinctive ethos, due to circumstances of geography and history – to name the most obvious determinants – ours is on the whole a monochromic world that is shaped by universal myths which are the product of the Enlightenment and its successor, the scientific revolution. The shallowness and ego-centrism of so much of modern life are the direct results of our failure to replace the medieval and renaissance world-views and their in-built ethical programmes, with new and responsible alternatives that could seriously address in our own time the age-old questions of what is the good life, what is the nature of happiness, how and where can we find meaning in time and history.

This should not be interpreted as though I regard the advances of the Enlightenment and scientific progress as evil or to be rejected. Much has been achieved through the freeing of the human subject from outmoded, authoritarian structures that sought to control human thinking and acting in the world. It would be difficult to imagine even the possibilities of various feminist liberation movements today for example, without the understanding of human freedom and dignity that have been hammered out over the past two centuries. And who could deny the advances for human life in the world that science in its many forms has achieved over the past 150 years in particular. What has been wrong is not that such intellectual and scientific advances have occurred, but that we have allowed them to go unchallenged in terms of their meaning for all of human life in this world. The gloriously free and autonomous self of Kant, having failed in some of its more ambitious projects, has become the feckless, disillusioned and in the end irresponsible self of some post-modernist writers. The unbridled exploration and use of our natural resources that has followed in the wake of much scientific advance has brought us to the very brink of ecological disaster on a global scale. Nuclearism may have receded temporarily from our list of ideologies that have to be resisted, but nevertheless we are for ever doomed to live in the last age of the world. We and our children must always live now in the realisation that we have at hand the capacity to destroy ourselves irrevocably.

In the midst of such competing ideologies, many of them literally life-threatening, the Christian churches are faced with new challenges, but also new possibilities. Ecumenical hair splitting, debates about women's ordination and other inner church conflicts are almost obscene luxuries, by comparison with the tasks that confront us. Where the Christian messianic vision is being lived today, as in the third world countries, we can hear again, and more importantly, see again, the reality of Jesus of Galilee's prophetic critique and the transformative power for human living in the world of its radically alternative life-style. We have as yet hardly begun to discern what shape it might take in our own more affluent cultures or how we might begin to learn from the voices of the oppressed among us.

What if Christians in Ireland were to take seriously the messianic life-style of Jesus? What changes to church and society could we ex-

pect? A number of subsequent papers in this collection attempt answers to these pressing questions in the areas of justice for the poor,
especially for poor women, the ecology and politics. As background to those more detailed discussions it may be appropriate
here to recall that insofar as Ireland has experienced social revolutions in the past – Davitt's 'land war' of the last century and
Larkin's campaign for the urban workers in this – these never
coalesced to bring about a total revolution for all within our society.
Sectional interests still vie with each other while appealing in a
highly selective manner to a notion of justice that smacks more of
the 'I'm-all-right-Jack' philosophy of the middle classes than of
Jesus' vision of a justice that is biased in favour of the needy.

In attempting to envisage a new society inspired by such a vision
we might do well to recall the values that were embedded in the
old Irish notion of *muintearas*, a concept for which neighbourliness
is a rather bland translation. Mutual help, support and sharing
were the hallmarks of the peasant economy of the countryside. This
suggestion is not prompted by any nostalgic looking back to the
past, but by the awareness that any viable alternative to the current
dominant trends of our macro-economic practitioners must draw
on our own well-springs, while always for Christians also recalling
the radical challenge of Jesus' vision. Europe and 1992 is no pana-
cea for the deep-seated social ills that beset our society, despite the
increased affluence for those in the privileged position to avail of
the new opportunities.

In rural Ireland *muintearas* could be narrow-minded, inward-
looking and self-interested, yet its heart was in the right place. With
limited resources life's necessities had to be shared and mutual
help was based on mutual trust. As such it was grounded in social
realities similar to those that prompted Jesus' radical vision which
we have been exploring in this paper. His first followers attempted
some daring experiments in putting this ideal into practice in the
new urban environments of the Mediterranean cities, thereby providing a home for the homeless, status for non-persons such as
women and slaves, and a welcome for strangers. The conservative
moral economy of the peasant took on a radical dimension when
translated from the kinship society of peasants to the open and free
associations of the city. Were Irish Christians to embark on a similar
imaginative venture based on the memory of togetherness that our

forebears practised ('ní neart go cur le chéile' – 'Our power comes from our co-operation'), yet continuing to be challenged by the older memory of Jesus, they would certainly be a transforming force in our churches and our society.

One has the distinct impression that at present the 'alternative vision' which the churches have to offer is stifled by their own failures at the institutional level to take that vision seriously. They can hardly expect society, either north or south, to be too impressed by words when, with some notable individual exceptions, deeds of justice and caring seem to be lacking. One is reminded of the prophetic words of Dietrich Bonhoeffer, as relevant today for the European churches as when they were uttered in a German prison fifty years ago: 'Our Church that has been fighting in these years only for its self-preservation, as though that were an end in itself is incapable of taking the word of reconciliation to the world... Our being Christian today will be limited to two things – prayer and righteous action in the world ... We are not yet out of the melting pot, and any attempt to help the church prematurely to a new expansion of its organisation will merely delay its conversion and purifi cation.'

Further Reading:

W.D. Davies, *The Setting of the Sermon on the Mount*, Cambridge, University Press, 1964.

H.D. Betz, *Essays on the Sermon on the Mount*, Philadelphia, Fortress Press, 1985.

J. Lambrecht,SJ, *The Sermon on the Mount: Proclamation and Exhortation*, Wilmington, Michael Glazier 1985.

H.Moxes, *The Economy of the Kingdom: Social Conflict and Economic Relations in Luke's Gospel* , Philadelphia, Fortress Press, 1988.

Michael H. Crosby, *House of Disciples: Church, Economics and Justice in Matthew*, Maryknoll, Orbis Books 1988.

S. Freyne, *Galilee, Jesus and the Gospels. Literary Approaches and Historical Investigations*, Dublin, Gill & Macmillan 1988.

W. Meeks, *The Moral World of the First Christians*, London A.P.C.K., 1986.

D. Mieth & J. Pohier, *Changing Values and Virtues*, Concilium No 191 (edts), T. & T. Clark, Edinburgh.

R. Horsley, *Jesus and the Spiral of Violence: Popular Jewish Resistance in Roman Palestine*, New York, Harper & Row, 1987.

P. Ricoeur, 'The Golden Rule: Exegetical and Theological Perplexities', *New Testament Studies*, 36 (1990), 392-397.

CHAPTER 4

Conscience, Guilt and Sin

Gabriel Daly

'Two things fill the mind with ever new and increasing admiration and awe, the oftener and the steadier we reflect on them: the starry heavens above and the moral law within.'

Immanuel Kant's celebrated remark is a reminder of his distinguished place in the history of both astronomy and ethical theory. It was he who first suggested that nebulae might be galaxies. It is, however, with his insights into 'the moral law within' that I wish to begin my reflections here.

The first thing we should notice is that he does not simply say 'the moral law', but 'the moral law within'. What excites his wonder is first and foremost the sheer givenness of the human sense of right and wrong. People may vary widely in their estimate of what is right and wrong, but whether or not they accept the existence of a natural law, they agree that a sense of moral obligation is a universal feature of humanity. Kant focuses his philosophical gaze on this interior moral law and finds in it the source of its own authority. The source of ethical action for Kant is the will, by which he means the ability to bring oneself to act. He also calls the will 'practical reason', because it is reason devoting itself to deciding whether an act should be performed or not. For Kant nothing is radically good except the good will itself which acts only out of a sense of duty. He was reacting against the view, common in his day, that happiness is the true motive for human action. He was also reacting against the view, sanctioned by some kinds of religious faith, that good should be done and evil avoided because of divine reward or punishment. The motive for ethical behaviour is to be found not in any external source, even the will of God, but only in the inner sense of duty which exists in every human being. If I wish to know whether something I propose to do is good or bad, Kant tells me that I must ask myself whether I can will that the principle on which I am now going to act (which he calls my maxim) should become a universal law. For example, suppose I have the power and authority to switch off a life-support system and I am faced with the necessity of making a decision here and now in the case of this particular patient. The criterion which Kant places before me is whether I can recommend that any man or woman anywhere in the world faced with a similar situation should behave as I now propose to behave.

I need hardly say that philosophers and moralists have subjected Kant's teaching to a rigorous examination, and many of them have claimed to uncover flaws in it. I have chosen to begin with Kant's conception of conscience and ethics because his philosophy has been a major influence in shaping the modern world. Whether one agrees with it or not, one usually finds it necessary to define one's own position by some kind of reference to it, nowhere more than to his theory of ethics and moral experience.

This theory, then, is utterly dedicated to the conviction that the sources of ethical behaviour are to be found within the human mind and heart. Our moral imperatives must not be sought in some external authority. Kant is not attacking a religious interpretation of morality. He is attacking the idea that religion is the source of moral conviction. What he says is this: 'To be religious is to view our duties as divine commands.' Notice the order in which he places the two: They are duties before they are divine commands.

I draw attention to this aspect of Kant's moral teaching because it has an important bearing on any situation where a religion has played a dominant part in the shaping of consciences, especially if that religion emphasises authority as a source of teaching. In Ireland, for example, many people have traditionally experienced their ethical lives as predominantly tied to the authority of their church. They have, as it were, reversed the order of Kant's dictum that to be religious is to view our duties as divine commands. Instead, they have in effect acted according to some such dictum as: 'To be moral is to view divine commands as our duty.' Kant used the word heteronomy to describe a system of ethics which derives its maxims from any source other than each person's practical reason, or will. Heteronomy easily leads to a purely pragmatic attitude towards others, hence he advances another version of his categorical imperative: 'Act so that you treat humanity, whether in your own person or in that of another, always as an end and never as a means only.'

Kant's rejection of heteronomous morality is important in the formation of contemporary standards for two reasons. First, it is in keeping with a recognition of the blunt fact that there is in most of us an instinct to kick against regulations which are imposed upon us from outside and for which we do not see sufficient reason. Morality which does not arise out of inner conviction is scarcely more than the prudent conventions of the parade-ground. If the sergeant-major tells you to take two steps forward, you take them without a concomitant glow of virtue; indeed your inner feelings may be sulphurous, and the sergeant-major may know that they are sulphurous, but as long as you obey and keep your mouth shut, military discipline is satisfied. The parade-ground, however, provides a very poor model for representing ethical response, especially if that response is placed in a religious context which sees God as a loving Father.

There is another reason why Kant's rejection of heteronomous morality has a particular relevance to contemporary life. In a world which is undergoing increasing secularisation, it is vitally important for society that when people throw over, or at least distance themselves from, churches and religious traditions, they do not throw over ethical standards, merely because these standards have been closely associated with the religious authority that they are rejecting. Conscience has a crucial role to play in the practice of religious faith, but it does not depend for its existence on religious faith. It comes with the human condition; and that is what excited Kant's awe. Once Kant has secured the principle of moral autonomy in advance of all other considerations, he is quite ready to argue from it to the existence of God as its guarantor. A large body of modern thought has not been content to follow him in this. A century after Kant had made his appeal to the law within, Sigmund Freud set about explaining the presence of the law within by reference to infantile experience.

Freud is rather hard on Kant:

> The philosopher Kant once declared that nothing proved to him the greatness of God more convincingly than the starry heavens and the moral conscience within us. The stars are unquestionably superb, but where conscience is concerned God has been guilty

of an uneven and careless piece of work, for a great many men have only a limited share of it or scarcely enough to be worth mentioning.

Freud, like Marx and Nietzsche, is a teacher of suspicion in that he places a large question mark over the content of consciousness itself. To anyone who points to conscience as the sign of a transcendent lawgiver Freud says 'I can explain the presence of conscience by reference to the psychological make-up of human beings and to early family relationships. There is no need to postulate the existence of God in order to account for moral experience.'

Freud quite simply undermines all transcendental theories of conscience by undertaking to explain what is happening when we experience the approbation or the rebukes of our ethical sense. He sees the human ego as being formed under pressure on the one side from the cauldron of instincts, drives, and desires within us which he calls the id, and, on the other side, from the restrictions imposed upon us from an early age by the external world, embodied principally by our parents, who prevent us from instantly satisfying our every desire. According to Freud, 'consciousness of guilt was originally fear of punishment by parents; more exactly, fear of losing their love'. He is startlingly unambiguous about the matter:

> The first renunciation of instinctual gratification is enforced by external powers, and it is this that creates morality which expresses itself in conscience and exacts a further renunciation of instinct.

When these initially external powers are internalised they become the super-ego or faculty whereby the ego observes, censors, and judges itself.

How is the Christian theologian to respond to this way of explaining the human ethical condition? Clearly it will not do simply to ignore it on the grounds that Freud was an atheist who was committed to showing that religion is an illusion and that all religious claims and practices can be explained by purely physical theories. There is obviously much in Freud which the theologian will wish to challenge, dispute, or modify; but before doing so, he or she will be well advised to allow Freud to place a question mark against those elements in our theology which bear on guilt, conscience and culpability. Like Marx, Freud teaches us at least to suspect the content of our consciousness. We have to suspect that some at least of our sensibilities, our moral attitudes and judgements, have been affected, and possibly even shaped, less by grace and the Holy Spirit than by our unconscious needs and fears.

This kind of suspicion, far from being a threat to faith, can actually be a liberating experience. Take for example conscience as depicted by Thomas Aquinas or Immanuel Kant and the super-ego as depicted by Freud. Freud identifies conscience with the super-ego. Most Christian theologians and psychologists will reject that identification as reductionist and spiritually dangerous. Before doing so, however, we should be ready to concede that it is all too easy for Christians to mistake the super-ego for conscience. It can indeed be liberating to realise that many of our guilt feelings have little or nothing to do with conscience understood as an adult should understand it.

Take for example someone who has been brought up in an atmosphere saturated with the work ethic. Such a person may experience a sense of guilt if he or she sits down to read a newspaper or watch television. Or think of the sense of guilt which can afflict us after the death of a close relative when we reflect on all we could have done for them but did not. Or think of the sense of guilt that some parents feel when their children fail to come up to their expectations, or when the children reject their parents' system of values. Freud's theory of the super-ego may in these cases be the best explanation of guilt-feelings for which there is no rational justification.

It was Freud's aim through psychoanalysis to relieve the pressure of the super-ego upon the ego. As Iris Murdoch puts it, Freud speaks within 'the context of a scientific therapy which aims not at making people good but at making them workable'. Clearly, a Christian theology of conscience will need to aspire to something more than that; though it should be grateful for being alerted to the punitive and sometimes vicious character of the super-ego, and for being warned to suspect theories which treat conscience more or less as a diagnostic machine which registers right and wrong in the manner of a computer. If, however, one insists on employing the model of a computer, one should remember that splendidly laconic dictum of an American computer expert: 'garbage in, garbage out'.

This brings me to the question of the educated conscience.

The individual conscience begins its life as pure potentiality. It is like Aristotle's *tabula rasa*, or blank sheet, waiting to be inscribed by the outside world. The early inscriptions will be simple, indeed crude, expressions of approval or rebuke, and it will not be until the lessons learned from these early expressions are internalised that one can properly speak of conscience. I recognise, of course, that individual consciences can function at various levels of maturity, and that is a topic I am glad to leave to psychologists. What I wish to consider here is the relationship between the individual conscience and the culture within which that conscience is educated. Under 'culture' I include, of course, religious influences and church traditions.

To speak of conscience is to speak of freedom. Freedom of conscience is universally recognised, at least in theory, as one of the most basic human rights. John Stuart Mill gave it its classical formulation when he wrote, 'The only purpose for which power can be rightfully exercised over any member of a civilised community, against his will, is to prevent harm to others. His own good, either physical or moral, is not a sufficient warrant.' The Second Vatican Council's *Declaration on Religious Liberty* reflected Mill's dictum when it taught that human freedom is to be 'respected as far as possible, and curtailed only when and insofar as necessary'.

Conscience functions through acts of interpretation. It must register norms, laws, customs and injunctions on the one hand, and concrete situations on the other. This is a difficult, complex and often wearying procedure. Hence there is always a temptation either to abandon the whole business and live an ethical hand-to-mouth existence, or else to leave to others the prerogative of deciding what is right and what is wrong. Whether this is done in state or in church, it is a profoundly unethical act. Hermann Goering once remarked, 'I have no conscience. My conscience is called Adolf Hitler.' Politically such a view makes the superman the super-ego of the nation. The leader takes on the conscientious burdens of the people. Religious men and women might be expected to be among the first to denounce this totalising of ethics along with politics. Unfortunately this has not always been the case. As Dostoyevsky showed in his story of the Grand Inquisitor, it is unhappily possible to do the same in the name of God and religion. Dostoyevsky's story within a story is one of the most powerful statements about conscience to be found anywhere in literature, because it does not concern itself merely with spiritual and political tyranny. Rather, it portrays freedom of conscience as a burden as well as a gift which is necessary for the following of Christ.

In the story, Christ appears in Seville at the height of the Inquisition's activities. The people flock to him and he is arrested and imprisoned. On the night of his arrest the Grand Inquisitor, an old man of nearly ninety, visits the prisoner in his cell. What follows is the Inquisitor's monologue, for the prisoner does not speak. 'Why have you come to interfere with us?' the old man demands of his captive. 'Was it not you who said so often in those days, "I shall make you free? ... For fifteen centuries we've been troubled by this freedom." Although there is nothing so seductive to man as freedom of conscience, there is also nothing more agonising. Man has no more agonising anxiety than to find someone to whom he can hand over with all speed the gift of freedom with which the unhappy creature is born. Instead of taking possession of human freedom you multiplied it and burdened the spiritual kingdom of man with its sufferings for ever. You wanted man's love freely given so that he should follow you freely, fascinated and captivated by you ... having only your image before him for guidance. But did it never occur to you that he would at last reject and call in question even your image and your truth, if he were weighed down by so fearful a burden as freedom of choice? ... We have [therefore] corrected your great work; for who is to wield dominion over men if not those who have taken possession of their consciences ...?'

The sustained and biting irony of this famous chapter in *The Brothers Karamazov* is an indictment of any system of government, civil or ecclesiastical, which attempts to take over the functions of conscience in the name of a higher authority. States have the right to impose laws on their citizens and to enforce their external observance. The state, however, is a secular body with no jurisdiction over consciences and no duties towards religion except to ensure its freedom. In the past the church was often either established by the state or else it worked with the state in an alliance of equals. Dostoyevsky's story envisages the latter case, in which the Inquisition acted with the authority of both church and state.

In a pluralistic society no one church has the right to act as a kind of official corporate conscience of the state. Politicians and civil servants have to work out their own moral standards in the actual carrying out of their duties. Churches and similar bodies have, of course, the same right as anyone else in a democracy to campaign for causes which they value. Churches which produced no pro-phetic voices ready, for example, to speak out on behalf of the poor and the neglected in society could hardly be said to be living up to their calling.

Any church which has peremptory views on certain moral issues and which is reluctant to admit shadings or ambiguities in these issues needs to take special care of the manner in which it seeks to influence public opinion. Some moral campaigns are marked by a ruthlessness and intolerance of dissent which are very far from Christlike. The campaigners seem to think that their heartfelt con-viction of being in the right licenses them to ride roughshod over the conscientious convictions of others. Freedom of conscience is meaningless unless it entails freedom to be wrong in the estimation of others. (I am of course speaking of matters not covered by the law of the land.)

Conscience has a right to freedom within churches themselves. Whenever freedom of conscience comes up for discussion in the Roman Catholic church, there will often be someone who says, 'Yes, but it must be an informed conscience.' Everything here de-pends on what is meant by the phrase 'informed conscience'. It is sometimes used to describe a conscience which happens to be in agreement with official teaching on some matter. The implication of this is that freedom of conscience is theoretical only; since the church claims to teach in the name, and with the authority, of God, it is the duty of conscience to bring itself into alignment with offi-cial teaching. The authoritarian view is rarely expressed quite as crudely as this; but even when it is expressed with more nuance and greater subtlety, it often manages to suggest a policy of having one's cake and eating it: certainly you have freedom of conscience, but you must see to it that your conscience comes up with the same conclusions as those of the Congregation for the Doctrine of the Faith.

Properly understood, an informed, or, as I should prefer to call it, an educated, conscience is one which has carefully pondered the conclusions and the arguments put forward, from whatever source, before it reaches its own authentic convictions. Public debate is an important educator of conscience. Everybody loses, therefore, when public debate degenerates into raw abuse, and when people's good faith is questioned. There is no cause so holy or so morally elevated that it can afford to dismiss the voices raised against it.

As Werner Jeanrond points out elsewhere in this book, our ethical situation in the modern world has become ever more complex. Technology, for example, is giving rise to moral dilemmas for which there are few precedents in the past. Dr Jeanrond's conclusion is that 'no approach to ethics which deserves to be called critical can escape participating in the public discussion of ethical principles'. The participation of which he speaks belongs to the very process by which we achieve our ethical standards (or by which we inform our consciences, if that terminology is preferred). Participation in discussion promotes the sort of moral autonomy which Kant believed to be so necessary. In terms of conscience it facilitates the educational process whereby we internalise what we are discussing.

In this connection we should distinguish, though not separate, ethical discussion from the education of conscience. Ethical discussion can remain detached, academic – in short an intellectual exercise; whereas the education of conscience is an existential business which involves me in making decisions that give effect to whatever ethical convictions I may have arrived at. I say this in full awareness of the Liberation critique which gives primacy to action over reflection.

Liberation theology is itself an excellent example of what happens when men and women allow themselves to be ethically confronted by the plight of the poor and the oppressed. They see what they have always seen and yet have not seen. The education of conscience is often a matter of seeing something familiar in a new light. This becomes possible only when we have freed ourselves from the neurotic demands of the super-ego or perhaps from the obsessive concerns of some religious traditions. A conscience is only as good and as true as its sensibilities and sensitivities.

Ireland in the first decades after the foundation of the state offers a case in point. Professor Joseph Lee in his recently published book *Ireland 1912-1985* remarks that 'A morbid preoccupation with occasions of sin in dance halls [dominated] pastoral pronouncements through the twenties and thirties'. He goes on to make the important point that preoccupation with sex conveniently diverted attention away from other tenets of Christian morality. 'It was as if a rigorous sexual morality was felt to compensate for a more relaxed concept of other moralities' such as violence, perjury, and deceit in commercial and legal transactions.

Perhaps the most damaging feature of a conscience which is obsessively concerned with one restricted area of morality is that the obsession drains away the energies which are needed to power attention to other areas. The ethical complexities of life in the world today are such that we need all our energies not merely to respond to new challenges but also to preserve a balance of attention to all the competing challenges.

The Canadian theologian Gregory Baum has written a sobering and at times amusing account of a conference on 'Theology in the Americas: 1975' which was held in Detroit in that year. The original intention was to bring Latin American and North American theologians together. Preparatory discussion groups were set up, and in a very short time the agenda for the conference was in serious trouble, largely over its omissions. The upshot was that when the conference met, the participants included not merely North and South Americans but also Blacks, Chicanos and Feminists. The Latin Americans worked from the basis of class and economic analysis. The Blacks claimed that this overlooked racist issues. The Chicanos felt that the Latin Americans were too sophisticated to appreciate their simpler and more popular religion. The Feminists advanced the case against sexism. Each group had preoccupations which could be oppressive to the others. The Latin Americans and the Blacks were convicted of sexism. Some of the Feminists had black servants, and so on. Everybody had something to say about the white, male North Americans. Baum's comment is apt:

> It is a temptation for Christians, especially if they are heirs of a doctrine of total depravity ... of the human being, to fall into masochistic self-accusations and indulge in protracted convulsions of guilt. Some participants occasionally fell into this trap. They

were willing to identify themselves remorsefully as enemy and oppressor. A few men even wanted to get together to develop a theological theory appropriate to their own situation ... The wish of the few to sit together meant that they had not yet fully grasped the message of the conference that this is exactly what the American world is: the few white males sitting together and planning society.

Baum goes on to remark that 'the last thing the struggling communities want is to see us indulge in masochistic self-denunciations'. They want our solidarity in their struggle.

This is surely excellent advice; though I cannot help thinking that Baum is here giving an extrovert judgement suitable to the temperament of extroverts. The more introverted among us may not find it quite as easy to deal with our guilt-feelings so constructively. Political theologians of any kind, whether Marxist, Feminist or Black, occupy the high moral ground in relation to those they see as colluding, in however indirect a way, with an oppressive situation. In this respect they share a psychological advantage with fundamentalists. One instinctively quails before a prophet conscious of possessing a just cause who advances upon one with the light of rectitude in his or her eyes, proclaiming in a loud and peremptory voice: 'We talk, you listen.' Prophecy should be uncomfortable, but, as St Paul indicated, the discomfort should lead not to irritation, resentment or self-recrimination, but to conversion. We need prophets of every kind both to prime and to educate our consciences; but one must hope that the prophets will have learned from the mistakes of the past and will refrain from making unscrupulous appeals to the super-ego, no matter how just or urgent their cause may be. Deliberate attempts to induce guilt-feelings can be counterproductive, because they easily paralyse the will to change things, and they may actually promote an ethical opting out. After all, one well-tried way of dealing with a nagging conscience is simply to ignore it.

I have quite deliberately avoided using the word 'sin' up to this point. By introducing it now I intend to signal a change of direction and perspective. Unlike such words as guilt, crime, felony or misdemeanour, sin is an exclusively theological word and, moreover, one which when correctly understood is actually a very hopeful one. It has, I need hardly say, been secularised, sensationalised, and robbed of its own proper meaning. Tabloid newspapers like to use it because it somehow heightens the drama of the sleazy activities which they manage both to condemn and to describe with equal gusto, thus adding the spice of hypocrisy to what might otherwise be the banal recitation of unconventional sexual arrangements and antics. The fact that the phrase 'living in sin' is not normally used in reference to the habitual misuse of power or the habitual conduct of shady business deals is another reminder, should we need it, that obsessive concern with one area of morality is normally exercised at the expense of other possibly far more important areas.

Sin, then, is not a straightforward synonym for wrongdoing. It implies a damaged relationship with God which only God can put right. Christian revelation is centrally concerned with divine forgiveness and acceptance in spite of the worst that human beings can do. It accepts the human condition as fractured and it speaks of healing. It agrees with Pascal's estimate of humanity as the glory and the scandal of the universe. It sees all offence as remediable, and it locates the remedy in the life, death and resurrection of Christ. It proclaims that the Holy Spirit is sent into the world and into the human heart as an earnest of God's will to reconcile all things to himself.

Kant holds out before us the highest and purest of ethical principles; but he has nothing to say about where we are to find the supports and energies needed for pursuing our pure sense of duty. He has even less to say to us about failure, repentance, forgiveness and newness of life. He was a sworn foe not only of heteronomy but also of mysticism and devotion. God, for Kant, is encountered only through acts of the good will in pursuit of the fulfilment of one's duties. The most appropriate comment I know on Kantian moralism was made by the Scottish theologian John Baillie: 'Some people have just enough religion to make them desperately miserable.'

To Freud the word sin was meaningless. Conscience is a neurotic condition calling for relief. Freud was, however, well aware that in the process called transference which occurs during psychoanalysis, when the patient displaces on to the analyst the positive and negative feelings originally associated with parents and others who have had a significant influence on the patient's emotional life, there is often an implicit plea for forgiveness which, in Freud's own words, would be a call for unlimited transference. 'And now, just suppose I said to a patient: "I, Professor Sigmund Freud, forgive thee thy sins." What a fool I should make of myself.'

'Unlimited transference' is a thought-provoking metaphor for the doctrine of forgiveness which lies at the heart of the Christian experience. I say 'metaphor' because, important as the psychological dimension of forgiveness is, it is a by-product of something far more important. To ask for divine forgiveness is not simply to seek relief for a troubled conscience. It is a recognition that something is amiss which needs putting right. This is where the word sin contributes something which is absent in all the other words for unethical behaviour, such as crime, felony or misdemeanour. Its root metaphor in both Hebrew and Greek is 'missing the mark', 'falling short of the target', 'failing to find the right road'. The image is one of misdirection, with the implication that a return to the right road is always possible because God is a God of new beginnings.

The Christian doctrine of grace is first and foremost a statement that God takes the initiative in any process which makes human beings pleasing to him. Creatures can do nothing to put God in their debt. The sixteenth-century debate about the process by which men and women become righteous in the sight of God (viz. justification) does not divide Christians today in the way it did then. Martin Luther's controlling insight was the conviction that only grace, appropriated through faith, can give human beings their good standing with God. No deed, however good, can win God's saving love; for it is already given. Ethical behaviour is the result not the cause of salvation. Although Catholics and Protestants appeared in the past to disagree radically over the question of faith and good works, today it can be seen that the Reformers and the Council of Trent were approaching the question with different presuppositions and were using different types of language. What matters is the shared conviction that God forgives the sinner who repents and seeks forgiveness.

Divine forgiveness has been seen from the earliest days of Christianity as being utterly gratuitous. There is no contractual element attached to it. There is the injunction to sin no more and to forgive others as one has been forgiven oneself. Divine forgiveness of sin stems, not from God's omniscience, but from his love and compassion. It does not detract from human freedom and is not based on the slogan 'To understand all is to forgive all', which in the last analysis is an expression of determinism. It is not because God understands all that he forgives. The Christian doctrine of sin accepts the existence of human freedom and responsibility, in spite of the mysterious character of both. There is objectively something to be forgiven and not merely something which can in every case be explained and palliated by reference to genes, glands, conflicts with parents, and so on. As an anonymous reviewer in the *Times Literary Supplement* remarked some years ago about some sociological trends of the time, goats are not sheep from a deprived background.

Forgiveness is a radical act. It 'is not a forgetfulness of the past, it is the risk of a future other than the one imposed by the past or by memory'. That is why forgiveness is liberating. The Christian insight, so emphasised by Martin Luther, that forgiveness precedes virtue is psychologically as well as theologically sound. The classical scholar, Maurice Bowra, wrote somewhere that whereas it is sometimes said that the good person is a happy person, the Greeks believed that the happy person is likely to be a good person. Perhaps that insight lies at the heart of the difference between the super-ego and conscience. The superego produces misery and even sickness. A conscience which never loses faith in forgiveness can convict its possessor of guilt without destroying the peace and joy which are indispensable to beginning a new chapter. Indeed Karl Barth portrays the felt need of forgiveness as an indispensable prerequisite for encountering God. His words are quite startling: 'The mature and well-balanced man ... who has never been lamed and broken and half-blinded by the scandal of his life, is as such the existentially godless man.'

My eye was recently caught by a newspaper headline which proclaimed that athletes convicted of taking drugs 'should not be forgiven'. The writer appears to have meant that they should never be allowed to compete again in major athletic contests. I am far from condoning drug-taking by athletes, but I am often surprised by the finality and ferocity of the language used in condemnation of those who have offended and, what is possibly more to the point, have had the bad luck to be detected. The secular world often seems to be uneasy with the very notion of repentance and forgiveness.

By way of conclusion I would like to return to the subject of conscience, this time considering it in the light of the Christian revelation of sin and redemption. Not long ago I came across an article on conscience which stated that our aim ought to be to produce in ourselves a 'sensitively alert conscience, dependable in every question of moral significance, reacting quickly and weighing accurately all the factors involved'. I find that description as intimidating as it is unrealistic. The writer could be describing a state-of-the-art diagnostic machine straight from Silicon Valley, were it not for the phrase 'sensitively alert' which suggests that it should also be wagging its tail. What about the ambiguities of so many moral situations; and what about the ambivalence of so many of our moral responses?

We tend to talk about conscience as if it were a thing apart instead of being of a piece with our whole personality. Conscience is the mind and heart as they relate to conduct, and therefore it is linked to the imagination just as vitally as it is to the speculative reason. Wordsworth in *The Prelude* describes imagination as 'Reason in her most exalted mood'. Imagination is able to see behind and beyond what appears. It has a feel for metaphor, symbol, analogy and for many-levelled meaning. It can see the universal in the particular by intuition. It is sensitive to nuances and to conditions which discursive reason may overlook.

Moral response may be more profoundly influenced by how we picture the world around us than by how we reason about it. In war people are schooled to see some of their fellow human beings as enemies and to act accordingly. It is the imagination that sanctions the violence which in other circumstances would be judged barbaric. In warfare, conscience learns to follow imagination, and perhaps it is poets who can best see what is happening and who consequently cry out in warning. Whatever reason may say about the just war, a healthy imagination will warn of the corrupting influence of the violence which is entailed.

The savage beauty of Wilfrid Owen's war poetry, so magnificently reflected in the music of Benjamin Britten's *War Requiem*, gives a striking picture of conscience as imagination. Looking at the carnage around him Owen reflects on the burial of a comrade:

> Are limbs, so dear-achieved, are sides,
> Full-nerved – still warm – too hard to stir?
> Was it for this the clay grew tall?

In the poem *Strange Meeting* two soldiers from opposing sides meet after death on the battlefield:

> 'Strange friend,' I said, 'here is no cause to mourn.'
> 'None,' said the other, 'save the undone years,
> The hopelessness.'
> ....
> 'I am the enemy you killed, my friend.
> I knew you in this dark; for so you frowned
> Yesterday through me as you jabbed and killed.
> I parried; but my hands were loath and cold,
> Let us sleep now...'

In those poems we have conscience in its reflective, imaginative mode, piercing the carapace of militarised patriotism and reaching the inner and deepest truth of things.

War may seem a rather extreme instance of my point about the role of imagination in the function of conscience. Let me therefore take an instance nearer to everyday life. A blind man was begging in a city park. Someone approached and asked him what his takings were like. The blind man shook a nearly empty tin. His visitor said to him 'let me write something on your card'. The blind man agreed. That evening the visitor returned. 'Well, how did you do today?' The blind man showed him a tin full of money and asked 'What on earth did you write on the card?' 'Oh', said the other, 'I merely wrote, "Today is a spring day, and I am blind."'

The old saying that conscience is the voice of God can be interpreted in two ways. One can take it as saying that God the creator has endowed our species, *homo sapiens*, with the ability to tell right from wrong and thus to serve the creator. I do not think that that interpretation comes anywhere near doing justice to all the inner facts. With George Tyrrell I believe that conscience is a direct manifestation of the presence of God within every man and woman, whether or not they believe in God. Tyrrell frequently quoted a phrase from Matthew Arnold to the effect that God is primarily experienced as 'a power not ourselves that makes for righteousness'. Tyrrell, who once wrote that 'morality divorced from mysticism is a lean sort of religion', believed that conscience properly understood is far more than 'a merely moral or ethical experience'; it is also 'a religious and mystical experience'. That, in my view, is the true meaning of the statement that conscience is the voice of God.

Further Reading

C. Ellis Nelson (ed), Conscience: Theological and Psychological Perspectives, New York, 1973.

I. Murdroch, *The Sovereignty of Good* , London, 1985.

B. Mitchell, *Law, Morality, and Religion in a Secular Society*, Oxford, 1970.

C. Floristan & C. Duqoc (eds), *Forgiveness, Concilium*, April 1986.

CHAPTER 5

Ethics Human and Christian

Vincent MacNamara

Human and Christian? Human or Christian? Perhaps the title of this essay, like that of some others in the series, should have a question mark. There is a general assumption that Christianity does have a proper or particular ethic – designer ethics specially and uniquely spun from Christian beliefs and stories. A recent work begins with the assertion, 'The foundations of Christian ethics must be evangelical foundations; or, to put it more simply, Christian ethics must arise from the Gospel of Jesus Christ. Otherwise it could not be *Christian* ethics' (O'Donovan). When doubt is cast upon this, when a question is raised about a specific Christian ethic, the reaction, I find, is one of surprise. The query invariably comes: if there is no specific Christian ethic what is the point of being a Christian? That indicates the depth of the conviction of many Christians that the point of Christianity is that it has a special ethic for the world. Indeed we do, all of us, quite casually refer to Christian values or to the notion of a Christian society. We are much less sure, however, when we are pressed about what precisely we mean by this. Most of us struggle a bit then and often collapse into vague and fluffy talk about love or agape.

It has to be acknowledged immediately that there are difficult problems about the very terms 'Christian' and 'human' when applied to ethics. I cannot pursue the details of that here. I take it that what, roughly speaking, people are interested in is some reflection on the relation of the ethical tradition which is thought to derive from Christianity (and might be seen to be enshrined in church morality) and the ethical tradition and concerns of those who do not subscribe to any religious tradition. The distinction clearly is a rough one (whose Christian ethic? which human morality?) but I think it is manageable. (The terms 'ethics' and 'morality' have a technical meaning among philosophers. But they are used indiscriminately by Christian ethicists and I follow that loose usage.)

Many Christians consider what is called human morality to be inadequate. Barth declared that the very notion of human ethics corresponds exactly with the notion of sin. Bonhoeffer in a chapter which echoes our title – 'The "Ethical" and the "Christian" as a Theme' – contrasts ethical endeavour with the commandment of God. Richard Niebuhr classically set up the problem in his *Christ and Culture*: is it Christ against culture, Christ of culture, Christ above culture, Christ and culture in paradox, Christ transforming culture? Christian churches generally give the impression of regarding themselves as having some hegemony of ethics, some special proprietorship of it, and of regarding others as not doing it very well, not being really serious about it or merely seeking to legitimate permissiveness.

Humanists on the other hand frequently look on what has passed for Christian ethics as inhuman. Not so long ago in a volume on Christian ethics and modern philosophy, the philosopher Nowell-Smith began his article with the words 'The central thesis of this paper is that religious morality is infantile' – infantile not so much or not only in its content but above all in its meaning, structure and general conception and as favouring irresponsibility and destroying the rightful autonomy of the subject. And it comes as a shock to find that there were philosophers who regarded Christian ethics as cruel, harsh and unloving.

So, a Christian ethic? Perhaps we should pause on that very conjunction of words. We take so much for granted here and it might be useful to broaden the perspective. If there be such an animal as Christian ethics, it is an instance of a wider phenomenon – religious ethics. There are other religious moralities – Jewish, Moslem, Buddhist, animist etc. Should we expect the incidence of morality with religion? Religion and morality are formally distinct. They have different concerns, different objects. They deal with different clusters of questions. How do they encounter one another? What is the move from one to the other? In theory, at least, it is possible to be religious without being moral. And, contrariwise, it is possible to be moral without being religious – and that is something with which a Christian ethic must reckon.

The fact is that most religions do have an ethic, do in some way incorporate the ethical dimension into themselves. But they do so in quite different ways. They are greatly influenced by their general cosmogony. They have different views of the origin of morality. They give it a different significance. They incorporate it variously in their systems and weight it differently with respect to other elements of that system. All this is the concern of the discipline of Comparative Religious Ethics. To advert to such considerations sets our own question in clearer focus. It sharpens our wits. It questions assumptions that may have lain unexamined in the expression 'Christian ethics'. It might provoke us to pursue issues which greatly affect the contours of our lives. Why is Christianity an ethical religion? How, in what way and to what extent? Where does it get its morality from? How do we as Christians situate morality? How do we conceive of the relationship between God and morality? What is the significance of moral life for salvation? – and what salvation? Can we be moral and with what means? How does our Christian anthropology – and in particular our view of good and evil in our human constitution – affect our view of the whole moral enterprise?

It is because Christianity answers such questions in its own way that there is inescapably something that can be called Christian morality. It is a commonplace to say that biblical religion is ethical and biblical ethics religious. So too for Christians today the whole context of morality is religious or theological. It is shaped and interpenetrated by issues of origins, cosmogony, salvation. Such greatly affect Christian self-perception and enter into Christian daily life and conversation – I confess to Almighty God / I forgive you your sins in the name of the Father / If you love me keep my commandments / We love others in God / We see Christ in the neighbour / This murder is a crime against the sacred law of God / I have discerned this in the Spirit / I want to make my peace with God / Christ is the norm of morality. So much so that, on the one hand, Christians often have difficulty in allowing any autonomy to the moral dimension of life and, on the other, many virtually reduce religion to morality.

Such matters are not usually the focus when the question of Christian morality is mooted. The focus is usually the content of morality, moral norms, and whether Christianity necessarily proposes something different from other moral systems. But it should be obvious that the context – the particular way in which Christianity brings together religious myth and morals, as distinct from other forms of religious ethics – is of considerable importance. Christians live more fully and do a better service to both morality and religion if they are aware of how they modify and transform moral conscious-ness in their religion. If there is a charge that religious morality is infantile it may well be that it is in our general conception of the context of morality that we are most vulnerable.

So let me point a little further to issues in the general context of Christian ethics – language, symbols, conceptions – about which we need to be careful. The shadow side of morality is sin. That is a flash-point for many. Here each of us brings together elemental Christian notions in our individual murky brew. Failure, sin, guilt, alienation, punishment are dominant elements for many. We do have important things to say about God as the overall context of our lives and our morality – origin, sustainer, model, last end, sal-vation. How we say this, and the symbols we use to make our raids on the inaccessible mystery, may be more or less successful and life giving. Two great biblical scenes haunt us – the giving of the deca-logue and the final judgment scene in Matthew 25. They are attempts to say something about the curiously intricate and many-faceted relationship of religion and morality. But the tradition, generally speaking, read the symbol too sharply and produced an awesome system of God as Creator of the moral order, of morality as law, of sin as crime, of punishment as satisfaction to offended majesty, of heaven as reward merited by a life of moral rectitude. It is not surprising that it was along this particular fault-line of the relationship of God/morality/salvation that the greatest upheaval in the history of Christianity occurred in the Reformation. Not sur-prising. The deepest concerns of the human spirit do not easily yield their secrets to our puny thoughts – which is why it is enlight-ening and humbling to do one's ethics in dialogue with the great religious traditions. An overarching symbol for the wedding of religion and morality is not easily come to.

There were, of course, kindlier tendencies in the tradition – sin may be more sickness than crime and God more healer than judge – but in general they were choked off by a harsher element. What is important to remember is that our symbols are just that: they are in-accurate, incomplete, perhaps more distorting of the mystery than revealing. They are, of course, time- and culture-conditioned. And it can hardly have escaped notice how relentlessly and triumphantly male they are. They are not wearing very well. The Christian community, it seems to me, is doing its own rethinking.

What I am pointing to, however skimpily, are the implications of our understanding of a Christian ethic. We bring together here two sets of ideas, two languages, the language of ethics – right, wrong, duty, obligation, law – and the language of Christian salvation – grace, justification, sin. How we do so – in contradistinction to other systems – has immense implications for our sense of God, of morality, of ourselves. It is difficult terrain: it has been referred to as the theological frontier of ethics. It engages us in what Bernard Williams has called 'a baffling semantic task'. The stakes are high. If a question can be raised about whether Christian ethics enhances life and encourages responsibility it can be raised most fundamentally here – more so than on the issue of content.

I pass now to the issue of content. What are Christians to do? Is what is expected from them different from what is expected from others? What code of morality do we have? How do we know what to do? It seems to be a hankering of most religions that their morality should be esoteric – some special emanation from God. And one very entrenched version of Christian ethics is that we have a revealed ethic, that we have received from God by whatever process – however we understand revelation – moral information that is prescriptive and authoritative. Of this, it is said, the Bible is the primary depository. This – with greater or less emphasis – is a firmly held conviction of all the Christian churches. Much of their ethical thinking has been shaped by the simple syllogism, 'It says in the Bible ... therefore ...'

Why would we need a special revelation of morality? Two main answers emerge. The first is that because of our impaired and limited human understanding we cannot know the moral way. A qualified version is that we can go some distance in understanding but can do so only with great difficulty and without any kind of certainty – so we need a revelation to clarify and confirm our insights. The second reason adduced is that those who have been called to faith in Christ are called to a new, superior way of living which cannot be known without the special word of God. The first finds classic expression in Barth and Brummer. The second is a constant of Protestant thought but made an impressive appearance in the Catholicism of the forties and fifties.

The critical points about such a revelation ethic are that it can propose a teaching that by definition may not be available to those who do not accept the authority of the Bible, that it does not have to answer at the bar of reason, that it can be demanded although it does not commend itself to common ethical thought, that it does not in the end have to answer the question, why? It takes its stand on saying that 'we should obey God rather than men'. What is in question then is the issue of methodology, how one goes about moral discernment. And this has immense practical implications not only in inner Church life but in our culture and even in our legal decisions. In this country we have had appeal in legal judgements to the authority of biblical morality.

The appeal to the authority of a revealed ethic is some part of the moral methodology of all the Christian churches. And all of them are in crisis: I will not labour the details but will only say here that there are considerable and well-canvassed problems about the direct appeal to a revelation of morality. Problems of a general kind, of the very possibility of an authentic morality in such a context – relating to the charge I referred to earlier that such a morality, so to speak 'from beyond', is inimical to responsible choice. But also problems about plundering the Bible for moral prescriptions. One could easily quote the unease of theologians of all the mainline churches on this point. The net result is that there is a wide distrust of the ethical method of church morality and of talk about a Christian ethic. The consequence has been that some theologians say, in effect, a) that we should simply abandon the Bible as a direct source of moral norms because of the difficulties attendant on such an appeal, and b) that even if we could make such an appeal we would find nothing there that is not available to non-religious morality. Some call this the position of an autonomous ethics within Christianity. Note that this position is a particular way of construing the relationship of religious myth to ethics. It is saying that whatever one means by Christian ethics one does not mean that it is a code which issues directly from a revelation by the deity or that it can be derived solely from the particular world-view of Christianity. It does not deny that there is such a thing as Christian ethics. But the 'Christian' part of that conjunction of words refers rather to the context in which ethics is done, to the final significance of ethics and to the motivation which can be canvassed from the religious story.

This seems to me, as it has seemed to others, unduly pessimistic and a failure to take seriously the dynamics of moral discernment. If our religious myths are our most profound and ultimate framework of meaning, can they be so entirely unrelated to our understanding of action? Moral judgements are not made in a vacuum; they are made by people who see the world in a particular way because they are particular sorts of people. One's reading of the moral landscape, one's evaluative description of the field of action, the responsibility which one experiences in a particular moral situation, all depend on the sort of person one is. They depend on vision, on character – and these in turn depend on the beliefs, stories and symbols that shape one's consciousness and imagination. And so some Christian ethicists try to garner the beliefs which go into the making of the particular Christian consciousness or *Gestalt*: beliefs in a personal God, in human beings as created, in the death and resurrection of Jesus Christ, in the redeeming grace given to us in Christ, in the unity of the human family, in human stewardship, in the covenant love shed abroad in our hearts, and so on – our religious cosmogony. Or perhaps more successfully, they talk about the way in which Christian stories enter into our imagination.

The current rage of talking about Christianity in terms of story is, I think, more than a passing fashion. Dogmatic statements do not capture the imagination or engage the spirit as stories do. They do not get into the bloodstream of an individual or of a people in the same way. Our ballads and our songs are so much more powerful in creating a national consciousness than our Constitution. So too with faith-consciousness. The Jews did not hand down a set of beliefs. They told stories. It was a long story, recounted through the generations. It was a formative one. It made the people with a particular ethos, a common feel about themselves, an attitude to others, a way of looking at the future, a culture. Christians are the heirs to that story but the central event of which they could tell, the life/death/resurrection of Christ, was so strikingly different that they saw themselves as a new creation.

The task of the Christian, as I see it, is to do his/her morality in fidelity to that total story – as someone for whom the conviction has come true that the deepest reality is personal, accepting and forgiving, that life is a gift, that we are of more value than many sparrows, that one does not live on bread alone, that in the man Jesus going quietly to his death is our hope, that in the cross is resurrection. If we could receive all that we would be some way into morality. Some way not only to doing but to seeing. By seeing I mean understanding, judging what one should do, what shape of life is consonant with being a Christian.

These are only hints, a sketch of how we might go about doing ethics as Christians. The argument is that ethos affects ethics and that our particular ethos issues not so much in precise moral rules as in general perspectives, sensibilities, attitudes and awareness that translate themselves into choices in the individual moments of our complex lives. I can only tell you who I am if I tell you my story. And it is only if you can enter into my story that you can understand my stance on some of the basic issues – life, death, success, failure, wholeness, flourishing, love, hope, spirit, world. And all such can at times bear on moral choice.

We are not the first Christians, of course, nor the first who have tried to find the moral way. And so we carry on our discernment in continuity with those who have gone before us. The apostolic community too tried to think its faith into practice. The Bible gives us impressions of them. It gives us the possibility of entering into the imagination of those who experienced the inbreaking of the kingdom in Jesus, who first allowed the story to shape their vision. What is important for us is not that we scavenge in the Bible for moral rules but that we be able to enter into that world of religious and moral meaning, that we allow the biblical text to challenge and change us, to open for us the new and wider world of meaning that arises out of the experience of the divine irruption into history in Jesus Christ. And that we today creatively engage with the same story.

The heart of that biblical ethos, the great overarching metaphor there, is that the ground of our being is God the father of our Lord Jesus Christ, one who knows us thoroughly and loves us with a patient and forgiving love – each of us, all of us and together. Jesus Christ was anchored in that story. That was what shaped his perspective and the natural outcome of it was the highest point of biblical ethics, the Sermon on the Mount. 'Kingdom ethics', as Seán Freyne said in his essay. To quote him: 'Ideals such as turning the other cheek, love your enemies, sharing beyond the call of duty all make sense only when they are striven for in the context of a group who share these values and provide the kind of supporting ethos that makes them viable.' Joachim Jeremias has suggested that the reason why the Sermon on the Mount seems odd and so highly idealistic to us is that we have torn it out of its proper context. That context is the story, the story of the kingdom, of the forgiving and faithful love of God. And so Jeremias says that before every demand of the Sermon on the Mount we should place the great story-statement, 'you have been forgiven by God'. You have been forgiven and it is only in the inner experience of and confidence in this that we can make sense of the suggestion that we might now find our happiness and flourishing in forgiving others. Or, as John puts it in his First Letter, since God has first loved us we ought to love one another. That is, since to be a Christian is centrally to believe in, to experience and to be emotionally changed by the conviction of that love, we might be rid of the loneliness and inferiority that make us a threat to others and make them a threat to us. That will clear our heads – or our hearts – and enable us to *see*.

I am not talking about the Bible as a source of moral norms or about the sermon as law but about the attitudes and qualities of mind and heart that are consonant with the kingdom. We can give meaning to the talk of kingdom values: they are the preferences, the goods – and then the choices – that fit with the kingdom story or with its family of stories. The overarching, though not the only, symbol is God's forgiving and long-suffering love. Perhaps talk of love can be too simple: it does not absolve us from the hard graft of trying to discover its expression in the particular light of our kingdom vision. Not only, and perhaps not principally, in the one-to-one relationship but in social and political action, in overturning structures that are antithetical to love, in creating a society and environment in which God's creative peace reigns.

What matters then is that Christians do their ethics in fidelity to their story. That is the task: even in terms of content that gives an acceptable meaning to the notion of a Christian ethic. Kingdom values may also be the values of a particular human ethic. That does not matter. Christians need not feel any compulsion to prove that they have a different or superior ethic – there is more in the great secular traditions of truth, justice, liberty and equality than we can contend with. But it seems to me right to say that if Christians discern in the climate of their religious vision they may at times find themselves making choices that are justified precisely in terms of such a vision and that may not make sense to some versions of secular ethics. But so much here depends on the term of comparison and even on such basic issues as how we understand the range of morality and define a moral act.

What then of human morality? There are obviously varieties of such morality: the history of ethical thought is the history of such variety. It is reasonable however to concentrate on what unites much of human morality rather than on what divides it. The great bulk of it arises out of a central concern about the person – something related to the dignity, inviolability and autonomy of the person with its related notions of equality, fairness and impartiality. Combined with at least some sketchy recognition that there is a structure of sorts to human beings which suggests the implications attaching to the recognition of such dignity and autonomy and which employs especially notions of welfare and harm. So we have ethical theories built on respect for the person, on human rights, on human needs, on impartiality, on benevolence, on the virtues necessary for successful and satisfactory community living. All of which say that life cannot be lived arbitrarily, or lived any way your fancy takes you but that our very existence with others is a claim on us and that there are elementary consequences of such a claim – what has been called the minimum content of natural law. And which say that beyond that there are responses of generosity and unselfishness which are at least to be admired if not always prescribed.

What matters for our purposes is that this recognition of the other – however it be elaborated in the different ethical theories – is sufficient to generate moral obligation and to indicate its main lines. This is one of the most precious insights of the human community. It is the central arch in our civilisation. It is the source of some of our most important institutions. It is listened to when we send food to Ethiopia, when we campaign for the end of Apartheid, when we question the cover-up of judicial institutions, when we support the self-determination of peoples, when we defend the rights of minorities, when we say (with the medieval canonists) that the king is under no man but under God and the law i.e. the moral law, when we say with Aquinas that unjust laws savour of lawlessness rather than of law, when we try to undo the vicious circle of power, property and privilege and create equality of educational opportunities and equality before the law.

This great spontaneous human thrust – the medieval Christian philosophers referred to it as our sharing in the reason of God – must be acknowledged by Christian communities. However they understand their moralities – and here I pick up the concerns of the early part of this paper – it must be in a way that does not ignore or impair or devalue this independent moral sense. That does not devalue what one may call the autonomy of morality. Religious people will find the ultimate grounding and significance of morality – as of all else – metaphysically. But morality, without religion, has its own internal structure and coherence. It makes its own claim. To acknowledge it is to be human, to fail to do so cannot be Christian.

Morality, human or Christian, then, is centrally about recognising the claim of the other and acting on it, responding out of the inner conviction of the value of the other. This is the very core, the guts of moral response. There are, as educationalists have well demonstrated, stages of moral development. It takes time to appreciate precisely moral considerations, to make a precisely moral response. It takes much less time of course to appreciate other considerations e.g. considerations of reward and punishment, of acceptance and rejection. They are at opposite ends of the moral journey. Few of us – human or Christian – reach a totally authentic morality. But it is important to know where we might be heading.

A particular tension may arise between human and Christian ethics about moral motive. Not all doing good is moral doing. To do good, to avoid evil is something. If people could be persuaded to help the underdeveloped, to give half of what they possess to the poor, to stop killing one another, it would be wonderful. That is some level of moral consideration. But if we are concerned not only about what happens but about those who make it happen, then why people act, out of what kind of consideration, with what reason or motive, is a matter of importance. It is because particularly in Christian ethics there is a danger that precisely moral considerations will be by-passed that I dwell on this. Reward, sanction, fear can move and deter. They may be necessary to prevent evil. They may be the only thing that works in some situations. But while one cannot say that they are inimical to morality – they may be the first move to it – they are not yet morality. It is here that the subsumption of morality into religion is most dangerous. It is here that religion can most easily gobble up morality and inhibit true growth. True Christian morality, I believe, can only be one in which this great, God-given architecture of moral understanding is experienced and respected. In this sense you can say that we must be human before we are Christians.

If then morality involves the notions of responsibility, of autonomy, if it is about seeing as much as doing, if it is about the recognition of a claim, there are important pointers for what might be called church morality. Morality cannot be about obedience. The claim of morality is the claim of the truth and a true moral response is some recognition of that claim. It is about learning respect. It is about the education of our desires.

Moral systems are precisely that – systems. It has been a concern of all of them not to be a collection of disparate commands and prohibitions but to find some unifying principle. The Christian tradition finds in love its central principle. If human morality is minimally a concern to treat others with respect, to acknowledge their rights and if, in some versions at least, it is about bringing about the greatest good for others, then they clearly have much in common. The search then is a common one. The questions are the age-old questions: what is it to be a human being, what makes life human, what is the true language of our total conversation with one another, how in our relations with each other can we comport ourselves so as to enhance one another, what kind of society facilitates human flourishing?

About the concepts of love, respect, welfare I make a few brief points. All of them have to be concerned about human goods and needs. Such are of the most varied and subtle kinds – physical, psychological, intellectual, social, religious. Needs of different depths, importance and urgency, needs that must at times yield to needs. But what makes and keeps life human cannot be derived from some metaphysical definition of the human being but can only be discovered in the richness of our common experience: that is why the widest possible canvass is desirable before any definitive statement is made on moral matters. Moral argument or 'proof' is a particularly subtle and sensitive form of argument. It does not admit either of the method or of the certainty of the natural sciences. So Aristotle told us and so it is. The moral appeal is an appeal to one's sense of what it means to be a human being. That is something to which some are more sensitive and finely tuned than others. But no one – no theologian, churchman, economist, doctor, lawyer – has a monopoly on it. It may well be that specialists in any technical field may be the least open to moral judgements in that field. More than anything else there is required human sensitivity and imagination (and I have suggested that there is a typical Christian sensitivity and imagination): the 'undeveloped heart' Mary Midgley has said, is a form of immorality. Nor can the human or Christian search ignore the fact that the ethical enterprise is a common and historical one which takes the past seriously but engages it in an authentic hermeneutic.

To exalt moral experience, however, is to tell only half the story. The slender shaft of moral perception is found in the midst of much else – of darkness, confusion, irrationality, prejudice. Indeed it arises out of the desire to cope with them. We have to face the inhumanity of human beings to one another, to reckon with our personal and institutional violence, to acknowledge with fright the catastrophic disorder that can overtake races and cultures, classes and creeds. We all know the intractability of our hearts, the crazy projections that not only prevent us from doing good but even more fundamentally and more disastrously from seeing right. 'Human beings', says Iris Murdoch, 'are far more complicated and enigmatic and ambiguous than languages or mathematical concepts, and selfishness operates in a much more devious and frenzied manner in our relations with them'. And we know it. It is not our fault. It is how we have been created. It is the human situation. The long and curious growth of our evolution, the very need to survive, the very success in surviving, has left its own dark rings in our biological growth – to assert, to fight, to defend, to claim our ground, to demand our share. Likewise the extraordinarily difficult task of growing from helpless infant to adult with its conflicting needs of independence and acceptance is never resolved. Nor the adult task of the intersecting relationships in which we find ourselves with their constantly attendant penumbra of hopes and fears, of needs and aspirations. So that we who need so much the society of others and who in some place of our spirit recognise that it is in openness to them that we find ourselves are nevertheless constantly threatened by the other. Where there are others, a piece of Eastern wisdom tells us, there is dread. Morality is no mystical matter. It is the struggle to become, to individuate, to allow the self to emerge in the company of selves. So that we can be in the truth with others. The truth, we are told, will make us free. But it is a long way to that harbour of freedom, hugely interesting but at times tortuous and frustrating. The weary on the journey might be assured more often that they are doing well to be as good as they are.

So the struggle that goes on for us is to let the light pervade us, our own light. There is an ancient tradition that being moral is doing what you really and most want to do, that our peace – happiness, *eudaimonia* – lies in dissolving our envies, jealousies and power-needs. I find connections here with the essay of Andrew Mayes and his comments on the proverbial wisdom: 'These men lie in wait for their own blood, they set an ambush for their own lives. Such are the ways of those who gain by violence; it takes away the life of its possessors' (Prov 1:18). 'The integrity of the upright guides them but the crookedness of the treacherous destroys them … the wicked falls by his own wickedness' (11:3,5). And echoes of the Sermon on the Mount. 'Happy are …' Pehaps goodness is not so much doing or getting as allowing – allowing our true selves to emerge. There is a confidence in the tradition to which I belong that grace does not destroy but perfects nature. That seems like a conviction that at the heart of us there is goodness but that it has been overlaid by so much, so much that is an inescapable part of the drama of finding our place in the sun – the fear and anxiety about security and power and possessions, the need to be best and best loved and best remembered. So we fret and crave and fawn and cajole and make fools of ourselves and lose our freedom and our peace. Happy are we if we can find some solvent for the blockages that prevent the emergence of our soul. But it may be that what we consider our demons cannot be cast out – if they are to be cast out and not acknowledged, integrated and redirected – by the difficult path of prayer and fasting but by the even more difficult one of coming to true awareness of ourselves, of befriending our shadows, of holding together the antitheses in our personalities.

As we make our way in the confusion of our lives we should know that reason/conscience is not an unfriendly alien power that is meant to crush our instincts and passions. It is the call of our own personality. It is our own self becoming aware of our underlying pattern: it is a name for organising ourselves, for integration. The best psychology knows that the development of the personaltiy itself imposes rules upon the ego, that the wholeness of the self demands that the ego make sacrifices. What ideally rules us is our own centre: it is our sense of how our nature – our natural structure of needs and desires – works. The life within us suggests the way and seeks to resolve our conflicts in our own favour.

The truth shall make you free. Truth and freedom. Morality involves freedom to see and freedom to do. That would lead us, if we had time, further in the direction of Gabriel Daly's essay. For if authentic morality is genuine appreciation of and response to the claim of others and if reasons and motives are important, there is involved the hope that we can be freed from the super-ego stuff, the pseudo-morality that not only spawns false conscience but coats the best-looking of our actions with the verdigris of false motivation. If the reason why we do things is as important as what we do, if it in fact determines how what we do is to be described from the moral point of view, then the project of morality must deal not only with overtly distorted motives, such as fear of punishment, but with the more insidious ones that operate below the surface of consciousness. But that takes us too far afield now.

Christians find it necessary to put their morality in the wider (religious) frame of reference that for them enshrines the total truth about life and to do their discernment out of that world-view. They are entitled to do so: everyone operates out of some basic religious or philosophical stance, acknowledged or not. They have a view on the ultimate origin, significance and end of morality and its institutions and have their own version of human wholeness and flourishing. Morality for them is shot through with religion. But it should emerge from what has been said in the preceding paragraphs that there is much in the very nature and structure of moral response that human secular morality and related sciences set in relief for us. Christian ethics cannot ignore that. To do so results in a split between religious life and the human growth that is necessary to personal morality and to the development of moral institutions and structures. It often ends in frustration for those who pray and worship well but attend little to the dynamic of the human person. But we can pray well if we are so unaware of who we are and why we are how we are and why we do what we do? Miracles of grace cannot be expected.

Christianity, it has been alleged, has given Eros poison to drink. I take Eros to include the spontaneous and imaginative thrust for all that fulfils the great desires of the human spirit. Remember Blake:

'I went into the Garden of Love
And priests in black gowns were walking their rounds
And binding with briars my joys and desires.'

It need not have poisoned Eros. The medieval Christian philosopher would have told you that there is no more fundamental desire, no deeper longing or Eros than the desire to reach wholeness or perfection, to become a person, to bridge the gap between one's actual and potential self. That for them was what morality was about. Law, obligation, duty – concepts that for us have become central – were for them strictly derived notions, parasitic on something more native, nearer to the human heart – the desire to flourish as a person in the community of persons. A Christian ethic interprets and contextualises that in its own way. To respond to that inner human thrust, to move towards that particular end, the Christian says, is – whether one is explicitly aware of it or not – to reach out to our total meaning and destiny, to yearn for God.

Further Reading:

J. Fuchs, *Christian Morality: The Word Becomes Flesh*, Georgetown Univ Press, Gill and Macmillan, 1987.

V. MacNamara, *The Truth in Love*, Gill and Macmillan, Glazier, 1988.

V. MacNamara, Faith and Ethics, Gill and Macmillan, Georgetown Univ Press, 1985.

M. Midgley, *Heart and Mind: The Varieties of Moral Experience*, Methuen, 1981.

B. Mitchell, *Morality Religious and Secular*, Clarendon, 1980.

O. O'Donovan, *Resurrection and Moral Order: An Outline for Evangelical Ethics*, Inter-Varsity Press, 1986.

G. Outka and J.P. Reeder, Jr, (eds), *Religion and Morality*, Anchor, 1973.

W. Spohn, *What Are They Saying about Scripture and Ethics?*, Paulist, 1984.

CHAPTER 6

The Person, the Patient and the Christian

K. Kearon

There is little doubt that one of the strongest and most persistent themes in the whole of the Christian tradition and back to the Jewish tradition has been the concern with the individual. Human life has always been regarded as sacred. We see it in the decalogue of Moses and throughout the Mosaic law. Any interpretation of the incarnation must at least admit that it expresses God's concern for humanity, expressed not just as concern with the human race, but with individuals, and this was to be a dominant theme of Jesus' preaching and teaching, and a feature of the early church.

So Christians must be concerned, not just with humanity, but with persons, individuals, created by God. Individuals are important, simply by virtue of being persons. This concern has been at the root of the Christian compassion and care for children, for orphans, the sick, the poor, the needy, the dying, those that we today call marginalised. All are special because all are important to God. No one needs any particular ability or gift or attribute to be special – all are important, simply by virtue of being a person.

I think it is true to say that this tradition has been most consistently expressed by Christians in the area of medical care. Hospitals and nursing care have been a constant within the christian tradition since earliest times.

It is on the person as patient that Christianity has focused its expression of care and compassion. Of course this isn't a uniquely Christian tradition – hospitals and care for the sick and dying are features of every major civilisation; in fact it could be said that it is only insofar as it does care for the sick and the dying that a people can be called civilised.

The Christian concern for the patient as person expresses itself across the whole range of medical ethics – issues like autonomy of the patient, consent, the treatment of psychiatric illness and so on are fundamentally concerned with respect for the person; but it is to another set of medical ethical questions that I wish to turn to in this paper – the question of respect for the person at the boundaries of life. When does life begin? When does it end? I propose to explore the question by looking at the state of the discussion first at the end of life, and then at the beginning, and I note and accept the limitations imposed by the title because each of these issues is an enormous field in itself. The title focuses on the issues as posed by and to medicine, and the Christian approach to these issues as found in the field of medicine. I will then conclude with some remarks about a distinctively Christian approach to these issues.

Determining the end of life

Traditionally the absence of pulse and spontaneous respiration was regarded as sufficient for deciding that death had occurred. This was reasonable, since the cessation of respiration and circulation always produced the prompt death of the brain and hence of the person, and similarly death of the brain resulted in the cessation of circulation and respiration. Quite simply, absence of pulse and breathing were sufficient criteria for deciding that death had occurred.

It is only more recently, with the development of medical technology, and particularly with the development of life support machines, that the whole question of determining when death has occurred has been opened up. It is now possible, as we know, to maintain blood circulation artificially, and to resuscitate and maintain breathing well beyond the point where previously death would have occurred. It is also possible to maintain circulation and respiration beyond the point when we would want to say that a person is 'for all intents and purposes' dead.

The new criteria for death that eventually emerged was that of 'brain death'. In 1968 an *ad hoc* Committee of the Harvard Medical School formulated a set of criteria for 'irreversible coma'. I quote a summary of the criteria:

(1) unreceptivity and unresponsivity to 'externally applied stimuli and inner need';
2) absence of spontaneous muscular movements or spontaneous respiration;

(3) no elicitable reflexes.

[A. M. Capron and Leon R. Kees, 'A Statutory Definition of the Standards for Determining Human Death: an Appraisal and a Proposal', in *Death, Dying and Euthanasia,* ed by Dennis J. Horan and David Mall, (Maryland, 1980) p 42-3.]

These brain death criteria are relevant when resuscitative methods have taken the patient beyond the point where death would otherwise have occurred. In other cases the traditional criteria of heartbeat and respiration continue to be used. So therefore, in the borderline areas we are now considering we accept that the absence of brain activity is sufficient criteria for declaring that death has occurred, even though some organic function can be artificially maintained beyond this point. In other words, what we are saying is that today in these areas it is for signs of life in the brain rather than in the other organs that we look.

These criteria have been widely accepted by the medical profession and also very readily by most of the Christian tradition. At least what has been said is that the determining of death is a medical, not a moral or theological question. For example, Pope Pius XII in 1957, while discussing patients who are terminally unconscious, said 'As to the pronouncement of death in certain particular cases, the answer cannot be inferred from religious and moral principles, and consequently, it is an aspect lying outside the competence of the Church.' [Pius XII, *Acta Apostolicae Sedis* 45, November 1957, pp 1057-1033, quoted in T.A. Shannon (ed) *Bioethics* p 179]. Bernard Häring, the Catholic moral theologian, was more explicit: 'I feel that the arguments for the equation of the total death of the person with brain death are fully valid' [B. Häring, *Medical Ethics,* St Paul, Rev ed 1974, p 136]. The conservative Protestant writer, Paul Ramsey, agreed. Accepting the use of brain-orientated criteria for pronouncement of death, he said that proposals for updating the definition of death are, in reality, 'proposals for updating our procedures for determining that death has occurred, for rebutting the belief that machines or treatments are the patient, for withdrawing the notion that artifically sustained signs of life are in themselves signs of life, for telling when we should stop ventilating and circulating the blood of an unburied corpse because there are no longer any vital functions really alive or recoverable in the patient' [Quoted in *Bioethics* p 179]. But if the absence of brain activity is sufficient to determine death, is the opposite true, that the existence of brain activity means that the patient is alive?

To approach that question let me remind you of a very famous court case in the United States – the Karen Quinlan case. Karen Quinlan was a 22-year-old girl who collapsed and ceased breathing for at least two 15-minute periods; she was taken to hospital and gradually became deeply comatose over the next few days. Over a period of time it became apparent that her case was hopeless and that she would never recover. Her father applied to the court to be appointed her guardian, with the power to authorise discontinuance of all extraordinary medical treatment which he was assured was sustaining Karen.

The case was obviously a crucial one. Here was someone who was not brain dead, but was in a very real way 'hopeless'. Her father, a practising Catholic, sought the opinion of his church and this was quoted in the opinion of the court. To summarise, it stated that since Karen 'had no reasonable hope of recovery from her comatose state by the use of any available medical procedures ... the decision of Joseph Quinlan to request the discontinuance of the treatment is, according to the teachings of the Catholic Church, a morally correct decision'. ['Quinlan Case' in *Death, Dying and Euthanasia*, p 503]. The court concluded that if all of the appropriate persons and bodies, after full consultation agree 'that there is no reasonable possibility of Karen's ever emerging from her present comatose condition to a cognitive sapient state, the present life-support system may be withdrawn and such action shall be without any civil or criminal liability' [p 521].

Now as you can imagine the discussion of the case helped fill many legal, medical and ethical journals for many years, and all sorts of details have been questioned, but I am not aware of any substantial body of opinion which questioned the correctness of the final judgement and the opinion of the moral authorities – in this case the local Catholic church, that on the evidence before them Karen's father was correct in requesting the withdrawal of the life-support system. There was an unexpected twist to this case. After the support system was withdrawn, Karen began spontaneous respiration and continued doing so for quite some time. I will return to this point in a moment.

This has been a long excursion to make a simple but important point – that it is widely accepted that while the absence of brain activity may determine that death has occurred, the existence of brain activity in itself is not to be equated with being a fully alive person. The court sought some evidence of the possibility of a return to a cognitive, sapient state. Such a position would find support from most moral theologians, such as Daniel Maguire, who wrote that 'in a case where the personality is permanently extinguished, one needs a justifying cause to continue artificial, supportive measures. To maintain bodily life at a vegetable level without cause is irrational, immoral, and a violation of the dignity of human life.' [*Bioethics* p 213]

So then we have seen that the Christian concern for the individual as a person created by God has been very consistently affirmed in the area of medicine. A particular problem which modern medicine has raised is the difficulty in deciding at what point this respect should cease – in other words when can we say that a person has died. The Christian tradition has wisely left it to the medical profession to provide the criteria, and it is the evolution of this that I have tried to outline.

Brain death is the current criterion, not because to have a working brain is to be equated with being a person, but because it is the prerequisite for all those personal qualities that we equate with being human, yet one does not need to possess all of these abilities. No one in the Christian tradition to my knowledge, is suggesting that the mentally sub-normal or severely mentally handicapped are not persons. The Christian tradition in this area appears to be agreeing with medicine in saying that human life is not to be equated with biological life i.e. the functioning of the biological organism. Human life is more to be equated with the potential to express certain as yet undefined personal qualities.

A case in which some level of brain activity continues to exist, as in the Karen Quinlan case cited above, but without the required potential, prompts us to modify the way we regard the patient.

In determining death we often speak about establishing the 'moment of death'. This way of thinking would lead us to say that at one time the cessation of spontaneous breathing and circulation was the moment of death, and this was subsequently altered to the end of brain activity as the moment of death. Paul Ramsey, however, emphasises that death should be seen as a process, and that medicine's contribution is to establish a point at which we may be certain that death has already occurred. But this point is not the moment of death. This, in my opinion, is the significance of the fact that despite expectations Karen Quinlan did not die immediately after the treatment was withdrawn. The court opinion implies that we must recognise that Karen was well into the process of dying, and that the absence of any potential to return to a cognitive sapient state was a significant stage in that process, a process which presumably ended when spontaneous breathing and circulation ceased.

Paul Ramsey gives a rather blunt, but useful 'primitive' example which may be helpful since it takes the issue out of the area of medical technology and into a common-sense approach. A boy scout leader led a group of scouts into a remote area by the sea. Against orders, one of the boys decided to dive off the cliffs into the sea for a swim. Unfortunately the boy hit his head off a rock shattering his brain. No medical help of any sort was available. The leader applied mouth to mouth resuscitation and chest artificial respiration for some time. Eventually he gave up, declaring the boy to be dead. It would seem very strange for him to tell the family that he made this determination on the basis of the nature of the head injury and while the boy's heart was still spontaneously beating. Even more alarming would it be if the scout leader told the parents that he thought the boy was dead from the time he hit the rocks, while the assistant leader reckoned he died when the attempts to respirate him were stopped and his heart failed. No one can say when the boy died. He was probably 'hopeless' from the moment he hit the rocks. The attempts to respirate him were abandoned when it was clear that he was already dead.

It seems to me that one of the groups which has taken this idea of death as a process seriously is the hospice movement, whose philosophy recognises that there is a time when we begin to die; it accepts the inevitability of this process and alters its approach accordingly. More specifically it strives to improve the quality of life within the process rather than simply to lengthen it.

The Beginning of Life
Let us now turn from the question of trying to define the boundary

of life at the end, to the other boundary, that of the beginning of life.
And let us begin by reminding ourselves that there is no consistent
Christian tradition on the answer to the question 'When does life
begin?' A variety of answers has been offered throughout Christian
history – conception, implantation, quickening (when the mother
feels life) viability (when the baby would survive if taken from the
womb) and so on. Much of this discussion centred on the time of
ensoulment (when the soul enters the body). Augustine says that
the foetus is ensouled at 46 days; Aquinas that it happens at 40 days
for the male and 90 for the female. Abortion was still regarded as
serious before ensoulment, but amounted to homicide after ensoulment. But still despite the variety of answers and the debate about
them it is true that the Christian tradition almost always regarded
abortion at any stage as sinful, and usually as homicide after
ensoulment or after formation. The Christian tradition has always
been very strong in its defence of the unborn.

As in the case of determining the end of life, so too the demand for
more precision in the answer to the question of the beginning of life
arose quite recently, in this century. There were probably two factors which demanded a more precise answer:

(i) the general availability of a variety of means of contraception,
some of which prevented fertilisation, others which prevented implantation or destroyed the fertilised ovum;
(ii) the growing pressure for the legalising of abortion in some
countries, and the dilemmas that that posed for Christians.

The debate over the first, the various ways different contraceptives
worked was an issue at one time, but seems to have melted off the
ethical agenda, but the abortion debate as we all know is still with us.

The moral aspects of this debate are, as we know, very complex.
There are questions about the rights of the mother, who has the
right to decide, whether it is a personal decision or one for society
and so on, but central to it is the question of the status of the embryo – at what stage can we say it is a person? At what stage do we
accord it the same rights etc. that we accord to any other person?

The Christian response to this has been two-fold. The first has been
to reaffirm the long Christian tradition of respect for the embryo,
and as modern embryology has increased our understanding of the
process from fertilization to birth, to assert even more forcefully

that life begins at conception. For example the *Vatican Declaration on Procured Abortion* (1974) says:

> From the time that the ovum is fertilised, a life is begun which is neither that of the father nor of the mother; it is rather the life of a new human being with its own growth. It would never be made human if it were not human already.
>
> [SCDF Declaration on Procured Abortion 1974. *Abortion & Law*, Doctrine and Life Special, 1983, p 7]

Interestingly, the Declaration then goes on to make a distinction between human life, which it has said begins at conception, and being a human person. It states that the latter is a philosophical question, and admits that there is some doubt as to when this designation should be made. I quote:

> It is not up to biological sciences to make a definite judgement on questions which are properly philosophical and moral, such as the moment when a human person is constituted or the legitimacy of abortion. From a moral point of view this is certain: even if a doubt existed concerning whether the fruit of conceptus is already a human person, it is objectively a grave sin to dare to risk murder.

The second, alternative response approaches abortion differently.

The British Abortion Act of 1967 elicited from most of the Protestant churches some statement on abortion. There is a useful summary of many of these statements in R.F.R. Gardner, *Abortion*, Paternoster, 1972, pp 99-107. These reactions affirmed the rights of the foetus against wanton destruction, but did recognise certain limited circumstances where termination of the pregnancy might be an option. Always, when the life of the mother was seriously at risk, and usually in cases of such severe abnormality in the foetus which ruled out the possibility of meaningful life. Whenever abortion is being considered however, it should always be as the lesser of two evils, and always undertaken with a sense of sadness and tragedy.

The thinking behind this approach was, I think, well summarised recently by John Habgood:

> Biological processes are not amenable to the sharp distinctions that lawyers like to make. It seems to me that the conceptus is

neither simply a thing nor simply a person. It is an organism on its way to becoming a person ... The process of creation is a process of interactions going on during a period of development.

[John Habgood, quoted in *The Independent*, (London) 8 February 1990, p 2]

I have presented these two reactions to the issue of abortion in terms of response by the official churches for convenience. In fact when we look at the writings of various moralists the distinction among them on this is more easily drawn on conservative and liberal lines, rather than on different Christian traditions. So moral attitudes to abortion run across rather than along denominational lines.

From a moral point of view where are we? The first approach, as I have outlined it, makes a distinction between human life (or biological life as it is often called) and being a person. Human life begins at conception. There is doubt as to when to attribute the status of person, which is a philosophical question, and because of this doubt we must attribute full respect due to a person from the very beginning. That, to my mind, is the force of the statement 'even if doubt existed concerning whether the fruit of conception is already a human person, it is objectively a grave sin to risk murder' (*see above*). The approach emphasises the continuity of the person, continuous, before as well as after birth. This continuity before birth, must stretch back to conception, since there appears to be no other point at which it might begin.

The second attitude is more reluctant to attribute the status of person to the embryo, at least in the early stages. It demands respect from the beginning but not the same respect due to a person. Noting the universal favouring within this approach of the life of the mother versus the life of the embryo, we can conclude that it does not wish to attribute personhood from the earliest stage. This position might be expressed by saying that at conception a process begins which results in life, and so this process must be treated with respect; it does however, appear to avoid the question of when it is to be accorded the status of a person.

Let me introduce a final and even more topical area in this mapping out of the scene.

The Warnock Commission in Britain was set up in 1982 to consider recent developments in human fertilisation and embryology. Its report in 1984 raised a whole flurry of debate which has been with us ever since, and has risen to new levels again as legislation has been introduced in Britain to put its recommendations into law.

Its terms of reference were:

> To consider recent and potential developments in medicine and science related to human fertilisation and embryology; to consider what policies and safeguards should be applied, including consideration of the social, ethical and legal implications of these developments; and to make recommendations.
> [*Warnock Report* Par 1.2)

It is of course a totally secular report.

Basically it examines the techniques of artificial insemination and *in vitro* fertilisation both by husband and by donor, surrogacy, and research on embryos. The particular issues relevant to this paper are *in vitro* fertilisation and research on embryos.

Here I must divert slightly in order to outline the technique called *In Vitro* Fertilisation, and since I have no particular expertise in this area, I will simply summarise the description given in the Warnock Report (Paras 5. 1- 5.3).

The technique can be used in situations where a woman can produce healthy eggs or ova and has a normal uterus, but whose fallopian tubes have been damaged or diseased. IVF involves removing a ripe egg from the ovary, mixing it with the semen *in vitro* from the husband, and then if and when fertilisation has occurred, transferring it to the mother's uterus. However, for a variety of reasons the technique is more successful and also less stressful to the mother if a number of eggs are collected and fertilised with the hope of achieving a successful fertilisation and replacement.

The aim of course is to achieve one successful fertilisation and replacement. But what if more embryos are produced than can be transferred to the uterus? If more than two are produced all the risks associated with multiple pregnancy are introduced. One option is to freeze them, so that if the implantation is unsuccessful a frozen embryo can then be used without repeating the whole gathering and fertilising procedure. But what if more embryos are produced than are required? They could be donated to another infertile couple, though we must remember there are different moral questions associated with such donations. Can we allow them to die? or can we use them for research? The use of the phrase 'use them for research' always introduces instant emotional reactions, so let me just remind you that the fertilised ovum at this stage is smaller than a typed full stop on a page, and by research we simply mean sophisticated observation.

The Warnock Report, as you know, recommended that IVF should continue to be available subject to certain licensing and inspection requirements (5:10), and that research should be permitted for up to 14 days after fertilisation (11.22). I will look at the significance of the fourteen-day limit shortly. It seems that the main moral question centres on the existence of spare embryos. Is it morally acceptable to bring embryos into existence which will not be given the possibility of realising their potential?

How do we square this with what we have already seen of the Christian response to the question of the beginning of life? We saw these two responses, one arguing that human life begins at conception and so, even though there may be some uncertainty as to when the status of person is acquired, one must attribute full respect due to a person from the very beginning. From such a position it is clear, I think, that in theory IVF is an acceptable technique, but if spare embryos are created as part of the process, then this fact would rule out IVF in practice. If the technique could be done with one or two ova at a time, and all other risks are minimal, then in these circumstances the techniques, as far as the moral aspect is concerned at least, would be acceptable, and I understand that this is the practice with IVF in Ireland.

The second approach spoke in terms of a process which results in life; that this process must be treated with growing respect as it develops and should never be interfered with without good reason. The practice of IVF pushed for a greater precision. When should this respect begin? Does talk of respect preclude the practice of IVF?

Here I must return to the biology lesson and explain, as I understand it the early development of the embryo. Again I am summarising the Warnock Report (11.2 to 11.7). At fertilisation one cell is created, from which then two, four, eight, etc. identical cells are formed. This cluster of cells goes through a number of changes until the first recognisable features of the embryo proper appears (11.4) 'The first of these features is the primitive streak', and sometimes two primitive streaks may appear which means we have a case of identical twins. This is the latest stage at which identical twins can occur (11.5). This is, I think, a significant stage – the latest stage at which twins may occur, called individuation, and the first at which recognisable features of the embryo proper appear. This happens at 14 or 15 days after fertilisation. Throughout all this implantation is taking place. 'The development processes are identical for both *in vitro* and *in vivo* embryos.' 'There is a very high wastage rate for both as a result of their failure to implant' (11.7). The emergence of the primitive streak marks the start of a period of very rapid change. 'By the seventeenth day the neural groove appears and by the twenty-second to twenty-third day this has developed to become the neural folds, which in turn start to fuse and form the recognisable antecedent of the spinal cord' (11.5).

It appears that if the process gets beyond the 14-day stage it has a good possibility of continuing on through the usual stages of pregnancy and ultimately birth. About the same point changes in the embryo occur in which the first recognisable features of the embryo proper appear. Many do not reach this stage. The Warnock Report chose this point as its recommended limit on research, and some within the Christian tradition have argued that this is the point at which the respect must be said to begin. This was one of the arguments put forward in the Church of England response to the Warnock Report entitled *Personal Origins*.

Having outlined the first approach, the continuity argument, the response then goes on to expand the process argument, arguing that persons are valued, not because they are instances of a particularly important or special life form, but because they demonstrate certain 'personal' qualities. To be human is 'to be the subject of powers of mind and soul which set human kind apart from other forms of life' (par 89). It continues:

> At the foot of these powers is the phenomenon of consciousness, and it is as the subject of consciousness ... that we value the human being most fundamentally. It is important not to suggest that human beings must exercise some specific degree of intelligence or emotional maturity before they can properly be regarded

as human persons. Yet, if we are to draw a morally relevant distinction between humans and other animals, we seem compelled to define the human in terms of a sort of nature able to exercise rational, moral and personal capacities. We need to assert that all members of this species possess such a nature, even where, through some impediment, it cannot properly be exercised in many particular cases (para 89).

In summary then this argument posits that it is as subjects of consciousness that persons are valued. To be a conscious subject is dependent on certain physical states associated with the brain. So in looking for the earliest beginning of what will ultimately result in a human person we shall be looking at the 14-day stage, the development of the primitive streak, and of individuation. This is not to imply that the process from conception to 14 days has no value; but the process takes on significant moral value from 14 days. It may also be of some significance that this is also the time at which the woman begins to suspect that she might be pregnant.

The issue of embryo research at this very early stage may also have been decided by choosing this 14-day point, but we should recall that the process is not without some respect before this. Some would argue that genuinely necessary and unavoidable research may be undertaken under strict controls (as the Warnock Report itself recommended); others argue that all research is unacceptable (as the expressions of dissent in the Report have argued).

So then there are two major streams of thought over the question as to the beginning of life. The first, that life begins at conception and must be accorded respect as a person from the beginning, stresses continuity of the person before and after birth, and that all other features of the future person are latent in the fertilised ovum. It appears to act from a position of safety. Since there is uncertainty as to when to ascribe personhood, we must do so from the earliest possible point. In support of this view, it is worth considering one's own emotional reaction when one first heard of embryo research – it is to recoil from it in distaste; people are certainly very uneasy with the notion.

The second approach sees the development from conception onwards as a process which becomes more important as the potential is realised. When pressed by the possibility of IVF to define a point when respect must begin it looks to the appearance of the earliest traces of what will ultimately be a brain, which is the pre-requisite for a subject of consciousness.

In support of this approach consider two factors: (a) the way we treat a naturally occurring early miscarriage. We do not bury this product, nor do we regard it as a death; and (b) talking of the earliest traces of a future brain as the pre-requisite of the person mirrors almost exactly the language of determining death by seeking evidence of brain activity, not because brain itself is important but because without it we can have no sense of meaningful life.

Before moving on to my concluding remarks, let me make four comments on the discussion so far:

1) It is quite remarkable that the discussion within the Christian tradition on the beginning of life has been conducted virtually in isolation from that on the ending of life. Very few writers have made the connection and drawn conclusions from one area to the other. And yet both discussions are basically concerned with the same issue – that of defining when the status of person is to be attributed and when withdrawn. These separate discussions have been very different in both their methodology and their conclusions. The future of medical ethics will undoubtedly benefit from closer collaboration between the two.

2) The Christian tradition has treated the two areas very differently. Deciding the point of death has largely been seen as a matter for medicine, with Christian ethics happy to follow scientific evidence. No such openness is to be found in the quest for the beginning of life. That has been of central concern for theologians and church leaders alike. In fact it often seems that the voice of medicine has been largely ignored in the moral debate.

3) I have not discussed the nature of the respect due to a person. I have instead concentrated on establishing when this respect might be attributed and when withdrawn. My inclination is to say that we begin to establish the nature of the respect by looking at the respect due to every person in ordinary life, and then work to find appropriate means to express this respect in areas where the person is most vulnerable.

This quickly brings us into a discussion of the word 'potential'. We can talk of a 'potential for life' or a 'potential life' in the early stage, or at the end of life 'losing the potential' for example 'to return to a cognitive sapient state'.

'Potential' can have at least two meanings in the area. Potential may mean 'already there, latent', as in 'the potential person is already latent in the genetic code from the earliest'. On the other hand 'potential' may mean 'not yet present, lying somewhere in the future, not yet realised'. I said these were two different meanings, but in fact they may only be different emphases within the same meaning. However the distinction is crucial in the area we are discussing.

4) Outlining the various arguments in this area is not the same as answering the question, but I hope that in so doing I have shown that a number of positions on these various issues are held within the Christian tradition, and each of them held with sincerity and with good moral arguments behind them. So irrespective of the position we ourselves decide to take, we must at least recognise the integrity with which others, who may differ from us, approach these issues.

I have said that the discussions about the beginning of life and the ending of life have proceeded quite separately, but that does not mean there are no connections to be made. In the discussion of the beginning of life I outlined the diverging approaches – one which emphasised the continuity of the person from conception through to birth and onwards, and the other that spoke in terms of a process of coming to life. At the ending of life there has been no similar divergence. Discussion has centred on determining that death has occurred. This has often been expressed as trying to establish the moment of death. This, in my opinion, is consistent with the continuity approach seen at the beginning of life. I went on to say that perhaps a more helpful way of talking might be to regard death as a process, and to speak of seeking a point at which we can be certain that death has occurred, but not equating this with the moment of death. There are obvious parallels between this and talk of process at the beginning of life.

So we can, I think, characterise the discussion at either end of life as being in terms either of continuity or of process. But which way of speaking is more appropriate? A consistent theme of these essays so far is the need to take the reality of the human situation seriously. Dr Jeanrond writes of a dialogue between the Christian tradition and our understanding of particular situations. It seems to me, from a limited understanding of biological sciences, that the language of process is more appropriate in the area we are considering, though I doubt if this can be said with a strong degree of certainty or finality. If we accept this then Christians ought to reflect this in their approach to these questions.

Finally, how does this whole debate fit into the Christian story we have been examining so far in these essays – the story which laid down markers in the Ten Commandments and the Sermon on the Mount, which roots itself in the total and radical commitment to the other, which concerns itself centrally with the person?

I want to say that important though the discussion of the beginning and ending of life is, it is not of central concern to the Christian faith. These issues are important issues for society, of central concern for medicine and medical ethics, and it is important that there be a Christian input into these issues. But we are betraying the Christian tradition if we imply that this is all Christians have to say in this area, and sadly I think, this is often the perception.

So let me conclude by briefly outlining where I think the main Christian contribution in this area might lie.

Two major elements in the Christian tradition have been recovered and revitalised in recent years – the centrality of justice as a model for understanding our faith, and the sense of community for understanding the church.

In a study prepared for the World Council of Churches H.H. Sehrey states 'it can be said without exaggeration that the Bible, taken as a whole, has one theme: the history of the revelation of God's righteousness' (*The Biblical Doctrine of Justice and Law*, SCM, 1955, p 50). Whether or not this is regarded as exaggerated, the fact remains that righteousness or justice is one of the central themes running through the Bible.

This justice is not the narrow legal forensic type of justice we speak of today. It is justice in its widest sense, expressed in terms of right relationships with God and with each other. John Donohue describes the biblical idea of justice as 'fidelity to the demands of a relationship' (*The Faith that does Justice*,   ed J.C. Haughey, 1977, p 69).

It is through our relationships with others that we come to a relationship with God. The rich young ruler asked Jesus how he might obtain eternal life. The reply, 'If you wish to be perfect go sell what you have and give it to the poor', implies that relationship with God be expressed in relationship with others. Christians have often tended to break faith and justice into stages. First believe in God, and then go and do justice. Today we are beginning to understand that they are two aspects of one reality. Faith in God means justice (right relationships) with our neighbour.

The church is the community of relationship where justice is to be found and where it is to be preached. Again the preaching of justice is not to be separated from doing justice. The church does not just tell society about justice in the hope it will change its way; the church is the body which lives justice in society and in so doing hopes to transform society.

The issues of relationship and community are central to the Christian approach to the beginning and ending of life. A new life is the beginning of a new relationship, a new member of the community. Both are events to be celebrated. Baptism is not just a day when a new baby is brought along to join the church. It is the focus of a whole period of celebration of the beginning of a new relationship with God and within the community. Similarly a funeral and the various rites of passage surrounding it marks a change, not an end, in relationship with God and the community.

Yet we live in a society which speaks a very different language. When we talk of death we use the imagery of battle. We admire the fight for life, a fight which draws in all the weapons of modern medical technology and pharmacology. We speak of losing the battle for life, and significantly, of a person who accepts the inevitability of their own imminent death as having 'lost the will to live'. Those who surround a dying person will talk innane trivialities rather than mention the patently obvious fact that one of them is dying. We admire grieving relatives who stoically and in isolation face the public without betraying their inner feelings.

Death is seen as a failure, a loss, and possibly one of the most isolating experiences, even when surrounded by family and friends. The Christian contribution must be to reclaim death as a central event in life, and to address it in terms of relationship and community. The life that is ending is to be celebrated with thanksgiving, as well as with sadness and a sense of loss.

So too at the beginning of life. For a Christian any new life is to be celebrated as a gift from God. Yet our society does not welcome all children as gifts, nor does it even try to ensure that they will be cherished and nurtured in their early life. We cannot fail to be aware too that often it is the fear of hostility and alienation from family and society that lies behind our abortion statistics.

At both the beginning and ending of life the key Christian concepts of relationship and community are often absent. It is along these lines in my opinion that the Christian church must make its main contribution. This does not mean that the debate I outlined earlier is unimportant. It is a major concern for medicine and society and Christians like the rest of society must face the issues. But we fail in our responsibilities if we make that debate our central concern, and ignore the need to work to transform society in its attitudes and approaches at the beginning and ending of life.

Further Reading:

Paul Ramsey, *The Patient as Person* , Yale, 1970.

Thomas A. Shannon, (ed) *Bioethics*, Paulist, Rev ed 1981.

Mary Warnock, *A Question of Life*, Blackwell, 1984.

Jack Mahoney, *Bioethics and Belief*, Sheed & Ward, 1984.

Personal Origins, CIO, 1985.

R.F.R. Gardner, *Abortion*, Paternoster, 1972.

CHAPTER 7

Is There a Feminist Ethic?

Katherine E. Zappone

There is a rhetorical flair to the title of this essay. There are many ways in which contemporary ethicians are bringing together a feminist way of being in the world with the discipline of ethics. Indeed, there are several ways in which many women and some men live with a feminist consciousness as they engage in just, good and loving acts. And so, perhaps our question should be *what* is a feminist ethic, rather than *is* there a feminist ethic.

Because of the extraordinary dynamism of the global women's liberation movement, there exists today a pluralism within feminist ethics. This diversity can be characterised along socio-political lines, namely, how feminists analyse the historical and contemporary causes of women's oppression. Carol Robb, an American feminist ethician, identifies four kinds in this regard: a radical feminist ethic, a feminist ethic rooted in an analysis of sex-rolism, a Marxist-Leninist feminist ethic and a socialist feminist ethic. (See her essay in *Women's Consciousness: Women's Conscience: A Reader in Feminist Ethics.*) The variability could also be depicted according to the religious or philosophical interpretive framework that feminists bring to the ethical enterprise. We could speak about a Jewish feminist ethic, a Christian feminist ethic, a liberal feminist ethic, the meta-ethics of radical feminism (Mary Daly), a Wiccan feminist ethic (Starhawk), etc. At first glance, the pluralism may appear then, to fit into neat categories. Not so, I'm afraid. Sometimes those using similar religious and philosophical orientations, choose different socio-political analyses, and vice versa. What this indicates above all, I think, is the importance of fluidity and dialogue in the birth of a new form of doing ethics.

In the first essay of this series, my colleague Werner Jeanrond argues that our interpretive framework affects the ethics we do and the ethical lives we lead. I agree very much with this position, and wish to make a further proposal in the light of it. I think it is most productive to explore the question – what is a feminist ethic? – from the viewpoint of my own framework, namely, a Christian feminist liberation theology. While this theological position utilises insights discovered within other spiritual traditions, I want to focus on how a Christian feminist liberation perspective affects the method and content of ethics. As I have written and spoken elsewhere, an essential feature of Christian feminism is its willingness to dialogue with other feminist viewpoints. And so, a Christian feminist ethic will share some common ground with the other kinds of ethical positions already mentioned. Though my primary intent is not to focus on the similarities and differences – rather, it is to offer an exploration within one line of vision – I think it is important to mention at the outset that this vision emerges within a conversation between several feminist positions, as well as within the dialogue between women's experience and the Christian tradition. Such conversations, I hope, help me to be a self-critical Christian feminist. It is essential that those of us who are fired by a passion for justice and love remain humble enough to know that we always have something to learn from the 'other'. I will return to this point again.

Let me now map out our exploration. First, I will mention some key features of a Christan feminist theology within the context of the ongoing discussion of how religion affects ethics. This introduces some of the philosophical and theolgical foundations for what follows. Second, we will consider the methodology of a Christian feminist ethic. To conclude, I want to offer a brief sketch of the method at work. My choice of topic is much affected by the uniqueness of a liberation method. A Christian feminist liberation ethic prompts me to ask: 'Why are so many women in Ireland poor?' and 'What ought we to do about it?' These are two complex questions, therefore we may not reach definitive strategies within the scope of one essay. However, they are on my mind and heart a lot these days, as I continue to benefit from living within the twenty-seventh richest nation in the world.

Christian Feminist Liberation Theology

In their essays for the present collection, both Gabriel Daly and Werner Jeanrond make reference to the Enlightenment's challenge to religious ethics. Through the work of philosophers such as

Immanuel Kant, we know that one can make choices between the good and the bad thing to do even if she or he is not a religious person. Likewise, an individual's religion does not mean that the person must relinquish her or his own critical capacities for determining what is right and wrong. Even as we accept both of these insights, it is still important to insist that religious traditions do make a difference to our ethics. How is this so? I have already indicated that our interpretive frameworks – the ways we perceive the world and understand all its goings on – affect our thoughts and actions in relation to ethical dilemmas. Further, a chosen religious heritage is a primary source for shaping that vision through which we interpret reality. Thus religious world-views (as well as humanistic ones) will affect our ethics.

There is a second way to talk about the relation between religion and ethics. This has been brought to our attention by ethicians such as Stanley Hauerwas who insist on the importance of story or narrative for the ethical life. Vincent MacNamara, another author in this collection, discusses at length how the biblical narratives shape a distinctive lens within which Christians see the world. Christian stories – and symbols – will affect what Christians value, what motivates their choices, how and when they act. 'What is needed', MacNamara says, 'is that Christians do their morality in line with their story.' (See his article in *The New Dictionary of Theology* , p 687.)

A Christian feminist theology makes a substantial contribution to this discussion. To begin with, it claims that interpretive frameworks are rooted in our experiences of living in relationship. Relationships – with self, one another, God and the natural world – shape our critical capacity to see the world in one way rather than another. They affect how we hear the sacred stories and understand the sacred symbols. The interpretive framework of a Christian feminist liberation theology is grounded, above all, in a revolution at the level of living relationships. As Christian feminists attempt to live in relation to a powerful (effective) self, in relationships of mutuality and equality with others, in a co-operative and co-creative relationship with God, and in a reverent relationship with the earth, a unique world-view is sculpted. As we act our ways into new relationships, a distinctive vision is generated. We often call this a world-view or paradigm of interdependence. It affects and is affected by the way we hear and retell our sacred stories, the way we critique and refashion our sacred symbols. So, relationships affect hermeneutics; hermeneutics guide ethical acts.

What about our second concern? What does Christian feminism have to say about sacred stories, symbols and ethics? Let me suggest the following. If we are going to do ethics in line with Christian stories and symbols, then those stories must be reinterpreted and our symbols need transformation, *if* we are to be ethical. What do I mean by this?

The feminist critique of Christianity initiated in its identification of the sexist bias of this world religion. Feminists such as Mary Daly, Rosemary Radford Ruether and Elisabeth Schüssler Fiorenza outlined how the female has been suppressed within the deity (the primary sacred symbol), and how her stories have largely not been told within the biblical narratives. These scholars persuasively argued that exclusive male God-talk and the supremacy and centrality of men within stories deemed sacred has two major effects: (1) it provides divine legitimation of male rule within the public, social realm ('When God is male, the male becomes god', Mary Daly) and (2) it creates inner psychic conditions so that men (consciously or unconsciously) feel superior to women and women (consciously or unconsciously) feel less valuable and more powerless in relation to men. Thus the Christian religion promoted interpersonal and social patterns of relationship which feminists now view to be unjust and unethical.

Feminist theology squarely faces this incisive critique. It claims, however, that Christianity need not – ought not – encourage unequal power relations within our world. For this to be the case, though, the stories and symbols must be transformed radically. Christian feminist theology takes up this precise project. Such work is rooted in a faith-stance that the heart of the Christian vision is about 'making love and making justice' in our world.

With this belief, Christian feminists turn to the Hebrew and Christian scriptures. Rooted in the contemporary experience of struggling for women's liberation, some of the most important feminist biblical scholarship asserts that many biblical narratives are not sacred stories for women today. Instead they re-present the patriarchal prejudices and destructive tendencies hidden underneath the texts, and they must be remembered as such. Other feminist biblical theology discovers the powerful agency of women struggling against a male-dominated socio-political milieu. It charges that this is the way we are to remember the stories of Mary Magdalene, the Cannaanite woman, the Samaritan woman and the woman of Bethany. The important work of Elisabeth Schüssler Fiorenza interprets the Jesus story as one that invites a discipleship of equals to incarnate the justice vision of Sophia God. These are just a few examples of the ways in which Christian feminists are remembering the stories of their tradition so that they promote the full personhood and agency of all women. Only in this way will the stories continue to shape behaviour that is good and just.

When feminists turn to the sacred symbols, they argue that a radical reconstruction is in order. The traditional symbols of God, Jesus, Church, redemption, etc. have not been fashioned from women's experience of living in the world; they have been based on men's experience. In the past, women's experience was not considered revelatory of the truth about God, humanity or the world. In order that Christianity affirm the truth and value of woman, and become a religion that encourages gender justice, its symbols must change through an incorporation of women's experience. Feminist liberation theology re-images and re-conceives the Sacred so that the well-being of all women becomes central to the ethical agenda.

Though the reconstructive work of sacred symbols is extensive, I want to mention two areas that I consider to be the most pertinent for our ethical enquiry. The first and most obvious one is the symbol 'God'. Within the confines of this essay, I certainly cannot do justice to the extraordinary proliferation of Christian feminist writings on 'God'. I do, however, want to point out three key features of the reconstruction.

(1) The Sacred is one who resides within woman and man and the natural world, as well as the one who moves between each part of creation, sustaining the interdependence. Therefore 'God' ought to be called 'she' as well as 'he', and the Sacred one rightfully may be named 'Goddess' as well as 'God'.

(2) The Holy One, the Creative, Prophetic spirit envisions, supports and needs human activity that struggles against the acquisition of privilege within the status quo. Liberator God sides with those who are not free; she challenges humanity to co-create a society where there are no excluded ones. This is the heart of the salvific process.

(3) The Comforter – sometimes as Mother or sometimes as Friend – suffers with humanity and the natural world as both gasp for breath in the midst of oppression and exploitation. She feels pain. Out of these emotions, she provides the fire, water, earth and air necessary for our survival.

Each of these dimensions of the One whom Christian feminists call many names, is crucial for an ethical Christian ethics.

The second and perhaps just as obvious symbol pertinent to a feminist liberation ethic is 'Jesus'. Again, within the confines of this essay, I cannot delineate all the intricacies of feminist Christological reflection. But again, I do want to highlight two of its central aspects. First, Jesus healed and saved others, not because of his maleness, but because he lived relationships of mutuality and equality with others. In his mutual, equal relations with others he found the power to heal and to be healed by others. Jesus challenged the dominant-subordinate patterns of relationship during his time. He also allowed himself to be challenged by the wisdom and vision of those whom society had 'cast away'. Jesus' – and his community's – activities of mutuality and solidarity incarnated God's presence among them. In this way, Jesus demonstrated that redemption is a collective process. Salvation is a community enterprise; one whose membership must include the rich and the poor, the sick and the well, men and women, varied races and ethnic groups. Those who have been separated and unequally divided must struggle together, in community, toward individual relationships and social structures that enable the wholeness of every person.

I think that Seán Freyne in his essay hints at something similar. He argues that we can only 'understand the ethical vision of the Sermon on the Mount in the context of Jesus' life and story of practicing the demands he issues'. Freyne also asserts that Jesus' ethic was a communitarian one. Therefore, 'to attempt this ethic on our own may be foolhardy, perhaps even unethical'. If Jesus' vision was one of a communitarian ethic, and if Jesus practised what he preached, then we could argue that the Jesus story is not one of a heroic individual. Rather, as Rita Brock develops in her recent book on Christology, (*Journeys by Heart: A Christology of Erotic Power*), Jesus' salvific power was effective only in and through mutual relations with others. God's power resides in the common life.

Our second aspect of the feminist reflection on the Jesus symbol flows from the first. Jesus' vision of the good life for all (no doubt effectively taught to him by his prophetic mother) centred in a praxis of radical love and radical justice. The radical justice which Jesus practised was not about giving each person his or her due. The radical love which Jesus lived was not an agape of selfless disinterest. Rather, Jesus attempted to know intimately the interests of the other. He risked love and friendship with those who were considered not worthy. Because he loved them – and because they loved him – Jesus was willing to challenge the politico-religious powers which did not give the marginalised their due. In this way he began to restore right relations in his own time. As Kenneth Kearon rightly remarks in his essay, biblical justice is understood as the restoration of right relations between God, others and the world. Christian feminist theology accepts this definition of justice, and views Jesus' praxis as an embodiment of such a lifestyle.

What we have seen thus far are some of the ways in which feminist theology reinterprets the sacred stories and reconstructs the sacred symbols so that they hold the potential to shape an ethical vision and praxis that promotes the well-being of all people, especially women. Amidst this work, it is important for us to acknowledge that previous interpretations of the same stories and symbols have upheld a sexist church and society. Present-day society and the churches are sexist. Christianity continues to have a lot to answer for in this regard. Let us make no mistake about that. At the same time, I believe it is crucial for some of us to remain Christian and feminist.

I often ask myself, will I remain Christian? Though a pain-filled question at times, I am grateful to possess a loyalty to feminism so that my self-critical process of being Christian remains intact. Yes, I do want to 'try to be Christian' (as I heard Paolo Friere once say). At the personal level, I continue to find the Jesus story most compelling. It lifts my spirit, engages my heart and spurs my critical/ imaginative intellectual abilities like no other philosophy or religious tradition. The story continues to spur me into a life-style that I find to be joy-full and life-filled, though not without historical contradictions. The story helps me to live with and through those contradictions. At the political level, I – like many other Christian feminists – am convinced that it is essential for women to claim the centre of Christianity. In so doing, we hope to obliterate the patriarchal, sexist bias of Christianity which continues to support the sexism in our society.

The Methodology of a Christian Feminist Liberation Ethic

It is already apparent, I hope, that feminist theology fashions a liberation ethic. It is an ethic which situates its concern in the freedom of all for self-determination. It is an ethic that promotes humanity's responsibility for the earth and the earth's community. As such, its method shares similar features with other liberation theologies. The method – or recipe – for doing liberation ethics follows a praxis approach. Praxis is a word that attempts to describe the process of gaining knowledge by thinking about one's actions, and having one's actions directed by that reflection. A praxis method for ethics means that our knowledge of the good and right thing to do cannot be gained apart from reflection on our activities within the world. Ethical theory arises from analysis of human experience and activity. A praxis method is decidedly different from some traditional ethical methods which begin with the identification of ethical principles and norms that are then applied to the concrete moral dilemma. Liberation theologians argue that the method of 'applying theory to action' does not do justice to how the historical and social circumstances of the moral problem direct the formulation and choice of the most appropriate principles to guide our activity.

Does this praxis approach really make a difference to how we do our ethics? Is it that different from how ethics has been done in the past? I think so. It not only radically challenges the way we do our analyses, it also shifts the kinds of concerns that are brought to the ethical task. But I also think that it is easier to see and hear this difference by considering the actual steps involved in a liberation method, as well as a sample of the method at work. Before embarking on this, I think it's necessary to point out that a Christian feminist ethical method not only insists on the importance of praxis, but it also recognises the centrality of relationship. Its method, then, moves us in and through relationship, praxis and theory.

To return to the analogy of method as 'recipe', I suggest that there are five main ingredients of a feminist liberation ethic. All are needed for the 'cake to bake', so to speak. Let's look at each one in turn.

(1) Participation within communities that resist suffering caused by

social oppression provides the places wherein a feminist ethic rises. Membership in these communities is foundational for 'acting-each-other-into-well-being' (Beverly Harrison). Relational support spurs us to frame the moral questions, analyse the depths of the problems and choose appropriate action. I think that the Jesus story provides an example of such a resistant community. His primary community of friends and disciples provided the place wherein the work of love and justice was fashioned. Though he travelled a great deal, and moved in and out of various social circles and towns, Jesus always journeyed with his friends. As we saw earlier, Jesus practised ethics within community.

What we find by participating in these communities is that love and respect for other members provide us with a source of moral wisdom that cannot be found anywhere else. Such wisdom is not gained without conflict. In fact, a prime testing agent for the truthfulness of our judgements and effectiveness of our actions, is the ability to respect each other during the conflicts within communities. As many of us know, feelings run deep when individuals gather to struggle beyond their own and others' oppression. How can we choose an action that violates no one if we step on each other in the process? What I am hinting at here is the importance of mutual, equal relationships if we wish to choose the good and just thing to do. These relationships are not instantaneous; our conditioning does not move us easily in the direction of mutuality, even within all-women's groups.

We may belong to one or several communities that resist human suffering. More than likely, one or two will be all that's possible if we are to be active participants. An ongoing loyalty and membership requires time; we need lots of time to learn the ebb and flow of mutual relationships. A feminist liberation ethic originates, then, sometimes in the kitchen as we make soup and scones together, often in a circle of people sharing convictions and ideas.

(2) Within the relational context of community, feminists analyse women's experience of living in a patriarchal world. This means first of all that we attend to the personal concerns and struggles of real women. We do not begin with a hypothetical moral dilemma that may never be encountered. We start with the particular circumstances of women's lives. Reflection on personal issues,

however, will not be adequate unless we take account of the socio-political milieu within which they emerge. As an Irish woman considers whether or not to leave a husband who beats her, an analysis of the roots and contemporary manifestations of women's oppression is vital for her decision-making process. Her personal well-being, either within or outside marriage, is deeply affected by the societal context of patriarchy.

A feminist liberation ethic calls for an analysis of the historical contradictions within the social order, and it needs a social theory to do this. Yes, individuals are said to have the rights to food, clothing and shelter, but women's widespread economic dependency on men often blocks their access to such rights. The personal dilemma of women with violent partners is best resolved as all of us come to a deeper appreciation of the extraordinary contradiction in several women having to choose between bodily violence or poverty. Three points could be highlighted in this analysis: (i) several women are blocked from choosing justice for themselves because of the social systems in place; (ii) these social systems must be analysed and changed by those who may never experience bodily violence so that others will be free to choose the good life; and (iii) analysis of women's experience within patriarchy identifies the interrelatedness of all oppressions. Gender justice cannot be achieved apart from economic and racial justice.

(3) Once we have some sense of the societal oppressions that lie underneath personal issues, we dialogue with the Christian tradition to determine how its principles, stories and symbols can inform our praxis. The dialogue consists of a two-way process. We bring the authority of women's analysed experience to the tradition; likewise we bring the authority of the tradition to women's analysed experience. As I have previously indicated, Christian feminist theology refashions sacred stories and symbols in the light of women's experience. They must be reshaped so that women's full humanity is not denied or distorted. In this way, women's experience contains authority to critique and reimagine the tradition. This theological work – plus the insights of non-professional feminist theologians who study it – furnishes authoritative religious guidelines for our future ethical praxis. For example, a God who shares power with us through her immanent presence, invites us to know that women are competent moral agents, especially with regard to ethical matters

which affect us directly, as in the case of reproductive choice. Feminists critique and re-create the tradition; the tradition critiques and re-creates us.

(4) The discernment towards decision has already begun. In practice, it is not always distinguishable how one step of the method flows in and out of the other. Perhaps this is the heart of its dynamism. And so, the discerned decision contains several facets. Though the decision may be made by an individual or a group, it is not made apart from the support and influence of participation within communities. Secondly, the social theoretical analyses not only pinpoint the systemic causes of women's oppression, but they also attempt to suggest alternative structures and strategies for creating them. Here is where it is particularly essential, I think, to ensure that some of the analyses are being done by those who bear the brunt of social policy and practice. How will I, as an economically secure, white, settled woman make the best judgement regarding what ought to be done for a woman on social welfare with an unwanted pregnancy? As Beverly Harrison suggests, an 'objective' moral decision, in this case, can only be made if we identify our privilege as well as listen to the experiences of those who suffer most.

Discernment continues as feminists turn to the Christian tradition in the ways previously outlined. The process is not complete, however, without the use of what Ann Louise Gilligan calls our 'mystical imagination'. Creative decision-making regarding the right and just thing to do is empowered through stillness. We must quiet ourselves – individually or within groups – to discover imaginatively the truth within. Some of us call this prayer, others call it meditation. Regardless of how we name the 'quiet', it spurs us to image the interrelatedness at the heart of all reality. As we image and feel oneness with the Source of Life and all creation, we are better prepared to sift through each source of discernment so that the decision made will benefit the common good. Paradoxically, it is often the stillness that moves us to act after judgement.

(5) Is this how we find, then, the creative power to do radical love and radical justice? By 'power' I mean the ability to effect change. Radical love and justice means change that effects the personal and social well-being of an individual – which could be ourselves –

and/or a group of others. Yes, stillness does help us to do truth and justice in love. The depth of quiet conviction and the image of oneness propels action. However, the activity is sparked also by the extraordinary energy that is unleashed throughout the entire method of a Christian feminist ethic. There exists a tremendous experience of release throughout the whole process of consciousness-raising, social analysis and theological reflection. Such dynamism stays with us as we come to do the hard things that we ought to do. This is not to say that action follows decision every single time, for that would be incorrect. What I am trying to point to, though, is the inherency of energy within a liberation ethic.

Why is this so? I think that it has much to do with the relational setting and the new relational possibilities of a feminist liberation ethic. As we form relationships of mutuality within community, and as we act for a social order wherein more mutuality can occur, we not only feel supported but we also grow in our own confidence to effect change. Relationships of mutuality and equality, especially with those whose social background is different from our own, nurtures the self in a variety of ways. As others respect our inherent dignity, treat us equally and expect reciprocal fidelity, we cultivate a self-integrity that breaks the paralysis of self-doubt. For women, this is especially crucial in our movement from judgement to action. Finally, for many of us, we sense the energy of divine presence as we act for love and justice. We meet the transcendent in the immanent experience of reaching out for life. In sum, spirituality invigorates the ethical life. We act because we are in relation.

The Method in Praxis
Why are so many women in Ireland poor? What ought we to do about it?

From our discussion on method, it should be apparent that the ethical agenda of Christian feminism centres on economic, racial, sexual, ecological and gender justice. This is a big agenda! Ethicists are currently exploring topics such as 'A Woman's Work is Never Done: Unpaid Household Labour as a Social Justice Issue', 'Our Right to Choose: The Morality of Procreative Choice', 'Feminism and Peace', 'While Love is Unfashionable: An Exploration of Black Spirituality and Sexuality', to name but a few. I want to join this list by briefly outlining an ethical concern for women's poverty in

Ireland. I offer it as simply one way, knowing that there are several other ways presently going on in this country.

(1) In 1985 my colleague and friend, Dr Ann Louise Gilligan, and I decided to purchase a property in the Dublin mountains. This was the first step in gathering a community that would resist human suffering caused by social oppression. As we prepared to move, we wrote the following to our friends and families:

> For some time now we have dreamed of founding an educational centre. At the beginning of the summer we came upon 'The Shanty', an old cedar home in Brittas, Co Dublin. At the back of the house a previous owner had built a four-car garage that we hope to convert into this centre ... Our long term goal would be to form a small community of people who are committed to the work of the centre. We hope that both the communal and educational setting could promote freedom from sexism, classism, and any other kind of social inequality. Because of this, we choose to direct much of our energy and educational skills to women who, for varied reasons, experience societal injustice. We understand this to be a religious as well as educational venture. Our inspiration for this work comes from the prophetic and liberative strand of the Jewish and Christian scriptures, as well as the lives of other women and men who have had similar goals. We hope that the centre will become a place of worship, education and social praxis. Above all, we want to try to have a table that is open to all – for food, drink, compassion, merriment, visioning, storytelling and decision-making. This is our dream.

In 1986 Ann Louise and I invited a Tallaght Women's Studies group to come to 'The Shanty' so that we could share our dream with them. We were convinced from the very beginning that we could not do it by ourselves, and we wanted a small community of women – with a mixture of classes – to join us in shaping the dream toward an effective praxis. Ten women joined and we began the process of birthing what is now known as 'The Shanty Educational Project'. The single most important factor for us was the mixture of classes. We wanted to learn from those who experienced educational and economic disadvantage. As we struggled toward relationships of mutuality, we hoped that our growing love for one another would provide the well-spring for action that would make a difference in the lives of Irish women who are poor.

(2) We spent the first year together, meeting once a fortnight, analysing our own experience of living in a patriarchal Ireland. For much of the time, we simply told our own stories. As our trust grew, a bond developed that allowed us to 'hear each other into speech'. We discovered common experiences as women, and we (tensely) explored our differences due to class and educational background. The meetings were filled with laughter, conflict, pain and tentative love. During the past two years, we have slowly begun to realise the importance of coupling analysis of our own experiences with the sociological analyses of documents such as the 1988 ESRI report on *Poverty and the Social Welfare System in Ireland*, the CMRS publication of *Poverty and Family Income Policy*, the TCD report by Drs Pauline Lee and Michael Gibney on *Patterns of Food and Nutrient Intake in a Suburb of Dublin with Chronically High Unemployment*, and the recent study by Mary Daly on *Women and Poverty*.

Though we have a lot more social analysis work ahead of us, exploring the root causes of women's extensive poverty in Ireland has led to certain convictions. We are keenly aware of the relationship between domestic unpaid work and the present economic system of advanced industrial capitalism. We are also cognisant of how women's 'special place in the home' ensures women's economic dependency on men. Mary Daly reports that 'less than a third of Irish women earn an independent income through paid work, compared with 60% of men' (p 16). She also draws our attention to the fact that 'nearly 700,000 women of working age in this country are based full time in the home' (p 21). Such analyses assist us in answering the ongoing question: why are so many women in Ireland poor? From a United States context, Beverly Harrison asserts that 'the single most powerful source of women's sexual subjugation remains women's lack of deep and genuine economic equality ...' (*Making the Connections*, p. 96).

(3) These are the analyses, life stories and convictions that we bring to our dialogue with the Christian tradition. The Management Committee of the Shanty Educational Project is also a women's spirituality group. From its inception, we studied together the fruits of feminist biblical and theological scholarship. We did not have to do much research to discover the vision of the Christian story that no one ought to be poor. But did it tell us what to do about poverty? Were women active agents in bringing about God's

'Kingdom' (as they called it then)? Does God need us to participate in the liberation of humanity? These are just a few of the questions that we studied and continue to explore with one another. Though we have gained extensive direction in the dialogue, I want to note one particularly stunning insight that has helped us considerably.

One evening we were examining the narrative of the Samaritan woman. After listening to the story and considering Elisabeth Schüssler Fiorenza's exegesis regarding it, one of our members – Mary Sweeney – offered her interpretation. Mary suggested that the nameless Samaritan woman must have had extraordinary authority in her local community in order to convince Samaritans to hear the good news of a Jewish man. So, far from being a prostitute or 'loose' woman, she was most likely an important leader with the trust of her people. Second, Mary mused that Jesus was probably aware of her authority – and his need for someone of her stature – which is what prompted that famous conversation at the well.

Remembering the Samaritan woman in this way provides us with a story of the effective leadership of women. We have a picture of a strong woman, with lots of courage and self-confidence to speak in the public forum. Our group knows that it needs to be formed by narratives like this one in order to continue speaking publicly against women's poverty. We also have a story of Jesus' need for the assistance of a woman. The mutuality exhibited in this narrative provides us with a glimpse of God's need for our creative co-operation in the liberation of history.

(4) So, what ought we to do about the poverty of Irish women? Our discernment and decisions are ongoing. The dream kernel that Ann Louise and I had over five years ago has been shaped and reshaped by those who have joined us along the way. New horizons continue to surface because of a collective mystical imagination. With meditations and rituals, personal, socio-economic and theological reflection, we continue to decide that education is at the heart of freedom for women who experience poverty. It is not the only ingredient. But substantial, systemic change in the political, economic, religious and social spheres will never come about unless an increasing number of people are enabled to design and implement collectively a just and loving alternative. To do this, they must be able to read, write, and speak publicly, they must possess self-confidence and

an inherent sense of their own worth so that the paralysis of poverty is broken. 'Education is key', said Nelson Mandela in an interview given to *The Irish Times* (24 February 1990).

(5) The Shanty Educational Project has been offering courses to women of West Tallaght for three years now. The curriculum planning has tried to take account of Mary Daly's analysis that the effects of poverty are not simply lack of money. Poverty has personal, social, cultural and political effects also. Our literacy, personal development and assertiveness training courses attempt to address the personal effects of low self-esteem and a poor self-image. The social effects of poverty are evident when people are forced to live in a neighbourhood environment where everyone is coping with similar circumstances. In bringing women to a space that is beautiful, a space that encourages bonding in solidarity, we hope to confront some of the social effects of poverty. The cultural effects need little explication. If one is challenged to feed five adolescents and two adults on £49 a week, the sum left from the dole payment of £127 when everything else is paid, there is little time for developing one's creative or cultural interests. Our call to women artists to furnish the walls of the new centre with art is one response, and in the coming terms we hope to offer weekends on the creative arts. Finally, at a political level, poverty makes people feel powerless in the face of structures and systems that determine their lives. The course on local leadership training empowers women with an awareness of their ability to effect local transformation and political change.

Throughout the three years many other people have joined our community effort. Numerous course participants, well-qualified tutors and several committed volunteers have joined us. We established a Building committee of men who converted the four garages to what is now known as 'The Shanty Muse'. We are assisted by a Development committee of women who ensure that the project, which charges minimal fees for the courses, will continue to develop. Again, it has been very important to us that the entire community is made up of the full spectrum of class backgrounds. We have held several functions that invite all to gather, so that the experiences of everyone are utilised to plan an ongoing and effective praxis. This, we believe, is the heart of our creative power.

The Shanty Educational Project is just one effort to respond to the question: what ought we to do about women's poverty in Ireland?

It is one example, I think, of a Christian feminist liberation ethic at work. But will it make a difference? We know that it has made a difference to the individual course participants, as well as to those who administer and plan the project. This reality enables us to hope that it will make a difference – along with several other projects – to the social order of Ireland. We yearn for gender, economic and racial justice. Our relationships, praxis and theory keep this hope alive.

Further Reading:

Barbara Hilkert Andolesen, Christine E. Gudorf and Mary D. Pellauer, eds, *Women's Consciousness, Women's Conscience: A Reader in Feminist Ethics*, San Francisco: Harper & Row, 1985.

Elisabeth Schüssler Fiorenza, *In Memory of Her*. London: SCM Press, 1983.

Carter Heyward, *Our Passion for Justice*, New York: The Pilgrim Press, 1984.

Beverly Harrison, *Making the Connections: Essays in Feminist Social Ethics*, edited by Carol S. Robb, Boston: Beacon Press, 1983.

Mary Daly, *Women and Poverty*, Dublin: Attic Press, 1989.

CHAPTER 8

On Not Jumping On The Green Bandwagon
Denis Carroll

Even the briefest acquaintance with radio, television or newspaper discloses a shift towards ecological concern. To cite the British ecologist, Fred Pearce, 'cranks, kings and chemists have taken up the message'. The world cannot long survive as it is going. Our technology has conferred undreamt-of benefits on some people. It has presented all people with undreamt-of problems. Ecological irresponsibility damages the innocent as well as the guilty. Every day a new product or facility is announced. Every day, too, a new, problematic spin-off from yesterday's acclaimed discovery manifests itself. It is not in the scope of this paper to sketch the crisis which confronts our planet. The titles of well-known works sound the tocsin of alarm: *Silent Spring, Turning up the Heat, The End of Nature.* Perhaps the words of the Irish anthropologist, missionary and environmentalist, Seán McDonagh, summate it best: 'the industrial revolution ... in its engineering chemical, electrical, nuclear and microchip phases, has brought an exponential leap in the catastrophic impact of human beings on the other life-systems of the planet.'

Much talk about ecological responsibility is patently self-interested. Allegedly ozone-friendly products, touted by high-powered advertising, are presented for profit rather than virtue. 'Eco-labelling' is to be viewed with considerable scepticism and, at present, it is so viewed by fifty per cent of Irish shoppers. The claim now made by the nuclear industry that it is clean, limpid, innocent and environment-friendly is, at best, suspect and, at worst, a sickening piece of cynicism. Rightly are the attitudes struck by major politicians mistrusted. We suspend judgement until we witness a readiness to pay the cost of implementing fine-sounding programmes. Money is still the engine of growth. The needs of people are well down the priorities of world leaders, in the main. It may be that a green bandwagon is gathering momentum. On board clamber the rich, the powerful, the great and the good. However, the great and the good, the rich and the powerful cannot be fully trusted. They are still too committed to old ways of exercising power. With Gore Vidal one might wish to say 'do not let your movement be corrupted by the powerful ... co-opt the many and then convert the few'. Hence I gladly adopt for the title of this paper the suggestion 'On not jumping on the green bandwagon'.

Has theology a *locus standi* here? In particular, has Christian theology a credible voice given its long silence on responsible living as co-inhabitants of God's creation? With some justification it is said that Christianity has been inimical to cherishing the earth, its inhabitants and its resources. From the cultural right comes the accusation that the rich, abounding, joyful aspects of nature have their most virulent enemy in Christianity. Thus Nietzsche, with his affirmation of the will-to-power and his contempt for Christianity's entertainment of a 'platonism of the masses'. Thus, too the apologists for nature-myths, for witchcraft, for the repressed traditions of an ancient paganism.

A strong critique has been mounted by writers Alan Watts and Lynn White. Watts attacks the architectonic mind-set of the Christian meaning-system. This mind-set sees nature as an artifact. Its dominant metaphor is the transcendent God who allows us to be no more than puppets, dependent, fearful and joyless. All sacrality is driven out of nature. Nature becomes a flat, lifeless matter to be exploited or an enemy to be battled. Lynn White focuses on the lethal consequence of the biblical injunction to increase, multiply and have dominion over the earth. Humankind has indeed increased and multiplied – some would see this multiplication as itself a major threat to a sustainable future. Humankind has subdued the earth – by raping and plundering it. Here – at the very commencement of the Bible – the licence to despoiation seems to be conceded. Only 'man' is of account. A mentality of domination is anointed. Destruction, competition, and cruelty receive a compliant wink. Some would say that, given the harsh monotheism of the Bible, the outcome could not be otherwise: the sky god is by nature totalitarian (Gore Vidal).

Thus can be listed the charges as they are frequently made: the dualism of nature (to be exploited) and super-nature (to be cherished), the establishment of an other-worldly hope indifferent to the condition of the earth. Perhaps the most telling charge is forgetfulness of justice, mercy and *shalom* (integral peace). 'By your fruits you shall know them' run the words of Jesus. The Christian centuries at best yield a mixed harvest. At the heart of Christendom slavery flourished. There, too, imperialist exploitation was tolerated, sometimes even blessed. The cross was made to follow trade – shamefully and in arrant self-contradiction. Popes, bishops, clergy of all sorts, rested easily with the depredation. In return for institutional advantage exploitative practices were sanctioned. There were noble exceptions: Las Casas, Montesinos, Peter Claver. Yet, these ran a dangerous course at the margin of an official Christianity which provided a chaplaincy to British, Spanish and Portuguese colonialism. The accusation stands that the dominant streams in historical Christianity have for long underwritten sexism, racism, colonialism and oppression. Thus say the theologians of liberation whether they speak of economic, racial, or sexual liberation.

Theology's entry on to the ecological scene has been late. As Anna Bramwell has recently shown, the history of the ecological movement is not peopled with theologians or ecclesiastical figures. That movement stems from the zoologist Ernest Haeckel, the geographer Alexander Von Humboldt, the ethologist Konrad Lorenz, the economist Kenneth Boulding. Second and third generation names then occur from diverse sciences and disciplines. It is only with the Lambeth conference (1968) that ecological concern received explicit attention from church leadership. In the seventies, both the Roman Synod (1971) and Pope Paul VI take up the issue. In the eighties, the encyclical of Pope John Paul II, *Solicitudo Rei Socialis*, follows through the concern with valuable paragraphs. The nineties opened with an excellent New Year's Day message from the same Pope, *Peace With God, Peace with Nature*. Since 1979, the World Council of Churches has done major programmatic work on the themes *Towards a Just Participative and Sustainable Society* and culminating in the Seoul Convocation (March 1990) *Justice, Peace and the Integrity of Creation*. Also worthy of note is a comprehensive document from the European Ecumenical Assembly on *Peace with Justice* at Basel (Switzerland) May 1989.

In his study, *Creation and Redemption*, Gabriel Daly has insisted that 'genuine ecological concern is a spiritual condition and is not to be confused with cunning self-interest of the kind that recognises the diminishing returns ... of over-fishing the seas or of chemically dependent farming'. Enlightened self-interest is not to be despised. The grudging recognition of the imperative to alter patterns of production, distribution and consumption could be the beginning of necessary wisdom. Yet, we are entitled to expect more from theology than the endorsement of self-interest no matter how enlightened. Since Christian teaching, preaching and church activity still affect the broader community, a proper task for theological reflection is to re-examine the prevailing symbolisms in regard to God, persons and nature. Perhaps Gore Vidal is right: the sky god is inevitably totalitarian. Perhaps we worship and press upon each other this totalitarian god to our own detriment. Is this a god we can live with: the judge, the warrior, the master, the patriarch? Are there not other models in the tradition which we have not taken sufficiently to heart: the God of mercy and compassion, who would have us cherish the widow, the orphan and the stranger; the God of enduring faithfulness and love; the God of creativity and 'letting be'; the God who is intimately present to all that God has made.

Again, what do we mean by person? What are the rights and responsibilities of persons when related to global needs of both persons and of nature? Questions about biotechnology arise here, especially about genetic and social engineering. These questions bear in the first place upon the reverence due to each person. However, they also are about other species and the necessity to avoid the degradation of living beings, a degradation which rebounds on humanity and dishonours the creator. The words of Thomas Merton remain apposite: 'what we do to the least of His creation, we do to Him (God)'. Similarly, the reminder of St Thomas Aquinas is perennially valuable: to dishonour the creature is to dishonour the creator.

Finally, we have again to ask – as does McKibben in *The End of Nature* – what is nature? 'Nature' is a hold-all word with a multiple significance. It means different things to the artist, the philosopher, the ecologist and the theologian. Should we not begin to see nature as an *oikos*, a common home, the interdependence of which is to be respected, the systems of which require co-operation rather than blundering interference. We need to recover due humility in regard to our cosmos. Hitherto, we have – of necessity – viewed nature from a purely human-centred perspective. It now becomes possible to widen our purview taking into account the travail, billions of years in duration, which only yesterday (in relative terms) gave rise to our human day.

What is meant by dominion?

Let us return to Genesis 1, 26. The concept of 'dominion' is ambivalent. It can support the view that nature is to be subjugated, tamed, exhausted. Thus it is understood by Lynn White and the many others – all too frequently professing Christians – who find in the Bible the charter for patterns of action which cause the earth's destruction. It must be admitted that the tradition behind Genesis 1, 26 saw wild animals as threat and the desert as mortal peril. Nor can one deny that the text has provided a rationale for banishing the sacred from nature. Thereby – perhaps by misrepresentation of the text – the virtual plunder of nature receives an implicit biblical permission.

Yet 'dominion' is about responsible stewardship. It is about beneficent, merciful rule. Man/woman are not licensed to tyrannise over the rest of creation. They are charged to develop, maintain and extend the pleasure garden (Eden) as which the initial creation is mythically envisaged. The creation accounts are indeed to be situated within the experience of chronic water shortage, intermittent earthquake and threatening wild life. Nevertheless, there is also an awareness that the land has potential to flow with milk and honey. The texts (P and J) are not what a later time would make them – licences for profit and unlimited growth. They set forth a task to be attained under the blessing of God. The task is difficult yet possible, and – as emerges from the accounts of the Fall – dogged by rapacity, violence and greed. The *dominium terrae* – the subduing of the earth (Genesis 1, 28) – means 'tilling the soil with the aim of winning food from seed and growing of useful plants'. It certainly does not mean exploiting the earth to the point of exhaustion: let us remember the many purposes of the Sabbath, purposes which include giving rest and rejuvenation to the earth. The text does not mean poisoning the habitat. Dominion over the animals is about fostering life rather than destroying it. In passing one might notice that the Bible is not confined to pastoral or agricultural images; the New Testament culminates in an urban reference to the 'new Jerusalem'.

A Chastened Anthropocentrism

Undoubtedly, Genesis 1, 26 shows humankind to be pre-eminent in

God's creation. Man/woman show God forth in an altogether special way through their ability to know, to love, to respond to their creator's address or word. Augustine's distinction of image (man/woman) from vestige (the rest of creation) is apt. These insights are at the root of the medieval axiom *res sacra homo* (man/woman are sacred, or better, man/woman are sacredness). I would argue that the perception of man's/woman's sacredness is in need of reinforcement rather than diminution. The rights and needs of millions of people call for reiteration rather than de-emphasis. Nevertheless, there is danger of an anthropocentrism where man/woman are considered to the exclusion of all other inhabitants of creation. This would impede any recognition that there is a 'soil community', a 'cosmic confraternity' (Boff), with close interdependence of needs and service. The German moral theologian, Bernard Haring, speaks of a 'chastened anthropocentrism'. Yes, the needs and rights of persons must be acknowledged rather than ignored. On the other hand, the wants and claims of a pampered minority must be relativised in order that the world may survive. A chastened anthropocentrism recognises that the earth is a common home, an *oikos*. Archbishop Desmond Connell in a recent pastoral on reverence, calling for respect for the environment, spoke of 'a fundamental equality' between all creatures which roots in their very creaturehood. There is a 'soil community' which comprises the whole chain of being. Within that community man/woman have especial rights but they are also charged with especial responsibilities.

For the first time, humankind is able to put an end to all life as we know it. We have opened a box or jar of Pandora releasing great power for good but also a truly awful capacity for destruction. The selfish use of power can now lead to death for all creation. A chastened anthropocentrism would urge that what we can do (or claim) we sometimes ought not do (or claim). Every day, it is said, one species is forever destroyed because of a model of 'development' which is dominated by motives of short-term profit.

As long ago as 1929, the American Jesuit John A. Ryan argued that the only life worth living is one where our needs are few, simple and noble. There is an overtone of social responsibility here, even of asceticism. More concretely, Barbara Ward asked if our world can survive as a rich world: the rich must become poorer if the poor are to survive. As things stand, is not a rich world an unjust world?

Are not its riches enjoyed at the expense of many, many others. As we reconsider the Judaeo-Christian tradition we discover valuable guidance in facing such questions. One of the symbols which may be of help is *shalom*, the peace spoken of by the Old Testament. This is not the peace of quiescence, much less of acquiescence. *Shalom* is about healthy, healed, happy relationships of people – with each other, with their world and with God. Only when justice is done, when fair play is accorded, when patterns of domination are changed, will *shalom* be on the way to achievement.

Some Recent Documents from Ecclesiastical Authority
(1) The World Council of Churches

In recent years the World Council of Churches has presented remarkable formulations on reverence for creation. Two such formulations are especially noteworthy: *Towards a Just, Participative and Sustainable Society* (1979) and *Justice, Peace and the Integrity of Creation* (1990). These formulations are both aspirational and programmatic. They remind us that justice and sustainability belong together. An unjust society is radically unsustainable. Built upon selfishness, it carries the seed of its own dissolution. The injustice within a society erodes its very cohesion. Likewise, an unjust society wastes both natural resources and people. Poverty, claims the British politician Chris Patton, is still the greatest enemy of the environment. This is not to say that western models of development spell any large hope for justice or environmental sensitivity. It does concentrate our mind on the ecological imperative to social justice. To cite Pope John Paul II, 'the proper ecological balance will not be found without directly addressing the structural forms of poverty that exist throughout the world'.

The WCC also speaks of participation. No longer can the direction of our world be left in the hands of elites. Elites are normally self-serving. They have at their command experts to manage information, conceal risks, whitewash failures and present optimum scenarios. Despite the appearance of plural choice the really significant choices are made by the few – and normally for the benefit of the few. The diffusion of power or even of participation seems to remain a large threat to leaders in both church and state. Participation requires generous leadership in initiating moves to facilitate it. It also requires hard work, self-discipline and sacrifice on the part of those who enter its process.

It is necessary to bring forward together social justice, ecological responsibility and participative politics. The flourishing of people and the well-being of the environment must not be put in opposition. Such an opposition would be fatal to both values. There is a self-serving ecology which denies the benefits of technology to those who suffered most in technology's establishment. A steady-state ecology would be as selfish and unjust as steady-state economics.

The Seoul convocation of the World Council of Churches (March 1990) has endorsed a major affirmation on *Justice, Peace and the Integrity of Creation*. Its final document enjoins a programmatic action to tackle injustice, violence of all kinds, and the prevalent degradation of nature's systems. Refusing to separate issues of justice and ecological sustainability, it emphasises a fundamental interconnection between injustice, violence and massive wastefulness of the earth's non-renewable resources. It is clear that the convocation refuses to jump on any 'bandwagon'. Rather, it proposes a covenant to enter the process of conversion to just, transformative and peaceful patterns of action. Space does not permit longer analysis of this major document. Its significance lies in its ecumenical nature – from the standpoint of ecumenical action, it embraces global issues on a near-global scale. In the best sense, its content is both radical and realistic.

(2) Pope John Paul II
A letter of Pope John Paul II to mark world peace day (1-1-90) centres on the theme: *Peace with God the Creator: Peace with all of Creation*. One should associate the letter with the convocation at Seoul (Korea) of the World Council of Churches (March 1990). The New Year's Day message develops earlier references to the environmental issue in *Solicitudo Rei Socialis*. Main emphases of the document are here presented in punctual form:

(a) There is a moral crisis of which ecological destruction is but a symptom (par 5). This crisis spawns an insecurity which itself leads to collective selfishness, disregard for others, dishonesty and a lack of respect for life.

(b) Notice the letter's title: *Peace with God the Creator: Peace with all of Creation*. The Pope speaks of inter-connectedness in many dimensions. In particular, he calls for solidarity between developing countries and those societies which have been industrialised. Developing nations must not be asked to carry burdens which industrialised nations are unwilling to bear. At the same time, the Pope invites people to avoid mistakes already made: industrial pollution, radical deforestation and unlimited exploitation of non-renewable resources (par 10).

(c) Justice and sustainability belong together: 'the proper ecological balance will not be found without directly addressing the structural forms of poverty ...' (par 11).

(d) There is need for agreed public policy: 'the right to a safe environment is ever more ... a right that must be included in an updated charter of human rights' (par 9).

(e) A serious look at life-style is called for by the Pope. Instant gratification and consumerism are set against simplicity, moderation, discipline and a sense of sacrifice (par 13).

(f) It has been noticed that the Pope's message does not refer to population policy. Commentators have mentioned the necessity for the church to face this issue. It is worth remarking that such examination should be situated within the demand for social justice. After all, it is the 'first world' – where birth rates are falling – which is responsible for much of the destruction wreaked on the natural environment. Further, the issue of population should be addressed in tandem with that of effective land reform.

A Call for Conversion

Justice, participation and a sustainable use of the resources of God's creation will not be brought about by big business, Toryism, Stalinism or the many forms of social organisation which lie between these extremes. Nothing less is required than a recoil from unjust, exploitative, wasteful, violent ways. In effect, one is speaking of a new morality, a new spirituality. To adapt the remark of Thomas Berry, such a morality will extend its concern to the biocide and geocide which are now taking place around us. For a morality of this kind to eventuate, a conversion is required in our thinking and doing. Our thoughts, attitudes and actions should forsake (turn from) wasteful, uncaring patterns of consumption. They should embrace (turn towards) the values of justice, sharing and the fraternity/sorority that St Francis of Assisi marked out so well.

The requisite spirituality is one of compassion, of interconnection, of reverence.

Nevertheless the locus for conversion is not primarily the private sphere. For too long the sins of small people have been enumerated and condemned. The place where conversion is most required is the public domain in which issues of equality, justice and redistribution are decided for good or ill. For the Christian, ecological concern brings him/her up against intellectual/spiritual issues which transcend mere conservation. These issues go far beyond 'greenery' or romantic nostalgia for a lost paradise. The issues are about values and action directed towards justice, sustainability and integrity of creation. Such values and such action are central to the prophetic thrust within Judaeo-Christianity. They sound a challenge – if we take them seriously – to the greed of the affluent, the pride of the powerful and the destructiveness which resides in us all. They also sound a challenge to the 'new right' – this arrogant, apparently value-free and ultimately unjust system that seems to be gathering strength around us.

The issues thus opened up make us reconsider personal, social, and even cosmic morality. Teilhard de Chardin wrote in his *Phenomenon of Man*: '... people often think they are honouring Christianity when they reduce it to a sort of gentle philanthropism. Those who fail to see in it the most realistic and at the same time the most cosmic of beliefs and hopes completely fail to understand its mysteries.' Chardin, as was his wont, spoke in terms of the ideal. In doing so he tried to push the church beyond its stances on several issues of the day. Now, however, the agenda is even more complex than in Chardin's time. There are especial difficulties to cherishing justice, peace and integrity of creation in our age of advanced technology and of grave social disparities. The challenge for contemporary Christian reflection is to recover from its tradition (and such practice as there is) the accompaniment of justice and mercy, beauty and efficiency, smallness and appropriateness of scale. In the context of the churches' contribution, one can say that they (the churches) have a pressing opportunity to use their energies, educational resources and spiritual disciplines in fostering an appreciation of our planetary interdependence as we share a common home or *oikos*.

Further Reading

Anna Bramwell, *Ecology in the Twentieth Century: A History*, Yale University Press, 1989.

Seamus Cleary, *Renewing the Earth*, CAFOD, London, 1980.

Fred Pearce, *Turning up the Heat*, Bodley Head, London, 1989.

Sean McDonagh, *The Greening of the Church*, Geoffrey Chapman, London, 1990.

Bill McKibben, *The End of Nature*, Viking, 1989.

John Paul II, *Peace with God the Creator, Peace with all Creation*, Message for World Peace Day, 1/1/1990

Final Statement from the World Council of Churches Convocation on Justice, Peace and the Integrity of Creation, (Seoul, March 1990).

Final Document of the European Ecumenical Assembly: Peace with Justice (Basel, Switzerland, May, 1989).

Andrew Christiansen, SJ, 'Ecology Justice & Development', *Theological Studies*, March 1990, Vol 51, No 1 pp 64-81.

CHAPTER 9

The Christian and Politics

T.P. McCaughey

We are probably all quite familiar with the kind of evening spent in some place of public resort, during the course of which one of the company raises a question or expresses a view which is ruled out of order by the dominant people present on the grounds that religion and politics are not to be allowed to disturb their evening's fun. Either of them may be expected to cause what is called 'offence'. This ruling is given by someone who knows as well as most of those present, that a particular stance in the religious realm often in this country presupposes a particular stance in the political one, and vice versa. In the north of Ireland a Protestant may be expected to be a unionist, but if not, the effort to explain why not is itself liable to generate as much heat as light. On the other hand, Free Staters and Republicans of an earlier time who had disagreed on the Treaty may be expected to have sharply divergent views on the church and very sharply divergent experiences of its hierarchy's discipline.

The affable person who wants a good night out in pleasant company and cause no 'offence' in doing so, will simply avoid what is called 'religion' and 'politics' – especially those areas of 'politics' in which 'religion' is considered to have an interest or a view. The Irish pub philosopher will state – not without a strain of dogmatism – that a person's religion is a private matter between themselves and God. The pub philosopher, for his part, claims to take people as he finds them and asks no questions.

The fact is, however, that as the pub philosopher knows perfectly well, the leadership of the church to which he belongs, and of every other church in Ireland, is up to its collective neck in politics, both overtly and covertly. He knows that the leadership constantly represents to local and national government and public servants what church leaders take to be the church's interests in this or that sphere. The average citizen is usually satisfied to go along with the leadership's representations even if, in business and social life and for practical purposes, he himself takes the view expressed with some irony by one of Seán O'Casey's characters that religion is fine as long as it is kept out of as many things as possible.

Most Irish people have in fact belonged to what the pioneering German historian and sociologist of religion, Ernst Troeltsch, called a 'church' rather than to what he termed a 'sect'. Troeltsch defined 'church' as follows:

> A church is an institution which has been endowed with grace and salvation ... it is able to receive the masses and adjust itself to the world, because to some extent, it can ignore the need for subjective holiness, in favour of the objective treasury of grace and redemption.

This is in contrast with the 'sect' which he defined as 'a voluntary body of believers, living apart from the world and usually excommunicating both society and state'. Born into 'churches', in this sense, Irish people have assumed that the church should be the *cultus publicus*, the official public cult, which holds up the hands of the community and the state. Historically, they have taken it for granted too that the state should broadly speaking, reflect the values of a church, which in turn could include within itself the widest possible variety of adherents. People who by this definition belong to a 'church', assume that the church will have views on the ordering of society which, through its structures, it will of course promote.

However, the trouble historically in Ireland has been that we have had two or three competing national religions – each of them with pretensions at one stage to be the comprehensive/final solution to the religious question, the authentic public cult.

(i) The Roman Catholic Church – even when reduced in penal times to the status of a mission – still knew itself to be the one, holy Catholic and apostolic church.

(i) The Church of Ireland (and England) was by law established, even though at no time nor in any part of the country did it command a majority following.

(iii) The dissenters (mostly Presbyterians) who were neither established nor in a majority, except in certain restricted areas of the north-east.

Each of these churches was forced in the nineteenth century to concede that the others existed and were likely to continue to do so. By the nineteenth century the British Government, which had not been innocent of the sin of encouraging their mutual hostility, now under the liberal impetus, sought to hold the ring as these religious groups jockeyed for position in an effort to divide Irish life between them into various spheres of influence.

It is of course this uneasy jockeying for position that ever since has engendered the nervousness of the pub philosopher with whom we began. For even if, for instance, he never followed the debates which led to the disestablishment of the Church of Ireland in 1870, he knows in his bones that the churches in Ireland were never disestablished in spirit, and that the official disestablishment of the minority Church of Ireland in 1870 was in effect the recognition in official circles that Ireland would only be governable if the administration tried fairly to share out its official recognition among a plurality of more or less mutually hostile churches – each one of them with pretensions to being the *cultus publicus*. In many areas of Irish life in the nineteenth century (and even in the twentieth century in a diminished number of areas), ecclesial allegiance and socio-economic interests were so closely associated as to be almost impossible to unravel. The partition of the country in 1922 confirmed unofficial *de facto* establishment without needing to give it legislative form on either side of the border.

Our pub philosopher, of course, reflects the widespread realisation of many (at least since the end of the nineteenth century) that, if I am to continue to belong to my church, and to do necessary and profitable business with others outside of it, I must learn to relate to them as individuals at a level which somehow contrives to leave out of account – or at least, out of explicit mention – two things that have been essentially constitutive in making them and me what we are, i.e. politics and religion.

Of course, there are parallels elsewhere, but certainly in Ireland in the nineteenth century, religion can be discovered as fulfilling two functions:

(1) It provided, through the various churches, a shared vision. It was, to change the metaphor, the social cement of community. Even though not everyone behaved themselves, people were in broad agreement about how one ought to do so.

But (2) it enhanced the sense of the value of the individual person, for both Catholic and Protestant spirituality in this period were of a highly individualistic kind. Post-famine Catholicism in Ireland, like post-clearance protestantism in Gaelic Scotland or north-east Ulster, concentrated attention and anxiety on the individual soul in the face of cultural and social dislocation and even disillusionment. Both spoke of this world as a 'vale of tears', and encouraged the faithful to leave judgement of the oppressor to God in the next. No doubt this often led to supineness and political conservatism. But it should be said that both Catholic and Protestant pietism did allow the oppressed to sense their individual value before God in a way that nothing in their present circumstances otherwise encouraged them to do.

In conclusion, it could be argued that today we are the heirs to a situation in which it is taken for granted that church leadership will energetically promote interests which ordinary believers recognise are not wholly religious ones. At the same time, however, committed Christians will leave the leadership to get on with all that, while they themselves get on with the 'real' Christian life of prayer and good works, while perhaps also involved in philanthropic or charismatic groups. For practical purposes, then, there have developed two worlds: and 'religion' has entered the public arena as 'the religious factor' in an overall situation, to be taken into account according to the support it can command, along with an increasing number of other interest-groups. As far as the generality of the faithful are concerned, 'real' religion has been a private affair, conducted of course within the wider context of that shared experience which the sacramental community provides and maintains.

The idea that Christianity is essentially and was originally a religion with a primarily personal and individualist ethic is of course deep-rooted – particularly in post-Kantian Protestantism, but certainly not only there. From time to time it is alleged that Christian history is the account of an unlovely slide from individual or at least small-group purity and spirituality to the worldliness of a power-hungry institution. Of course the substantiating evidence for such a view is not hard to come by in the history of Christianity. But contemporary New Testament studies would tend to set a question mark against the starting point of that slide. Does the evidence on Jesus and the earlier communities support the picture of a group with a purely individualistic ethic or of political non-involvement?

Seán Freyne, in his paper, speaks of Jesus as proposing 'an alternative way of organising human social relations based on a rather specific social programme'. As he demonstrated, this included a radically inclusive attitude to women, e.g. the explicit inclusion of Mary of Bethany among the number of his disciples and the presentation of Mary of Magdala in John's Gospel in the role of apostle. It also included a flouting of the purity laws in the interests of liberation and healing, as instanced in the touching of a leper which itself is a challenge to those who exercise social control by operating those laws. Or one thinks of the social significance of the table-fellowship of those meals of his or the implications of the disturbance in the Temple which seems finally to have brought the house down on his head. Whatever actually happened that day, it was seen as a direct challenge to those who controlled the Temple and had painfully negotiated a most-favoured-nation treaty with the Romans.

Contemporary scholars who set about the task of categorising Jesus may quite defensibly opt for labelling him as an eschatological prophet, as charismatic leader or as holy man. But the evidence is that at the time the Sadducee priesthood and the Roman pro-consul, without prolonged study and reflection, quickly identified him and his counter-culture disciples as a threat to political settlement and social equilibrium. It is after all a stubborn fact that Jesus was executed on the orders of the pro-consul, Pontius Pilatus, by a method reserved for slaves and rebels. And this can hardly be because Pilate could not bear to be invited to consider the lilies of the field. No evidence is available either, which suggests that Jesus was executed on a misunderstanding, or that his arrest was a case of mistaken identity. Undeniably he dealt often with individuals, but it was the socio-political significance of these encounters which nailed him.

In the same way, it was the social and indeed universal significance of all this that led the early community to hail as 'Lord' one cornered by the successors of Moses and Aaron and executed by Caesar. His resurrection was hailed as first-fruits of that universal re-creation which some Jewish piety spoke of as the general resurrection of the dead. Certainly, as they moved out of the Palestinian homeland to the cities of the Empire, they were discernible first as a sect of Judaism, and then later as a religious sect in their own right. In these cities they adapted to some extent to the pluralist culture around them, and from the point of view of the imperial administrators, were indistinguishable from other more or less exotic oriental groups. At first they were seen as a Jewish sect, doing their own thing in the quiet of the synagogue, the guild meeting in a household, an initiatory cult or sometimes a little school. As time passed and new problems arose, the little communities often sought to solve them by borrowing from others – the Cynics, the Pythagoreans, the Sophists and others who had been longer in the field. As they settled down to life in the cities in the second century, we may also say that they lost a good deal of the radicalism and eschatological urgency which had characterised Jesus. But certain things prevented them from complacently settling down only to that 'incipient bourgeois quietism' which Martin Dibelius detected in those second century writings we called the Pastoral Epistles. These factors could be described as follows:

(1) an 'internal drive toward unity and even uniformity of belief which, however often frustrated, nevertheless persisted right across the Mediterranean';

(2) an undimmed sense that the death and resurrection of Jesus the Messiah had inaugurated a new and decisive age in human history;

(3) a persistent notion that the one God was calling all people on the same set of terms to God's self to form, not a new people but a new humanity.

Convictions such as these made it impossible for the Christians to take one another to court, to join the imperial army, to burn a pinch of incense to the 'divine emperor' or fulfil any other even of the minimal duties expected of all imperial subjects in acknowledgement of the divine origin and sanctioning of the Empire and the Pax Romana.

Quite remarkable about the early Christians is the persistent conviction which reappears again and again in the New Testament, i.e. that they are citizens of another state, a commonwealth (*politeuma*) which actually already exists. In the existing political Empire, which they saw both as overstepping itself, and as failing to be what it was called to be , they sometimes saw themselves as a kind of alien community, a *paroikía*. But this perception of themselves as aliens or sojourners in a strange land did not encourage in them the idea that it is the church which constitutes the new age. Quite the contrary! It is the city. Or, to put it again as Karl Barth does, 'the church sees its future and its hope, not in any heavenly image of its own existence, but in the real heavenly State'.

Like Antigone in Sophocles' tragedy of that name, the Christians were obliged to an authority more basic than that of city or empire, and were committed to breaking the equation Patriotism = Piety where necessary.

It is because they did so that they were actually called 'atheists'. By the mid-third century, when the then emperor came to see Christianity as a threat to public order and undertook to break its organisation he lacked the power to do so. When the Emperor Constantine decided to join the Christians, the two empire-wide organisations were co-terminous. In the art of the period Christ appears as *pantokrator*, emperor of the universe, and Eusebius (264-340) could write:

> By the express blessing of the same God, two roots of blessing, the Roman Empire and the doctrine of piety sprang up together for the benefit of the human race ... [With the reign of Constantine] a new and fresh era of existence had begun to appear, and a light hitherto unknown suddenly dawned ... all must confess that these things were entirely the work of God who raised up this pious emperor to withstand the ungodly. (*Vita Constantini* 2.1)

How different this position from that of Tertullian (c.160-222) a hundred years before, who could say:

> There is nothing more alien to us than politics.

He went on:

> The fact that Christ rejected an earthly kingdom should be enough to convince you that all secular powers and dignities are not alone alien to but hostile to God ... Your citizenship, your magistracies, the very name of your curia is the Church of Christ.

But who knows how Tertullian would have reacted if his generation had been offered the opportunity that Eusebius' one was of co-

operating fully with the rulers of this world or even of becoming
the religion of the Empire itself?

The Emergence of Christendom

Clearly transitions had taken place, and we today live in their after-
glow: the transition from sect to church and from church to Christendom. A recent writer has succinctly delineated the term 'Christendom' as follows:

> At its best, Christendom was the exploration of a question
> which had not occurred to the earliest Church i.e. How may
> Christian rulers responsibly and piously use their power to the
> glory of God and the welfare of God's people? At its worst, it
> would appear that Christendom was not so much the establish-
> ment as the subversion of Christian faith (Forrester).

Of course, now since Paul's time Christians had been committed to
the view that God is a god of order, not chaos, and that God's justice is what the rulers of this world are either co-operating with
(*Romans* 13) or working against (*Revelation* 13). But now that there
actually were Christian rulers, Christians were driven to seek answers to new questions wherever they could find them and, of
course, a primary source of enlightenment was the Hebrew Bible
itself.

The sixteenth-century Protestant reformers faced the question as to
how to order godly rule within the various emergent nation states.
Martin Luther (1483-1546) has been accused of having de-
politicised the faith. This may not be entirely fair or accurate; what
is true is that he believed and taught that the church's proper function is distorted when it meddles in the political world. He certainly believed, however, that the political realm is also God's, and that
in it the ruler exercises a function for God, even when he 'hangs,
beheads, slays and fights'. Calvin (1506-1564) for his part, also
believed that there are two kingdoms, but for him the distinction
was by no means so clear. It is noteworthy that in countries where
the Reformation was Calvinist, church involvement in civil and
political matters has traditionally been strong, even to the extent of
hankering after a theocratic settlement, as in Scotland post-1603.
On the whole, however, Calvinists were in this regard outstripped
by the Enthusiasts, Anabaptists and other sectarians. These groups
sought to, and occasionally did manage to set up 'godly common-

wealth' – manifestations on earth of the new Jerusalem. But, in the end of the day, they most often had to be content, like the Moravians, the Waldensians and the Catholic orders, simply to give expression to what they took to be the pristine Christian vision behind enclosing walls and closed doors.

Meanwhile, in the world outside, the Enlightenment was teaching people to exalt the individual, enlightened reason. The national religion which this produced was, however, as J-B Metz has critically observed, for the most part a privatised one, 'specially prepared for the domestic use of the propertied middle-class citizen ... a religion of inner feeling ... which does not protest against ... the definitions of reality, meaning and truth of the middle-class society of exchange and success'. It is at least arguable that a good deal, though clearly not all, of the so-called 'secular' Christianity of twenty-five years ago stood in a direct line of succession from the bourgeois, privatised religion of two centuries before.

On the other hand, the political theologies of today – black, feminist and liberation – appear as protests against the northwestern, middle-class, individualistic WASP-ish presuppositions of a very great deal of what was recognised as radical theological writing in the first half of this century e.g. in the work even of such great men as Karl Barth and Rudolf Bultmann. The work of the black, liberation, feminist or generally contextual theologians may itself be of uneven quality, but these theologians attempt to 'do' theology from the bottom, to contextualise it – not just in the study, but in the streets and shanties of the humble and the meek.

What now?

I take it that, even in Ireland, we are at a stage in history in which it is less and less an open option to be the public cult any more. Christians are not the powerless and scattered sect of pre-Constantinian times and, even if they were, they could not pretend that the centuries of Christendom had never happened. On the other hand, however tenaciously the vestiges of former establishment hang on, it is true that the processes of government have achieved autonomy and been fairly thoroughly secularised. It may be that the choice between 'sect' and 'church' as modes of Christian presence is still there but, if it is, it has been considerably transformed.

In the time that is left to us we may profitably consider what characteristics that presence might arguably have if Christians are to fulfil any political obligation. Ideally they should comprehend both that care for the whole of society together with a desire to be a sign in it of the transcendent reality of God's justice which characterises 'churches' and that passion for personal and collective holiness which characterises the 'sect'.

We may perhaps mention three such characteristics:

(i) Solidarity

I take it to be the case that those who announce a kingdom such as Jesus spoke of, heralded and anticipatorily made present, proclaim something which is not identifiable with any institution visible here today or there yesterday. They are committed to what Christians speak of as the justice of God which is thought of as a future reality pushing its way into our present. Whatever a commitment to this transcendent justice might mean in political terms, it is certainly more than a commitment to ameliorative action. Even though ameliorative action may at certain times be the only action possible, Christians and Jews are thirled to the movement for radical change. If that change is ever to begin to be God's kind of change, then it cannot be prescribed by the rich or thought of as something which the privileged in some way concede to others. Of course the rich, the privileged, the intellectual and the well-instructed ideologue may be set to work for radical change, but their contribution can in the end only be beneficial when they put themselves at the disposal of those who are oppressed, deprived and suffering and learn to endure the consequences when the judgement of those who have suffered much seems to those who have suffered less to be lopsided or even unbalanced. In solidarity with the oppressed, there is implicit a critique both of the sect model, which basically attempts to withdraw its members from the world, and of the church model which historically has most often sought either to control or to prescribe.

(ii) Conformation

Solidarity can scarcely be dissociated from conformation. Christians are necessarily called into the political world like Moses, who had to be taught that a surreptitious and impetuous blow against a task-master on the building site was not enough. At the burning bush he was sent back to the world of Pharaoh's court which he knew so well, but feared to return to. Our predicaments are of such a kind that neither shows of indignation nor philanthropic answers are enough. At best, they are no more than pledges of commitment. Political questions require political answers and the formulation of those answers is necessarily going to involve Christians, like everyone else, in dirtying their hands, in co-operation with others whose motives we suspect. On occasion it will involve us in collusion with the morally suspect. Certainly it will involve Christians in a realm of ambiguity, as it did their Master, and it will not necessarily be desirable or even possible to clear oneself or one's own reputation in the course of all this (Cf. Matt 12.24).

But, as Dietrich Bonhoeffer repeatedly pointed out, ultimate responsibility, final statements and ultimate decisions are not ours to make. Our obedience has to be worked out precisely in the interim period between that decisive action of God in Christ and the ultimate resolution of all things in the general resurrection of the dead. But conformation involves two things – conformation to Christ and conformation to the world, and the two of these must be held together. Christians who have opted for the sect-model have opted exclusively for conformation to Christ, and this has tended to take them out of the world. Those who opted for church-model have attempted to comprehend the world within themselves but have run the risk of being conformed to it. The calling today is, as it always was, realistic conformation to the Christ who is himself conformed to the world so closely as to share the ambiguity of human living. Only thus does he overcome the world, or enable us to share his triumph.

(iii) The endeavour to form a shared consciousness

I take it to be a most important part of what the Christian community is all about that it should seek to form what it is probably rather dangerous to refer to as a 'collective conscience', but quite correct and helpful to call an ever-expanding 'shared consciousness'.

The prophets of old Israel did not use the term 'conscience', but the whole thrust of their proclamation was in the direction of ever and again widening the consciousness of the people and drawing ever wider implications and conclusions from the people's nominal or real commitment to Yahweh. So every time the people settled down to their 'way of life', a prophet came along and said 'That's fine. But what about the poor? the alien? the children? the women? the creation?' When they rejoiced in what Yahweh had done for them as a people, the prophet asked about God's dealings with the Philistines in their history. Christianity would appear to be committed from the beginning to the widening of consciousness since, in essence, Christianity is the proclamation of the good news of God's universal call through the crucified one to all on the same terms, regardless of race or sex.

These three characteristics are essential if we are to fulfil the obligation, so often laid upon us, of speaking out in the political domain.

It is generally agreed that the church should 'speak out' about things that matter in a particular community or state or even that it should have something to say at the international level. That is easy to agree to, but even when it is, the question arises as to how it is to be done. Just at the time when the churches in Ireland are losing some of the prestige and position they once held as institutions with political clout, they find that they are being called upon to pronounce on very complex issues or are being forced to decisions on matters of which they have only an imperfect understanding. Rather than leave these questions to those, both Christian and non-Christian, who are at the pit-face, the leadership has taken expert advice and has of recent years produced some excellent and courageous statements, e.g. on poverty. These efforts must be commended, representing as they do the conviction of Christians that the church of the crucified Jesus cannot rest content to play the role of sect on the periphery of life or be no more than a cell for the cultivation of personal holiness.

But history has made it difficult for us to find a way in which to take common Christian action for justice without generating seriously damaging misunderstanding. David Hollenbach puts it well with reference to the, admittedly different, situation in the United States. He says:

> If common action is to be effective in a bureaucratic society, it must be organised action. There is a strong cultural bias present in our society which results in the misrepresentation of any public or political activity by the Church as a violation of the separation of Church and State ... Cultural pressure to keep the Christian community's action in society non-institutionalised also leads to

the fragmentation of Christian efforts to bring greater justice to social organisations. It often leads to the view that religiously-motivated actions by individuals are legitimate expressions of religious liberty, while such actions by organised groups or churches are attempts at re-establishment.
(*Faith that Does Justice*, p 237)

A trio of theologians in Germany, belonging respectively to the Reformed Lutheran and Roman Catholic traditions, i.e. Jürgen Moltmann, Wolfhart Pannenberg and J-B Metz, take the view that the Christian churches are by definition engaged to be participant in the struggle for the transforming of society and the liberation of humankind. Like us in Ireland, they belong to a country in which the churches have never been entirely disestablished, but which is nevertheless considerably more secularised than Ireland is as yet. In their view the churches are committed to the promise of God's rule and, because they are, they resist the institutional stabilising of things. By raising repeatedly the question of meaning, they make things uncertain and keep them moving and elastic in the process of history. In line with Karl Barth, they see the church as working for the revolution till it happens, and then quitting so as to start working for the next one. Metz, in particular, seems to assume that energetic social critique is an end in itself which holds the church together in social engagement. But the question arises as to whether this is so. There is, after all, a long Christian tradition which, while it recognises that here we have no abiding city, nevertheless seeks certain provisional or penultimate norms by which we might at least regulate our social life.

David Hollenbach has referred to a number of 'extremely thorough theological questions which are urgently being debated within the church today'. He is talking primarily about the Roman Catholic Church and his experience in North America, but there can be no doubt that what he says applies to other churches and, with obvious differences, also to Ireland. They include:

(i) the extraordinary difficulty [particularly on the part of the Roman Catholic Church] in dealing with any kind of social pluralism. The Roman Catholic Church in Ireland during the nineteenth century had to opt for pluralism. At the same time, by means of its role in the educational system and by the medical and social care-services, it minimised the pluralist impact. Now that that system is breaking down or cannot be afforded, real theological and practical problems arise.

(ii) the problem shared by both Catholics and Protestants in finding a sound basis for the claim to teaching authority outside, and perhaps sometimes inside, the realm of doctrinal matters. Knowledge has become increasingly specialised and the faithful know that not even highly intelligent clerics are able to operate in every specialism within which serious moral problems arise.

(iii) There are problems about the actual ecclesiastical structures themselves and their adequacy in coping with questions of political or social ethics.

The Roman Catholic Church is still hierarchically structured and, in the end of the day, the bishops are more powerful than the Conference of Major Religious Superiors or any other power-group within the church. The other representative bodies set up under the influence of the Vatican Council have no real power and appear to have only very slight influence on those who do.

The structures of the other 'main' churches in Ireland appear at first sight to be a good deal more democratic, but in fact those lay persons who can afford the time to participate in the courts of the church are not always representative of the church membership. They are often either retired, well-heeled or, very occasionally, unemployed.

They will almost all be middle-class, to a man or woman, and this repeatedly shows up in the wording and the underlying prejudices of the resolutions they pass. But there is a question concerning the appropriateness of the decision-making process itself. The proceedings of the General Synod and the General Assembly are quasi-parliamentary. Resolutions are brought forward either by Boards of the Synod or Assembly which [like sub-committees of a larger committee] have been working away at the particular question throughout the year. They are seconded and debated and eventually voted upon. The problem certainly arises, once something has been passed, as to how binding it is upon church members. Clearly some things are more binding than others. When, for instance, the Presbyterian Church in Ireland terminated its membership of the World Council of Churches, it made a difference to all members of the church. But when the 1988 General Assembly threw out a resolution in favour of sanctions against South Africa and substituted one which called on the Irish and British Governments to give aid to the Botha regime, no member of Assembly who believes in mandatory comprehensive sanctions slackened for a moment in their efforts to have such sanctions universally implemented. It is not to be supposed that those who voted for the resolution ever expected that they would! So what was the whole exercise about? What was happening was that two groups of people with differing convictions on what ought to be done about South Africa and apartheid, sought in the interests of public relations and the canvassing of world opinion, to get this little Irish church to row in behind their particular position. One lot failed and the other lot succeeded. Those who failed did not feel themselves in any way bound by the terms of the successful resolution, in the way that they would necessarily have to be bound by a decision on ministerial pensions or the termination of membership of the WCC which involve the church as institution, its structures, finances or external relations. Decisions on the really important issues, e.g. poverty, racism, sanctions, the Anglo-Irish Agreement or Articles 2 and 3 of the 1937 constitution, are in the realm of exhortation to the church's own members or to the world outside, issued by a majority of the members of that particular year's General Assembly or Synod or Conference.

All this is at the national level. At an international level we find the universal church, both through the organs of the World Council of Churches and the Roman Catholic Church, attempting to grapple with the great social, political and economic problems of our time. Many of these attempts have been courageous and intelligent and deserve to be defended against those who suggest that, since questions of peace and war, nuclear power, poverty and development or the terms of world trade are complex, they should be left to the experts. But the tendency of Christian world bodies on occasion to be rashly and prematurely specific in their directions should not lead us to conclude that specific decisions or actions on these matters are not our business at all.

In fairness, however, we should ask whether there is not in the churches today a dangerous tendency towards justification by works which expresses itself in a desire to pronounce on everything or be seen to be involved everywhere? Is there a danger that bodies like the WCC or the world confessional bodies, may come to see themselves increasingly in papalist terms? They hear and see the Pope talking about everything everywhere, all the time, and they want to do the same. Instead of limiting themselves to statements which make certain general points, lay down certain general guidelines, sketch out the constraints inside which Christians believe this or that question must be worked out, these bodies [or important people within them] appear to hope to 'bind' membership by what is often a quite premature *status confessionis*.

One suspects that this premature specificity arises fundamentally from the desire to walk by sight where in fact we can walk only by faith. Perhaps it is of the nature of the Christian way that, most often when we meet together we can agree only on what Paul Ramsay has called 'directions', as opposed to specific 'directives' with a claim to universal applicability. Then, in a rather fragmented way, we must go back to the world in separate and one hopes perhaps mutually respectful groups, to work on the specifics of the problem in our own way. Then, as we work away in our separate groups, sometimes taking mutually exclusive lines on South Africa or the future of Northern Ireland, or whatever, we have to work out our obedience in faith not sight, tremblingly, but not expecting to be backed up by a legislative majority in any court, secular or ecclesiastical. We have to consider that small groups in disagreement is sometimes the only form the one, holy, catholic church can take in our day. We will not necessarily even have the satisfaction of being sure at any given moment that our little group really is the church in action at all. But while that is very disturbing, and even frightening, we must simply 'sin boldly', recognising that according to the Creed 'the church' is an item of faith, not an object of sight.

Further Reading

Juan Luis Segundo, *The Liberation of Theology*, Maryknoll N.Y. 1985.

Duncan Forrester, *Theology and Politics*, Oxford, 1988.

Dietrich Bonhoeffer, *Ethics*, English trans ed E. Bethage, London, SCM Press, 1955.

Johann-B. Metz, *Theology of the World*, New York, Herder and Herder, 1969.

David Hollenbach, 'A Prophetic Church and the Catholic Sacramental Imagination', in *The Faith that Does Justice*, ed J. C. Haughey, SJ, New York, Paulist Press, 1977, pp 234-263.

The Contributors

WERNER G. JEANROND teaches theology in Trinity College, Dublin. His publications include *Text and Interpretation as Categories of Theological Thinking*, Dublin, Gill and Macmillan, 1988; and *Theological Hermeneutics: Development and Significance*, London: Macmillan 1991.

ANDREW MAYES teaches Hebrew and Old Testament in Trinity College, Dublin. His publications include *Deuteronomy* in the 'New Century Bible' series; *Judges* in the 'Old Testament Guides' series, and *The Old Testament in Sociological Perspective*.

SEÁN FREYNE is Professor of Theology in Trinity College, Dublin. He specialises in Early Judaism and Christianity and has published a number of books and many articles on these topics, most recently, *Galilee, Jesus and the Gospels*, 1988. He is a member of the editorial board of *Concilium, An International Journal of Theology* .

GABRIEL DALY is a lecturer in Systematic and Historical Theology in Trinity College, Dublin. Author of *Transcendence and Immanence* and *Creation and Redemption* (1987).

VINCENT MacNAMARA lectures in Christian Ethics in Trinity College, Dublin, and is visiting professor at the Gregorian University, Rome. He is the author of *Faith and Ethics* (1985) and of *The Truth in Love* (1988).

KENNETH KEARON is part-time lecturer in Christian ethics in Trinity College, Dublin. He was Anglican chaplain in the College from 1984 to 1991, and has recently been appointed rector of Tullow Parish in Co Dublin.

KATHERINE ZAPPONE lectures in Practical Theology in Trinity College, Dublin, with special interests in the spiritualities and ethics of liberation theologies, as well as religious education. She co-directs 'The Shanty Educational Project' with Ann Louise Gilligan. Her book, *The Hope for Wholeness: A Spirituality for Feminists*, will appear in 1991 from Twenty-Third Publications, Mystic, CT.

DENIS CARROLL is a priest of the Archdiocese of Dublin. He is engaged in parish work at Kilnamanagh, Tallaght (Dublin). He has written on ecological questions. His publications include *Towards a Story of the Earth* (1987) and *A Pilgrim God for a Pilgrim People* (1987).

TERENCE McCAUGHEY is a lecturer in Irish at Trinity College, Dublin, and is a Presbyterian minister with special concern for prison ministry. He also lectures in early Christian literature at Trinity College. He is currently engaged in a study of *Church, Politics and Prophetic Theology in Ireland*, in the series *Theology of a Pilgrim People* (Gill & Macmillan, Dublin, 1987-).